THE EUROPEAN UNION AND HEALTH SERVICES

Biomedical and Health Research

Volume 50

Earlier published in this series

Vol. 15. N. Katunuma, H. Kido, H. Fritz and J. Travis (Eds.), Medical Aspects of Proteases and Protease Inhibitors

Vol. 16. P.I. Harris and D. Chapman (Eds.), New Biomedical Materials

Vol. 17. J.J.F. Schroots, R. Fernández-Ballesteros and G. Rudinger (Eds.), Aging in Europe

Vol. 18. R. Leidl (Ed.), Health Care and its Financing in the Single European Market

Vol. 19. P. Jenner and R. Demirdamar (Eds.), Dopamine Receptor Subtypes

Vol. 20. P.I. Haris and D. Chapman (Eds.), Biomembrane Structures

Vol. 21. N. Yoganandan, F.A. Pintar, S.J. Larson and A. Sances Jr. (Eds.), Frontiers in Head and Neck Trauma

Vol. 22. J. Matsoukas and T. Mavromoustakos (Eds.), Bioactive Peptides in Drug Discovery and Design: Medical Aspects

Vol. 23. M. Hallen (Ed.), Human Genome Analysis

Vol. 24. S.S. Baig (Ed.), Cancer Research Supported under BIOMED 1

Vol. 25. N.J. Gooderham (Ed.), Drug Metabolism: Towards the Next Millennium

Vol. 26. P. Jenner (Ed.), A Molecular Biology Approach to Parkinson's Disease

Vol. 27. P.A. Frey and D.B. Northrop (Eds.), Enzymatic Mechanisms

Vol. 28. A.M.N. Gardner and R.H. Fox, The Venous System in Health and Disease

Vol. 29. G. Pawelec (Ed.), EUCAMBIS: Immunology and Ageing in Europe

Vol. 30. J.F. Stoltz, M. Singh and P. Riha, Hemorheology in Practice

Vol. 31. B.J. Njio, A. Stenvik, R.S. Ireland and B. Prahl-Andersen (Eds.), EURO-QUAL

Vol. 32. B.J. Njio, B. Prahl-Andersen, G. ter Heege, A. Stenvik and R.S. Ireland (Eds.), Quality of Orthodontic Care – A Concept for Collaboration and Responsiblities

Vol. 33. H.H. Goebel, S.E. Mole and B.D. Lake (Eds.), The Neuronal Ceroid Lipofuscinoses (Batten Disease)

Vol. 34. G.J. Bellingan and G.J. Laurent (Eds.), Acute Lung Injury: From Inflammation to Repair

Vol. 35. M. Schlaud (Ed.), Comparison and Harmonisation of Denominator Data for Primary Health Care Research in Countries of the European Community

Vol. 36. F.F. Parl, Estrogens, Estrogen Receptor and Breast Cancer

Vol. 37. J.M. Ntambi (Ed.), Adipocyte Biology and Hormone Signaling

Vol. 38. N. Yoganandan and F.A. Pintar (Eds.), Frontiers in Whiplash Trauma

Vol. 39. J.-M. Graf von der Schulenburg (Ed.), The Influence of Economic Evaluation Studies on Health Care Decision-Making

Vol. 40. H. Leino-Kilpi, M. Välimäki, M. Arndt, T. Dassen, M. Gasull, C. Lemonidou, P.A. Scott, G. Bansemir, E. Cabrera, H. Papaevangelou and J. Mc Parland, Patient's Autonomy, Privacy and Informed Consent

Vol. 41. T.M. Gress (Ed.), Molecular Pathogenesis of Pancreatic Cancer

Vol. 42. J.-F. Stoltz (Ed.), Mechanobiology: Cartilage and Chondrocyte

Vol. 43. B. Shaw, G. Semb, P. Nelson, V. Brattström, K. Mølsted and B. Prahl-Andersen, The Eurocleft Project 1996-2000

Vol. 44. R. Coppo and Dr. L. Peruzzi (Eds.), Moderately Proteinuric IgA Nephropathy in the Young

Vol. 45. L. Turski, D.D. Schoepp and E.A. Cavalheiro (Eds.), Excitatory Amino Acids: Ten Years Later

Vol. 46. I. Philp (Ed.), Family Care of Older People in Europe

Vol. 47. H. Aldskogius and J. Fraher (Eds.), Glial Interfaces in the Nervous System – Role in Repair and Plasticity

Vol. 48. H. ten Have & R. Janssens (Eds.), Palliative Care in Europe – Concepts and Policies

Vol. 49. T. Reilly (Ed.), Musculoskeletal Disorders in Health-Related Occupations

ISSN: 0929-6743

The European Union and Health Services

The Impact of the Single European Market on Member States

Edited by

Reinhard Busse

Matthias Wismar

Philip C. Berman

On behalf of

The European Health Management Association

IOS
Press

Ohmsha

Amsterdam • Berlin • Oxford • Tokyo • Washington, DC

ISBN 1 58603 209 7 (IOS Press)
ISBN 4 274 90495 4 C3047 (Ohmsha)

Publisher
IOS Press
Nieuwe Hemweg 6B
1013 BG Amsterdam
The Netherlands
fax: +31 20 620 3419
e-mail: order@iospress.nl

Distributor in the UK and Ireland
IOS Press/Lavis Marketing
73 Lime Walk
Headington
Oxford OX3 7AD
England
fax: +44 1865 75 0079

Distributor in the USA and Canada
IOS Press, Inc.
5795-G Burke Centre Parkway
Burke, VA 22015
USA
fax: +1 703 323 3668
e-mail: iosbooks@iospress.com

Distributor in Germany, Austria and Switzerland
IOS Press/LSL.de
Gerichtsweg 28
D-04103 Leipzig
Germany
fax: +49 341 995 4255

Distributor in Japan
Ohmsha, Ltd.
3-1 Kanda Nishiki-cho
Chiyoda-ku, Tokyo 101
Japan
fax: +81 3 3233 2426

LEGAL NOTICE
The publisher is not responsible for the use which might be made of the following information.

PRINTED IN THE NETHERLANDS

Foreword

Philippe BUSQUIN
European Commissioner for Research

It is with pleasure that I introduce and commend the publication of the final results from the project: "The Impact of European Union Internal Market – Regulations on the Health Services of Member States", financed under the European Commission's Biomedical and Health Research (BIOMED2) Programme 1994-1998.

The project's results come at an important time in the policy debate over healthcare and the role of the European Union, particularly in the light of European Court cases on healthcare and the EU Internal Market. Its findings provide a significant contribution to policy-making in this field.

The project's success demonstrates the importance of a coherent policy-oriented research effort at the European level in the field of public health. That is why the Commission has proposed to include such research as a subject in the next Research Framework Programme (2002-2006).

In the next Framework Programme, such research is foreseen under the heading "Anticipating the EU's scientific and technological needs".

Research under that heading will focus on emerging issues and on issues of relevance to Community policies. I expect it will help to create, over time, a more efficient environment for policy research in the EU, in line with the objectives of creating a true European Research Area.

It should provide policy actors throughout the EU with a facility to access relevant Community research. It should make the link between research and policy stronger, more responsive and more coherent than before. And it should provide opportunities for research support to a wider range of policy areas than has been the case in the past.

Foreword

David BYRNE
European Commissioner for Health and Consumer Protection

Over recent years, health issues have assumed increasing prominence at the European level. Since the formal public health competence was defined in 1993, more recent decisions of the European Court of Justice have drawn attention to the fact that health care is affected by other policy domains – particularly the EU Single Market. Indeed, the Commission Communication for a new health strategy for the European Community recognises that the Single Market has important consequences for both health and health systems. Importantly, the Court's role in bringing health services under the umbrella of the Single European Market (SEM) will provide new opportunities and challenges for health policy-makers throughout the European Union.

This publication, which explores the impact of the SEM on health services in the Member States, makes a significant and valuable contribution to helping policy makers both at European and Member State levels, as well as healthcare managers, to understand the effect that the SEM may have on health services.

The research team, led by the European Health Management Association, has reached a number of important conclusions. It is becoming increasingly clear that the relationship between health services and the SEM is highly complex, particularly because the patient is regarded, in the context of the SEM, as an individual consumer rather than as a citizen with collective rights and responsibilities. The European Court of Justice has addressed this issue in the Peerbooms case, but the relationship between the European social model and market forces is undoubtedly a matter that will require further consideration.

The researchers have developed a number of "futures scenarios" which have led them to conclude that "neither total integration of health services at a European level nor the exclusion of health services from the SEM are probable". They suggest that "the third option, 'muddling through', does not provide easy solutions, but doing nothing is not a sensible solution". The challenge facing policy makers is to develop a strategy to manage the relationship between the SEM and healthcare in a manner which will preserve the European social objectives and which will be for the benefit of patients throughout the Community.

The book also highlights that health services – as part of the SEM – function within a global market place. This is of particular importance in relation to supply and demand of health professionals – an issue which is likely to become increasingly significant.

I know that the work of this research group has already had a considerable impact on the work of the Commission's High Level Committee on Health and its Working Group on the Internal Market, and I am sure that the detailed analysis, together with the individual chapters which explore specific aspects of the impact of the SEM on health services, will provide a valuable basis for policy makers in the future.

Contents

Foreword, *Philippe Busquin*   v

Foreword, *David Byrne*   vii

Contributors   xi

Acknowledgements   xii

Abbreviations   xiii

The European Union and Health Services: Summary, *Calum Paton, Philip C. Berman,
   Reinhard Busse, Bie Nio Ong, Clas Rehnberg, Barbro Renck, Nuria Romo Avilés,
   Fernando Silió Villamil, Mona Sundh and Matthias Wismar*   1

Part I: Introduction

The European Union and Health Services – The Context, *Matthias Wismar,
   Reinhard Busse and Philip Berman*   17

The Single European Market and Health Services – The Research Design, *Philip
   Berman, Reinhard Busse, Matthias Wismar, Bie Nio Ong and Calum Paton*   31

Part II: Single European Market Legislation and Jurisdiction

Analysis of SEM Legislation and Jurisdiction, *Matthias Wismar and Reinhard Busse*   41

Transposition of European Directives into National Legislation, *Matthias Wismar,
   Reinhard Busse, Calum Paton, Fernando Silió Villamil, Nuria Romo Avilés,
   Maria Angeles Prieto Rodríguez, Mona Sundh and Barbro Renck*   49

Part III: Free Movement of Persons

The Mobility of Doctors and Nurses – A United Kingdom Case Study, *Clare Jinks,
   Bie Nio Ong and Calum Paton*   63

Scenarios on the Future Mobility of Doctors and Nurses, *Calum Paton and
   Bie Nio Ong*   91

The Mobility of Citizens – A Case Study and Scenario on the Health Services of the
    Costa del Sol, *Nuria Romo Avilés, Fernando Silió Villamil and
    Maria Angeles Prieto Rodríguez*   97

The Impact of the SEM on Data Exchange and Protection in the Swedish Health
    System, *Barbro Renck and Mona Sundh*   109

Part IV: Free Movement of Goods and Services

A Swedish Case Study on the Impact of the SEM on the Pharmaceutical Market,
    Clas Rehnberg   131

The Impact of the SEM on the Medical Devices Market in Sweden, *Mona Sundh
    and Barbro Renck*   159

The SEM and the Public Procurement of Goods and Services in the Andalusian
    Health Service, *Fernando Silió Villamil, Nuria Romo Avilés and
    Maria Angeles Prieto Rodríguez*   179

Consumer Choice of Medical Goods across Borders, *Matthias Wismar,
    Jens Gobrecht and Reinhard Busse*   213

Consumer Choice of Healthcare Services across Borders, *Reinhard Busse,
    Markus Drews and Matthias Wismar*   231

Scenarios on the Development of Consumer Choice for Healthcare Services,
    Reinhard Busse and Matthias Wismar   249

Part V: The Future

Scenarios on the Future of Healthcare in Europe, *Matthias Wismar and
    Reinhard Busse*   261

Author Index   273

Contributors

Calum Paton	Centre for Health Planning and Management, Keele University, UK (Scientific Director)
Philip C. Berman	European Health Management Association (Project Director)
Reinhard Busse	European Observatory on Health Care Systems, Madrid, Spain
Markus Drews	Medical Review Board of the Statutory Health Insurance Baden-Württemberg, Freiburg, Germany
Jens Gobrecht	World Health Organization, Geneva, Switzerland
Claire Jinks	Primary Care Sciences Research Centre, Keele University, UK
Bie Nio Ong	Faculty of Health, Keele University, UK
Maria Angeles Prieto Rodriguez	Andalusian School of Public Health (EASP), Granada, Spain
Clas Rehnberg	Centre for Health Economics, Stockholm School of Economics, Stockholm, Sweden
Barbro Renck	Centre for Public Health Research, Karlstad, Sweden
Nuria Romo Aviles	Andalusian School of Public Health (EASP), Granada, Spain
Fernando Silio Villamil	Andalusian School of Public Health (EASP), Granada, Spain
Mona Sundh	Centre for Public Health Research, Karlstad, Sweden
Matthias Wismar	Department of Epidemiology, Social Medicine and Health System Research, Hannover Medical School, Germany

Acknowledgements

Many people have made significant contributions to this project over the last five years (including the preparatory period). While it is impossible to name everyone, the contributors would like – in particular – to thank:

- *Hans Stein*, of the Federal German Ministry of Health, who was "godfather" to the project, encouraging its development, obtaining financial support from the German Federal Ministry of Health for the initial meeting of the partners, and providing advice during the course of the project;

- *Per-Gunnar Svensson*, formerly Director of the Centre for Public Health Research, Karlstad, Sweden, who was the original Scientific Director of the project and who co-authored the proposal before he resigned from the project on assuming the post of Director-General of the International Hospital Federation;

- *Bernie Merkel* and *Michael Hübel* of DG Health and Consumer Protection, whose advice has been greatly valued by the project team;

- The experts who took part in the working meeting in Celle, Germany, in January 2001, and whose advice helped to shape the final recommendations, namely *Rita Baeten*, *Nick Boyd*, *Penny Dash*, *Johannes Dommers*, *Kaj Essinger*, *José Manuel Freire*, *Otmar Kloiber*, *Willy Palm* and *Eva Sveman*;

- *Lisette Schermer* of DG Research who, as the Commission official with responsibility for this project, has been most helpful in supporting and guiding the project team;

- *Paul Belcher* who, as EHMA's Head of European Union Affairs, has played a significant role throughout the project; and last but not least

- *Stefanie Reich* who was responsible for the lay-out of this book.

Abbreviations

AHS	Andalusian Health Service
BOE	Official Journal of the Spanish State (*Boletín Oficial del Estado*)
BOJA	Official Journal of the Andalusian Regional Government (*Boletín Oficial de la Junta de Andalucía*)
CCST	Certificate of Completion of Specialist Training
CE (label)	"Communauté Européenne" label
CEN	European Committee for Standardization (*Comité Européen de Normalisation*)
CENELEC	European Committee for Electrotechnical Standardization (*Comité Européen de Normalisation Electrotechnique*)
CoI	country of insurance (or other social security) affiliation
CoS	country of service provision
CPMP	Committee for Proprietary Medicinal Products
CST	Certificate of Specialist Training
CWSs	Client Welfare Services
DoH	Department of Health (UK)
EC	European Community
ECJ	European Court of Justice
ECSC	European Coal and Steel Community
EEA	European Economic Area (i.e. EC plus EFTA)
EEC	European Economic Community (predecessor of EC)
EFTA	European Free Trade Association
EMEA	European Agency for the Evaluation of Medicinal Products
ETSI	European Telecommunications Standards Institute
EU	European Union
EuBasicBP	European Basic Benefit Package
EuHFiP	European Healthcare Finance Pool
EuHiRiP	European High Risk Pool
EURATOM	European Atomic Energy Community
EuSCAl	European Standardised Per-Capita Allocation
GMC	General Medical Council
HO	House Officer
HSS	Health Care Standards Institution (*Hälso- och sjukvårdsstandardiseringen*)
INSS	National Social Security Institute (*Instituto Nacional de la Seguridad Social*)
IT	information technology
ISO	International Organization for Standardization
JCPTGP	Joint Committee on Postgraduate Training for General Practice
LIV	County Council of Värmland (*Landstinget i Värmland*)
MRCOG	Membership of the Royal College of Obstetricians and Gynaecologists
MRCP	Membership of the Royal College of Physicians
NHS	National Health Service
NHSS	National Health Service Supplies
OJEC	Official Journal of the European Community

OTC	Drugs sold "Over-The-Counter"
PLAB	Professional and Linguistic Assessment Board
PWG	Permanent Working Group of European Junior Hospital Doctors
SEM	Single European Market
SGB V	Social Code Book V (*Sozialgesetzbuch V*)
SHI	Statutory Health Insurance
SHO	Senior House Officer
SLF	Swedish Healthcare Suppliers Association (*Sveriges läkarförbund*)
SMEs	small and medium enterprises
SpR	Specialist Registrars
Spri	Swedish Institute for Health Services Development (*Hälso- och sjukvårdens utvecklingsinstitut*)
STA	Specialist Training Authority of the Royal Colleges
SWEDAC	Swedish Board for Accreditation and Conformity Assessment
TBT	technical barrier to trade
TEC	Treaty Establishing the European Community
UCM	Union des Caisses de Maladie
UK	United Kingdom
UKCC	UK Central Council for Nursing, Midwifery and Health Visiting
VAT	value added tax
WTO	World Trade Organisation

The European Union and Health Services
R. Busse et al. (Eds.)
IOS Press, 2002

The European Union and health services: Summary

Calum PATON, Philip C. BERMAN, Reinhard BUSSE,
Bie Nio ONG, Clas REHNBERG, Barbro RENCK, Nuria ROMO AVILES,
Fernando SILIO VILLAMIL, Mona SUNDH and Matthias WISMAR

1. Introduction

This book presents the results and conclusions from a project financed by the European Commission's BIOMED2 programme. The purpose of the project was to analyse the impact of the Single European Market (SEM) on the regulating, financing and delivery of health services in the Member States.

The Treaty Establishing the European Community (TEC) defines several areas of competence for the European Union with potential impact on healthcare and health services. In addition to the establishment of the SEM, these include competition law, agriculture, social protection, environmental policy etc. This book is concerned only with the SEM, with its four freedoms for persons, goods, services and capital.

The project has been organised in three phases, to meet the following six objectives:

Phase 1
- To identify SEM regulations and directives as well as respective European Court of Justice (ECJ) decisions which explicitly refer to health services and which therefore are classified as having a potential impact on the purchasing, supply and delivery of health services.
- To identify both the methods used as well as the actual extent to which these EU directives have been transposed into the laws and rules of the Member States, whether at national or regional level.

Phase 2
- To analyse the factors involved in the extent to which EU regulations have been adopted.
- To evaluate the impact of these national or regional laws and rules on the purchasing, supply and delivery of health services (i.e. to what extent has policy in Member States been changed?).

Phase 3
- To identify outcomes, including both intended and unintended effects, of the SEM on Member States' health services and to develop futures scenarios exploring key issues identified in the earlier analysis and evaluation; and
- To produce an overall report highlighting and analysing the key issues.

2. Main issues and conclusions

2.1 Context and overall significance

- In political terms, there appears to be a contradiction between the purpose of the Single European Market (SEM) and the manner in which statements in article 152 of the Treaty Establishing the European Community are widely interpreted ("… excluding any harmonisation of the laws and regulations of the Member States. … Community action in the field of public health shall fully respect the responsibilities of the Member States for the organisation and delivery of health services and medical care.").
- This study investigated the impact of SEM regulations and directives as well as respective European Court of Justice (ECJ) rulings – taken together as "interventions" – on the health services of the Member States. It demonstrates that the relationship between health services as a major sector of Member States' economies and the SEM are intertwined in such a complex manner that it is virtually impossible to separate them. The argument, therefore, that subsidiarity applies to health services is not fully sustainable within the context of the SEM.
- Thus, the SEM may rightfully be seen as a challenge for health services, adding a further complexity to the principal driving forces such as changing healthcare needs, increasing patient expectations, the development of e-health, a regionalization of political decision making in a context of economic globalization. This is particularly true because the SEM inevitably regards the patient as an individual consumer rather than as a citizen with collective rights and responsibilities.

2.2 Markets and the European social model

- At a European level, the SEM requires health services to adapt to market rules, while at national level, governments seek to adapt market rules to ensure the effective delivery of health services within a social model.
- Differing views on the future structure of health services in Europe underlie much of the debate on health in Europe. These differences are based on two principal, divergent models – the European social model and market forces.
- SEM regulations and directives, while stressing the market, have not been exclusively aimed at achieving economic objectives – indeed some SEM interventions have a social purpose in terms of consumer and health protection (such as Directive 93/42/EEC on medical devices). Some directives are, arguably, even geared to regulating or limiting market forces (for example Directive 89/105/EEC on pharmaceutical price control and regulation). Nevertheless, there is a need to recognise that market forces and the European social model have differing objectives.

2.3 Intended and unintended effects

- SEM interventions have both intended effects (principally to create a single market with free movement of goods, services, people and capital) as well as unintended effects.
- Intended effects include providing the basis for a range of European activities in healthcare, e.g. a common public procurement system for goods and services, Europe-wide mobility of doctors and nurses, a common system for regulating medical devices, common licensing and market access procedure for pharmaceuticals as well as a European system to provide health services for tourists, and provisions to ensure healthcare coverage for persons working in other EU Member States.

–   Unintended effects on the purchasing, supply and delivery of health services often result from the fact that these have not been sufficiently taken into account when the regulations and directives were drafted. For example, SEM interventions have sometimes led to increased health service bureaucracy. Small and medium-sized enterprises were also effected negatively by such requirements. SEM interventions may also lead to patient/citizen movements from one country to another in order to obtain treatment, thus undermining attempts at priority setting within the publicly-funded systems of member-states. Movement of doctors and other professionals may create shortages in poorer – especially accession – countries.

–   The different political or organisational settings of health services, as well as countries' geographical settings within the EU, may lead to differing effects of SEM interventions within Member States. Policy-makers (and judges) should be aware such of differences.

2.4 Impact on health services

–   While the actual impact of some SEM regulations, directives and ECJ rulings on health services may currently be marginal, the inherent conflicts behind many of the directives and ECJ rulings may have a significant impact and may cause unexpected systems turbulence.

–   For example, should the cases which are currently pending at the ECJ be decided in favour of free choice of healthcare goods and services, then the patient-provider relationship would be more firmly embedded in the range of European activities in healthcare – with free choice of provider dominating other objectives. Should such free choice be permitted across national borders, it might also have to be mandated within countries – with potentially major consequences for healthcare systems.

–   The thrust of such policy is to emphasise individual rights as opposed to the collective priorities (and collective rights) of public healthcare systems. While it is generally the better-off who can currently take advantage of such individual rights, the extension of free choice to healthcare within Member States would make the benefits more widely available. On the other hand, collective priorities may be undermined by mobility which prevents effective national planning. Basic characteristics of Beveridge (NHS) systems in particular may be threatened.

–   Assuming that there is a triangular relationship between citizens/patients, third party payers, and providers (Figure 1), we can see that provider-citizen/patient and the provider-payer relationships (i.e. the supply side) have been the subject of the majority of SEM interventions (especially if competition laws are also taken into account).

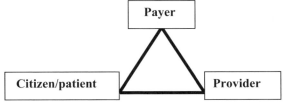

Fig. 1: The triangular relationship between citizen/ patient, third-party payer and provider

–   The relationship between citizens/ patients and third-party payers – the third side of the triangle – has not been subject to either EU regulation or ECJ rulings. This might entail, for example, either regulating citizen choice of third party payer or developing a European benefits package. If either of these were to lead to a market of third-party payers, it would constitute a powerful driver towards a European system of health services. However, such a development would certainly lead to substantial systems turbulence, again particularly in Beveridge systems, and would almost certainly be resisted by Member States.

2.5 Implications for policy

- Based on the future scenarios conducted as part of the study, neither total integration of health services at a European level nor the exclusion of health services from the SEM are probable. The third option, "muddling through", does not provide easy solutions, but doing nothing is not a sensible option.
- An honest and explicit debate on the advantages and disadvantages of "muddling through" must take place. This first requires an acceptance of the intertwining between the SEM and health services. Such an acceptance would enable the development of a proactive role for health policy-making – as opposed to the current decision-making which is all too often reactive, especially to ECJ rulings. While different objectives and interests will no doubt continue to be the subject of compromise, an overt healthcare strategy to manage the relationship between the SEM and healthcare should be developed.
- There is a need to continue to monitor the effects of the SEM on health services. This should be combined with the health information strand of the new EU health strategy.

2.6 A note on globalisation

- While this project focuses primarily on the SEM, it should not be forgotten that health services – as part of the SEM – function within a global market in which the demand for health professionals and the market for health products operates. The World Trade Organization is increasingly active in this area, and Member States will have to reconcile national interests with the European Commission's right to negotiate on their behalf (Article 133 TEC).
- The SEM is part of Europe's strategy to compete in the world global market place. The EU and its Member States should develop a strategy which would include its social objectives as part of this externally-oriented policy – emphasising a sustainable European social model alongside the Single European Market.

3. Background and methodology

3.1 Context and overall significance: the Treaty, the SEM and health services

According to Article 3 of the Treaty establishing the European Community, the European Union has, in principle, a broad policy mandate for health ("… the activities of the Community shall include … a contribution to the attainment of a high level of health protection …") including specific tasks which are set out in Article 152 and other articles. Nevertheless, according to the principle of subsidiarity and the widespread (but disputed) political interpretation of Article 152, the organisation and delivery of health services are argued to be excluded from this policy mandate.

The assumption, however, that European economic integration is separated from the purely national responsibilities for healthcare – which most commentators as well as policy makers have accepted as the reality – has to be questioned. Since a healthcare system is not only a part of the welfare state, but at the same time an important part of the economy, it is impossible to regulate one without causing effects on the other. Restricting health systems policy to the Member States while sponsoring economic integration at EU level does not create a tidy or even meaningful separation. Free movement of persons, goods, services and capital also means free movement of physicians, nurses, other professionals, patients, drugs, medical technology and healthcare services. The relationship between the European Union – including the Single European Market (SEM) – and the health systems and services of Member States is therefore becoming an increasingly complex area.

There have been different interpretations of the SEM. Clearly it is an "economy wide" initiative, not specific to social welfare let alone health. Accordingly, EU policy may have an effect upon these services mainly through generic, i.e. sector-unspecific, regulations. Some have portrayed the SEM as an attempt to regulate the (otherwise) free market, at least in part to ensure the protection of social objectives and social values. Others have tended to see it simply as a tool of economic policy. Even here, however, debate exists between those who see the SEM as a means of promoting competition both across the European Union and even within Member States, and those who see it as a means of allowing rationalisation and concentration (merger into large scale industrial sectors) against a background of globalisation. These debates provide an important context for understanding how SEM interventions might affect health services, and for determining whether or not the impact of these interventions was intentional or accidental.

It should be remembered that health policy exists in a wider environment, both within Member States or across the European Union. Health policy is concerned with the effective provision of a health service as part of the welfare state objectives. Health policy must also take into account the contribution of health and the healthcare industry to the economy as a whole. "Healthier workers" and workers employed in the health industry – as well as its profits – are the concern of most governments.

3.2 The project's methodology and terminology

The project's research has concentrated on the four freedoms of the SEM, i.e. the free movement of individuals; the free movement of goods; the free movement of services; and the free movement of capital. To explore their effects on health services, relevant categories were defined, taking both "supply" and "demand" factors into account (Figure 2). For example, the free movement of individuals comprises both the free movement of doctors, nurses and other healthcare professionals as "suppliers" of health services as well as of persons undergoing short or long term stays in other countries who may "demand" health services during those stays. In contrast, movement of consumers with the explicit intention to receive healthcare goods or services is classified under free movement of goods and services, respectively, to reflect the intentions of the respective SEM interventions (= SEM regulations and directives as well as respective ECJ rulings). The other important demand-side categories regarding these two freedoms relate to public procurement while regulations regarding the pharmaceuticals, medical products and health insurance market constitute the supply-side.

In summary, Figure 2 presents a typology devised to explore relevant legislation and issues. This typology is not the only possible way of organising the study, but is a robust means of reflecting on the impact of the SEM on health services.

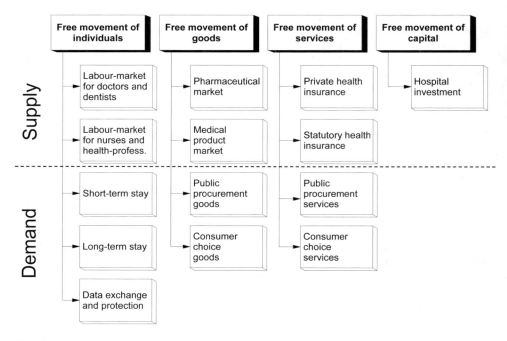

Fig. 2: Analytical categories used in the project

The categories of Figure 2 are not all treated equally in the project. The case studies and scenarios concern some but not all of the categories in Figure 2. The case studies have produced analyses of the impact of interventions on specific areas which were considered to be of particular importance – such as mobility of medical manpower and the free movement of goods and services (or consumers of healthcare moving across national boundaries as part of consumer choice of goods and services). Each case study has been led by one of the national project teams and focuses on the issues that are of particular relevance to that country. For example, consumer choice has been based in Germany; medical manpower has been pursued primarily in the UK; public procurement in Spain; and pharmaceuticals in Sweden. Where appropriate, the case studies have incorporated brief information from the other three countries to provide a broader picture of the impact of EU regulations and policy.

Some of the topics were developed into scenarios. The scenarios seek to depict – at a very broad and general level – "alternative futures", based upon different assumptions about the behaviour of key actors and events. The scenarios are not full-blown, data-based scenarios but attempts to provide a basis for future policy by EU and Member State policymakers – by drawing attention to the possible consequences of different courses of action or inaction.

A distinction is made between the impact of SEM interventions and outcomes in terms of effects on health services or healthcare. Impact refers to the effect of SEM interventions upon domestic legislation and the administrative rules of national or regional institutions. Impact on Member States depends on a number of factors, including the extent to which directives are transposed, and the extent to which health system rules of Member States are changed. The same EU intervention may have different impact in different countries. For example, one country may already have all the data protection legislation required, while another country may have to introduce a considerable body of legislation.

Equally, countries may transpose legislation more or less effectively (or, in extreme cases, not at all). Full transposition can be explained in a number of ways: a political culture of enthusiasm for Europe ("being a good European"); an "automatic" process of transposition of regulations; or the perception that regulations offer national advantage.

To explore whether duration of EU membership also has an influence on the impact of SEM interventions, four countries were selected for the project to represent the "four waves" of membership of the European Union. Germany represents the original membership group from 1952/58; the UK the first accession group of 1973; Spain the southern expansion in the 1980s; and Sweden the accession countries of 1995.

For each of the four countries, reports are available of the transposition of key directives (based on the application of the "four freedoms" to health services). The process of transposition differs from country to country – not least reflecting differences between unitary states (such as England); federal states such as Germany; and states such as Spain with varying regional autonomy. One must equally distinguish between formal transposition and implementation within the health sector. Equally one must distinguish between transposition and impact: it is possible to have full transposition but little impact and only partial transposition yet significant impact

Outcome refers to the effect of SEM interventions on health services and healthcare – in terms of management, finance, supply and delivery. Effects may be intended or unintended. The case studies and analyses pay particular attention to these effects and to the different perspectives of the EU and the Member States.

4. Main findings

4.1 SEM interventions referring to health services

The collection and analysis of all SEM interventions referring to health services (with potential impact on regulating, financing and/ or delivery of health services in the Member States) revealed that

- the European dimension in health services began directly with the formation of the EEC in 1958;
- the frequency of interventions relevant to health services has increased since the 1970s in particularly, and especially in the first half of the 1990s;
- in total, 233 regulations, directives, decisions, recommendations and rulings, which met the project's criteria, were issued between 1958 and June 1998;
- almost two thirds of these interventions emanate from European political decision-making process, but more than one third result from the judicial process at the European Court of Justice;
- the interventions which, potentially, have the most significant effects on the health systems of Member States are usually based on the more powerful instruments – directives and proceedings for preliminary rulings; and
- the distribution of interventions among the four freedoms is uneven with the vast majority focusing on the free movement of persons and goods. Approximately two thirds of the interventions are concerned with the supply-side rather than with the demand-side.

4.2 Labour market for doctors and nurses

Current EU policy on the free movement of labour requires that healthcare workers, who are EU citizens and meet certain training criteria, have the right to register to practice in Member States other than the one in which they trained. The case study focused on the movement into the UK of doctors from the EEA (European Economic Area). The reasons for European mobility are a result either of "push" factors (medical unemployment or lack of specialist training posts in the "home" country) or "pull" factors (the reputation of UK education attracting trainees).

Formally, there is mutual recognition of qualifications between Member States. However, at the informal level, there is considerable uncertainty expressed as to the content, comparability, and quality of the medical (and nursing) curricula of various countries. This affects assessment of doctors' suitability for training posts, which can result in inequality of training opportunity.

In addition, varying demarcations between the organisation of clinical specialties in different Member States may mean that it is difficult for a doctor from another Member State to find an appropriate position in the UK NHS. The "general physician's" work may have a different content in one country as compared to another. EU wide policies and directives are in place and have been transposed in the UK; yet their interpretation and implementation is variable – not only because of national "selfishness" but also because of genuine discrepancies in quality and suitability.

Scenarios for the future demonstrate that increased mobility may adversely effect the supply of medical personnel in the poorer countries of the European Union – especially accession states when they become full members. There may be a "perverse incentive" to rely on imports of doctors rather than educating and training adequate numbers (at undergraduate and postgraduate levels) in the home country.

Against this can be set the view that mobility will always be limited for cultural, linguistic and other reasons. Member States will continue to seek "national self sufficiency" in healthcare personnel, although the effects of the SEM, in terms of the free movement of doctors and nurses in particular, will continue to be felt, if only at the margin.

4.3 Pharmaceutical market and medical product market

These topics were explored with particular reference to Sweden. As well as the Treaty of Rome's general stipulation of free trade in goods, there are a number of specific directives aimed at facilitating single markets for pharmaceutical products and medical devices. Swedish domestic legislation closely follows directives from the European Commission and judgements from the European Court of Justice.

The EU legislative framework has mainly been concerned with the approval procedures, patent protections, standards for distribution and marketing, and with less influence on price regulations and the design of reimbursement and drug benefit systems. The centra-lized EU approval procedure, and co-operation between national regulatory authorities have increased the capacity of these agencies to deal with the growing complexity of the approval process for new chemical entities. By co-operating and sharing information and knowledge about the same new products, these regulatory authorities are on par with (or at least less inferior than) the multinational pharmaceutical industry. Supra-national regulation can thus be seen to increase capacity to deal with the multi-national pharmaceutical industry. Another important consequence is that the centralized approval procedure leads to a clear separation of the decision to approve a new drug and the decision to subsidize it.

A set of EU-decisions (directives about standardized packages, the ECJ verdict on parallel imports) has clearly facilitated the development of parallel importation of drugs –

drugs sold more cheaply abroad that can then be re-imported to the country of production to "undercut" the existing supply.

The results from the Swedish case study demonstrate that most EU directives and regulations concerning the pharmaceutical market have had influence on the supply side rather than the demand side (where questions of pricing, subsidies, availability of drugs, and services are regarded as national issues).

Regarding medical devices, it appears that larger companies have found it easier both to adapt to requirements of the directives and to derive benefit from the EU stamp of approval. For smaller companies, which did not have ambitions to develop exports, the directives have created problems but few benefits. While there has been general recognition of the benefits of common standards, smaller companies have also had greater difficulty and cost in standardising for sale outside their own country. Users have also had difficulty in influencing design and standards.

EU directives have also had an impact on medical technicians. The broader definition of medical-technical products has had the effect that medical technicians are now responsible for a larger area of responsibility. There are, currently, discussions within the profession concerning the responsibility for the repair and maintenance of medical-technical products.

An unintended outcome of Directive 93/42/EEC (which specifies the requirements and regulations for testing, certification and labelling of appliances and equipment) concerns the obligation to report serious adverse events. However, many countries within the European Union do not have national laws requiring users to report adverse events. The study indicates that accident reporting systems within the EU may not work sufficiently well unless the Swedish National Board of Health and Welfare (or the corresponding authority in other Member States) demands that users of medical products are obliged to report either accidents or narrow escapes both to the manufacturer and the supervisory authority.

An additional problem identified in the study is that ethical committees in the respective countries who evaluate applications for the commencement of clinical testing command varying degrees of knowledge and competency. This can therefore lead to significant variations in evaluations of applications for clinical testing. This weakness does not appear to have been sufficiently recognised.

4.4 Public procurement

This case study was carried out in Spain, and concerned the public procurement procedure in the Andalusian health service. The European Directive on public procurement is geared to developing a Europe-wide internal market. Public procurement, however, also has a potential influence on the evolution of the industrial and commercial structure of any Member State, and the European Directive on public procurement has clearly led to substantial changes in Spain.

The study detected an increase in the volume of purchases made using the method of official submission (calls for tender), with approximately 67 % of the total expenditure on public procurement of goods occurring through calls for tender in 1998. More than 89 % of these submissions were advertised in the official journal of the European Community.

On the positive side, the new legislation has led to an improved organisation of services and greater objectivity in specification. On the negative side, purchasing has become more bureaucratic; it takes longer to make a purchase; and large and multinational companies can adapt themselves more easily than small and medium enterprises (SMEs) to the requirements of the European legislation. There may also be perverse incentives to "break down" procurement into units smaller than the level at which European wide calls for tender must be made, in order to avoid the bureaucracy involved in a Europe-wide tender.

The study came to the conclusion the public procurement directive fails to take adequate account either of the specific nature of the health sector or of the EU's objective to create sustainable SMEs.

NB: In regard to public procurement in healthcare it is important to note that the project concentrated on applying public procurement rules by healthcare providers such as hospitals and not applying them to health services themselves, i.e. making them the subject of procurement by the public payer. This discussion has started recently in Sweden after St. Göran's hospital in Stockholm was sold to a private for-profit company – with the agreement calling for a procurement process of hospital services in Stockholm from 2004.

4.5 Consumer choice for healthcare goods and services

Regulation EEC1408/71 – which serves to coordinate social protection systems in the European Union to allow the free mobility of workers and citizens – also provides the basis for facilitating rather than restricting cross-border consumer choice of healthcare goods and services. It could even be argued that the ECJ's Decker and Kohl rulings, which made the free movement of goods and services applicable to social protection schemes, may not have been necessary if reimbursement procedures had been handled in line with this regulation.

The project identified four dimensions to consumer choice: i) access to the widest possible range of services; ii) access with fewest possible restrictions (restrictions being authorisation procedures or mandated referral patterns); iii) the maximum choice of provider; and, iv) full reimbursement for any amount charged by the provider. (It may of course be desirable to restrict some of them in pursuit of other social objectives such as equity.)

Potentially the impact of European legislation and ECJ decisions on cross-border consumer choice is high, although the outcome to date has been very limited. Four factors account for the limited numbers of patients actually taking advantage of cross-border choice: i) restrictive handling of the E112 procedure whereby care abroad has to be pre-authorised; ii) differences in the "healthcare baskets" across Europe; iii) lack of cost reimbursement provisions in many countries; and, iv) the nature of medical goods themselves and their distribution. The political impact of the Kohll and Decker rulings, however, was substantial, since the ruling resulted in the much-debated method to enable cross-border care (in addition to E111 and E112), namely the ex-post patient reimbursement of unauthorised goods and services.

Germany (the location for this case study) provides an illustration that there is potential for cross border consumer choice in prescribed medical goods. During the brief period when German legislation allowed free use of patient reimbursement instead of the usual application of the benefit-in-kind principle, there were reports from sickness funds that bills from abroad had been cashed in. Additionally, a strong claim in favour of the cost reimbursement principle for the purchase of prescribed medical goods and services was made by old age pensioners living abroad for long periods who did not wish to give up their German residency.

The Court ruling in the Decker and Kohll cases was restricted to: 1) ambulatory care services which are 2) included in the benefits' catalogue of 3) patient reimbursement systems. Cases currently pending at the ECJ challenge these three restrictions. If decided in favour of increased choice, there will be significant implications for inpatient care and benefit-in-kind systems.

An unintended outcome of European interventions has therefore been the challenge to the benefit-in-kind principle. While this principle has been favoured in most Member States' health services in order to protect the consumer from direct payments, it tends to restrict the sovereignty of the patient in relation to cross-border consumer choice.

However, even if the ECJ decided against increased choice, i.e. in favour of a continuation of the status-quo, this would raise the question whether – within a SEM – it is justified that existing alternative methods of social protection institutionalise different methods to gain access to different benefits, partially different providers and potentially different levels of reimbursement.

Unrestricted access to services and providers outside the borders of the individual's country of insurance, reimbursed by public payers, would pose serious questions for national policy. How could Member States deny choice inside their own country (for example, to restrict access to a limited number of contracted providers) if these limitations do not exist for cross border care? To what extent would such a new situation undermine national health policy measures, such as rationing/prioritisation, or (more generally) cost-containment?

Under these circumstances, Member States might seek to restrict access to a defined minimum standard benefits package. Yet this would not provide a real solution to the problems raised by free mobility or patients, if this was only implemented by individual Member States, as access to nationally excluded services would be available for patients willing to travel. This leads to the ultimate question: would Member States have to design a uniform benefits catalogue, apply uniform reimbursement rates and a uniform system of accreditation, contracting and payment of providers – in effect a "European healthcare system"?

5. Further considerations

5.1 Markets and the European social model: the market ruling – or ruling the market?

Inherent in many of the conclusions emerging from this report is a critical difference between the way that the European Union views the relationship between "the market" and health services and the way that Member States view this relationship. At a European level, the SEM requires health services to adapt to market rules, while at national level, governments seek to adapt market rules to ensure the effective delivery of health services within a social model.

However, what is known as the "European social model" embraces particular values concerning social policy. The relevance of these values to health services – for example, promoting both solidarity and equity in access to health services – should be explored and stated openly. Where SEM regulations have consequences that may conflict with such values, it would be desirable to ensure that SEM regulations are not interpreted in a manner which will damage the values inherent in the "European social model".

Clearly where the freedoms embraced by the SEM are basic human freedoms (especially mobility of individuals), they cannot simply be ignored in the case of health services. To that extent, there is no question of simply "exempting health from the Single European Market". There may however be significant cases where regulation of the market is required in order to achieve health objectives. Paradoxically, this requires a new coherence and prominence for EU health policy – not just to draw a sustainable rather than accidental line between Member State policy and EU-wide policy, but also to make the aspirations of both these actors more coherent.

5.2 Avoiding possible unintended SEM effects in the future

It is not the function of this report to trace potential unintended effects to their extremes. It is worth pointing out, however, that the basic policy choice at European level concerns how best to resolve the inherent conflicts between the SEM and health policy. Is continuing pragmatism enough? Or will it be necessary to develop an EU health policy so that the SEM avoids negative effects either in relation to equity or solidarity in public healthcare systems, on in relation to perverse incentives as regards the education, training and movement of individuals (workers and consumers).

A coordinated approach would facilitate an exploration of options and possibilities to avoid the following unintended effects which otherwise might occur:

- *Restriction of benefits?* It is conceivable that future decisions of the ECJ in favour of increased choice might motivate or force the European Union and/or Member States to move towards a "standard benefits package". This might occur in a manner to threaten comprehensive public coverage if done in a "political panic".

- *Privatisation of supply?* Emphasising individual rights (e.g. to mobility) over public objectives is likely to increase the role of the private sector, since public planning is less viable when factors of production and rules of consumption cannot be controlled. Yet increasing reliance on the private sector to correct imbalances or shortages of health personnel or facilities might be at the expense of equitable access to publicly funded healthcare systems. The accession states in Central and Eastern Europe might, for example, experience a shortage of doctors over time due to emigration (partly due to SEM freedom of mobility) to richer Member States of the European Union. The consequence would be increasingly private medical education to produce doctors for private suppliers of healthcare, and this healthcare would disproportionately be purchased privately by the better off. Medical students would only enrol if they had expectation of income adequate to pay off their loans – probably private healthcare.

  Affordability of public healthcare in poorer Member States would be called into question if there were a need to pay "market rates" for scarce doctors, nurses and other healthcare professionals. Additionally, the mobility of scarce professionals may have an unintended incentive in the light of the EU's social objectives: Member States have a disincentive to educate doctors and other professionals publicly if a significant number are likely to emigrate.

- *Concentration of companies:* The SEM may incorporate contradictory objectives – first, competition within Europe; but second, the competitiveness of Europe in the world.

  On the one hand, it is often the case that European Union policy is aimed at the promotion of competition both within Europe and within the Member States and, indeed, the promotion of Small and Medium Enterprises (SMEs). But it is clear, particularly from the public procurement study, that competition within Europe may damage SMEs to the ultimate detriment of health services.

  On the other hand, regulations start from the recognition of increasing concentration not only in European but also in global markets. European-level recognition of new drugs through the EMEA can, for example, be a means of streamlining in the context of a multinational market for pharmaceuticals. The European Union's logical intention to use the SEM to strengthen its competitive position in the global marketplace can lead to concentrations of companies which might have negative consequences for health services.

5.3 The future for health policy-making: driving or being driven?

Even if the impact of many SEM interventions is small in terms of numbers of patients or professionals affected by these interventions, the systems turbulence caused by these interventions, particularly those resulting from ECJ decisions, may be greater than the numbers involved. SEM directives and ECJ rulings have the potential – in a "worst case" scenario – to undermine Beveridge systems if "managed competition" in compliance with other aspects of European law leads to the spread of sickness funds in the context of the insurance model. Equally, there could be considerable turbulence in Bismarckian systems if the rules were to be changed away from a "social" health insurance model.

To address such problems, arising from the unintended consequences of European Union regulation on health services, it is therefore time to raise the profile of health policy at the European Union level – but in a manner consistent with the aspirations of Member States.

Part I

Introduction

The European Union and Health Services
R. Busse et al. (Eds.)
IOS Press, 2002

17

The European Union and health services – the context

Matthias WISMAR, Reinhard BUSSE and Philip BERMAN

Abstract. With some exceptions, health policy has always played a minor role in European integration. A formal policy mandate in the area of public health was introduced with the Maastricht Treaty, which came into force in 1993. As health services were explicitly excluded from this mandate, there appears to be a contradiction to the Single European Market. Not surprisingly, research has therefore investigated various aspects of European integration in regard to its impact on health services since the early 1990s. While this research has contributed towards the understanding of the relation between the European Union and health services, an overall assessment of the impact of European Integration on health services of Member States is still missing.

1. The European Union and health policy

Health policy has always played a subordinate role in the course of European integration. Nevertheless, in some specific cases, health issues have been addressed. Elements of a policy for the protection of workers' health and safety were already introduced at the beginning of the fifties within the framework of the European Coal and Steel Community (ECSC). Health protection was also given early consideration in the European Atomic Energy Community (EURATOM), particularly in regard to the protection against ionising radiation. Aspects concerning health policy can also be found in the policies of the European Community (EC), but their significance tended to be of minor importance and focused on public health excluding health services regulation, financing or delivery.

The current structure of the European Union (EU), as depicted in Figure 1, comprises the three Communities pillars, namely the ECSC, EURATOM and the EC; Common Foreign and Security Policy; and Co-operation in the fields of Justice and Home Affairs. The three Communities have common institutions: the European Parliament, the Council, the Commission, the European Court of Justice and the Court of Auditors. Common Foreign and Security Policy and Co-operation in the fields of Justice and Home Affairs are not governed by the common institutions, but are developed directly by the Member States. The EU is to be understood as encompassing all these areas, the Communities and the latter two fields of policy. The research findings gathered in the chapters of this book exclusively focus on the European Community and its predecessor, the European Economic Community.

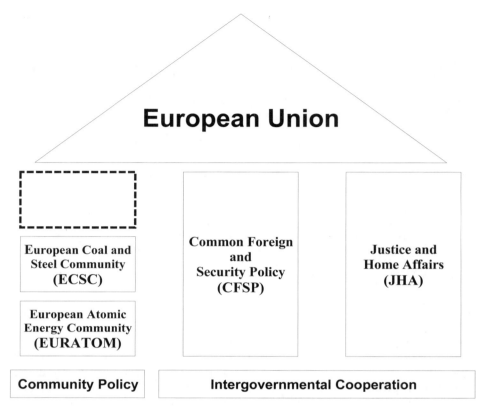

Fig. 1: The European "temple"

This institutional setting was established by the Treaty on the European Union (the Maastricht Treaty) which came into force in 1993. The objective of this Treaty was the fundamental reform of the existing Treaties and particularly the Treaty Establishing the European Community (TEC), which represents the core document of the European Community and contains the major legal provisions establishing the Single European Market (SEM). The SEM was established in its current form through the Single European Act in 1986, which aimed at the completion of the SEM by the end of 1992. The development of the various Treaties and elements of the European integration are represented in Figure 2.

In regard to health and health services, the Maastricht Treaty is of particular importance as it gave the Community concrete legal competencies related to health through two new provisions. First, Article 3(o) empowered the Community to "contribute to the attainment of a high level of health protection" for its citizens. Second, Article 129 repeated this objective ("Health protection requirements shall form a constituent part of the Community's other policies.") and outlined specific areas of competence to achieve such an objective, namely "the prevention of diseases, in particular the major health sources, including drug dependence" through promoting "research into their causes and their transmission, as well as health information and education" and "encouraging cooperation between the Member States and, if necessary, lending support to their action".

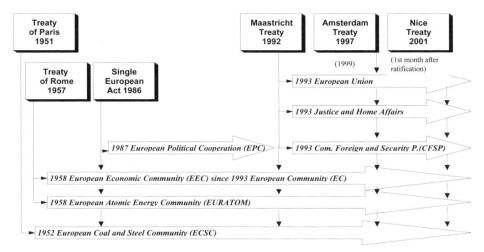

Fig. 2: Development of the treaties

This mandate on (public) health was renewed and slightly revised (mainly in response to the BSE crisis) in the renumbered Article 152 at the summit of Amsterdam in 1997. The "Amsterdam Treaty" was signed on 2 October 1997 and has been in force since 1 May 1999. Currently, the Treaty of Nice which will amend the Treaty on European Union and the Treaties Establishing the European Communities and certain related acts is in the process of ratification[1] and will come into force one month after this process has been finalised.[2]

Table 1 presents an overview on all articles in the Treaty in its Amsterdam and Maastricht versions which are directly related to health. With the exception of Article 137, none of the health related articles in the TEC will be changed by the Treaty of Nice. And, while Article 137 is both broadened and specified, the health aspect remains unchanged.

It should be noted, that the health related articles in the Treaty have differing characteristics. While Article 3, paragraph 1 (p) in particular, and to a certain extent Article 95, paragraphs 3, 6 and 8 as well as Article 186 formulate a general health related mandate, Articles 137, 140, 152, 153 and 174, paragraph 1 provide legal provisions for specific actions only. Other articles, however, refer to health as a reason to restrict other legal provisions in the Treaty.

What is basically a broad mandate on health policy, though, comes up against clear limits in the prevailing interpretation of the legal framework. The subsidiarity principle set out in Article 5 is invoked as a basic principle. In the areas which do not fall within its exclusive sphere of competence, the Community only becomes active if and when it is clear that their objectives cannot be realised by the Member States and can only be achieved effectively at a Community level.

---

[1] At the time of writing, the Treaty of Nice has not yet been ratified by Belgium, Greece, The Netherlands and Sweden. In a referendum on the Treaty, Ireland voted against ratification.

[2] Since the amended TEC is not yet in force, the general rule is that articles in the TEC will be quoted by the version of the Treaty of Amsterdam. Reference to other versions of the Treaty will be made when appropriate and indicated in the text.

Table 1: Anchoring the EU's mandate on health policy in the EC Treaty

Article, new version (Amsterdam Treaty)	Article, old version (Maastricht Treaty)	Contents/ significance for public health
3 par. 1 (p)	3 (o)	a contribution to the attainment of a high level of health protection
30	36	restriction of free movement of goods on the grounds of health
39 par. 3	48	restriction of free movement of workers on the grounds of public health
46 par. 1	56	restriction of the right of establishment on the grounds of public health
95 par. 3	100 (a)	attainment of a high level of health protection in the approximation of laws
95 par. 6	100 (a)	extension of the approximation period in the absence of danger for human health
95 par. 8	100 (a)	Member States obligation to notify specific public health problems in a field which has been the subject of prior harmonisation matters
137	118	improvement in particular of the working environment to protect workers' health and safety
140	118c	prevention of occupational accidents and diseases
152	**129**	**public health competencies**
153	129a	health protection as part of consumer protection
174 par. 1	130 (r)	protecting human health as part of environmental policies
186	135	including public health provisions to the provisions on the association of the overseas countries and territories

This general subsidiarity principle is specifically reflected twice in Article 152 of the TEC, namely in paragraph 4(c) ("... excluding any harmonisation of the laws and regulations of the Member States.") as well as in paragraph 5 ("Community action in the field of public health shall fully respect the responsibilities of the Member States for the organisation and delivery of health services and medical care."). This is often interpreted as a clear indication that healthcare is not the subject of Community policy and that any kind of intervention or harmonisation of the structures for regulating, financing and delivering medical care on the part of the Community institutions is to be categorically excluded.

In political terms, there appears, therefore, to be a contradiction between the purpose of the Single European Market (SEM) and the manner in which the statements in Article 152 are widely interpreted. However, the inherent dualism in the TEC between an integrated SEM on the one hand, and health services with their national borders on the other has to be called into question on theoretical grounds. After all, the free movement of persons, goods, services and capital, as established in the TEC, also involves the principle of unrestricted mobility of doctors, other healthcare professionals, patients, medicines, technical equipment, and direct investments into healthcare facilities in the EU. The allocation of health services to an area which remains impervious to EC legislation and judicial decisions concerning the SEM is therefore implausible.[3]

2. Research on European integration, health and health services

Academic research has only recently begun to turn its attention to the relatively new filed of EU health policy. The purpose of this section is to map European integration and health services as a field of research. The intention is to provide an overview of the research questions and issues in order to set the background for this study and to locate it in its academic context. It is not the intention, therefore, to provide a comprehensive review on the literature.

2.1 The completion of the SEM and health services

With the ratification of the Single European Act, the question of the impact of European integration on health services gained relevance on the scientific agenda. Various topics were highlighted, for example the harmonisation of taxes, in particular VAT, in terms of their impact on financing health services. Other studies focused on the free movement of physicians and nurses, the pharmaceutical sector, medical devices, the export of social benefits, health protection at the working place, and the possibility of cross-border hospital care at border regions. This early discussion of the impact of European integration on health services of Member States also raised concerns – depending on the country perspective – about the likelihood that integration might put pressure on social standards that had been achieved, leading to a reduction in healthcare benefits and health protection or, alternatively, that the integration would exert a nationally undesired upward pressure of social standards (Deppe 1990; Deppe & Lehnhard 1990; Lehnhard 1990; Deppe 1991; Ham 1991; Altenstetter 1992; Sachverständigenrat für die Konzertierte Aktion im Gesundheits-wesen 1992). Like an "overture", this research has introduced important themes which are still relevant for research on European integration and healthcare. Yet, while this research was being carried out, the SEM was not yet completed and important areas, such as data protection or medical devices, were at this time only partially regulated by European law, i.e. the research was necessarily theoretical rather than empirical.

2.2 Tracing the legal development Europe's role in health

Another body of literature attempts to analyse the political mandate on health issues introduced by the Maastricht Treaty in order to arrive at new political strategies for action (Mäder 1995). There are, in addition, studies which consider the mandate particularly from the perspective of administrative law, but also from a historical perspective (Schwanenflügel 1996; Berg 1997). These studies are of great value in providing, for the first time, an overview on health activities of the Community institutions in the field of health policy. However, since these studies approach the subject primarily from a juridical point of view, they are less sensitive towards the outcomes and effects of European

---

[3] It was only recently that the German Advisory Council for the Concerted Action in Health Care emphatically referred to the dual function of the health system as a welfare-state sector consuming the wealth of the nation services and, at the same time, a productive branch of industry. Thus the special reports for 1996 and 1997 (Sachverständigenrat für die Konzertierte Aktion im Gesundheitswesen 1996, 1998) bear the title "Gesundheitswesen in Deutschland: Kostenfaktor und Zukunftsbranche" (The Health Care System in Germany: Cost Factor and Branch of the Future). Admittedly, the special reports do not consider this dual function and its inherent tension in relation to European integration.

legislation on Member States. The analysis of a "hidden agenda" or the emergence of a policy in regard to healthcare is outside the focus of these studies.

2.3 Health as an horizontal issue in European integration

Shortly after the inclusion of the health mandate in the TEC, academic debate started (Ham & Berman 1992). Two strands can be distinguished, the first focussing on the areas and determinants of health (and possibly health services) that the EU should address, and the second looking in the other direction – on the impact of EU health policy on the Member States. A prominent example of the former is the book "Choices in Health Policy – An Agenda for the European Union" (Abel-Smith et al. 1995) which is based on a report for Health Ministers. Following that, systematic attempts by the Commission were made to integrate health requirements into all policies of the EC (Hunter & Hübel 1996). While these attempts were warmly welcomed, there has been criticism that these reports fall short in terms of rigour, because they had – unsuccessfully – to rely on the willingness of all parts of the Commission to provide the necessary information (Coghlan 1996). At the same time, the first publications focusing in the other direction began to appear (e.g. McKee et al. 1996).

Today, many conferences and publications by Member States and various organisations are trying combine the two perspectives. Examples include the conference proceedings of a large conference held in Germany when it held the presidency in the EU (Bellach & Stein 1999) or the annual conferences organised by the European Health Forum Gastein (e.g. Leiner & Schuppe 2001). This broader perspective has also been pursued in academic work (Theofilatou 2000).

2.4 The "completed" SEM and its impact on health policy

After "Maastricht", analysis also focused on specific elements of the SEM in regard to health and health services, especially in the areas of medical devices (Altenstetter 1996; Heppell 1996; Altenstetter 1998) and pharmaceuticals (Mossialos 1998; Keck 1999) but also on private health insurance (Bastiani 1995), health protection at the working place (Gerlinger 2000) and the labour market for health professionals (Jinks et al. 2000). One of the reasons that these research projects were undertaken was that new legislation was being introduced to harmonise various aspects of these sectors across the Member States of the EU. In some cases even new institutions, for example the European Agency for the Evaluation of Medicinal Products (EMEA), were being established.

2.5 Empirical studies on patient mobility

Prior to the ruling of the ECJ in the cases Kohll and Decker, the subject of cross-border patient mobility was addressed in terms of an assessment of the existing instruments which regulate and facilitate cross-border care within the EU. Empirical studies have focused on the "E 111" procedure which applies to emergency care during short stay abroad (Hermans & Berman 1996; Hermans & Berman 1998), on patient mobility (Hermesse et al. 1997) including case studies, for example on Italy (France 1997) and Greece (Kyriopoulos & Gitona 1998), and on patients' rights to cross-border care (Hermans 1997; Verschueren 1999).

Cross-border healthcare schemes which were set up in the "EUREGIOs" attracted especial interest. There are a number of useful published studies on these EUREGIO: Meuse-Rhine (Starmans et al. 1997; Hofmann & Kochs 1998; Grünwald & Smit 1999); Rhine-Waal (Lottman & Wilt 1999), and overviews on the various schemes (Ministry for

Women Youth Family and Health of the State of North Rhine-Westphalia 2000; Mountford 2000; Palm et al. 2000).

Research has not only focused on the actual cross-border flows but also on the administrative mechanisms that facilitate this cross-border flow. Some studies have sought to analyse citizens' and patients' knowledge, attitudes and experience of cross-border care within the EU (Calnan et al. 1997; Calnan et al. 1998; Gesellschaft für Versicherungswissenschaft und -gestaltung 2001).

2.6 Analysis of ECJ cases on cross-border care

In April 1998, two preliminary rulings of the European Court of Justice (ECJ) caused a stir among Member States. The two Luxembourg citizens, Kohll and Decker, had obtained goods and services in the field of medical care while abroad. Decker obtained a pair of spectacles in Belgium on presentation of a Luxembourg prescription, while Kohll took his under-age daughter across the border to Germany for orthodontic treatment. When they returned to Luxembourg, both citizens demanded reimbursement from their health insurance funds. This was refused on the grounds that no preliminary approval had been granted (i.e. the E112 form). The argument was that the European directives provided for reimbursement of costs through the competent institution only in cases of medical emergency while on business trips or on holiday, unless preliminary approval had been obtained. A journey with the explicit purpose of obtaining benefits abroad, it was argued, did not fall within the scope of the European directives. The Luxembourg health insurance funds did not therefore see themselves under any obligation to reimburse the expenses. The cases were brought before a Luxembourg court. As the plaintiffs invoked the free movement of goods and services in the EC, the Luxembourg court sought clarification from the ECJ on the interpretation of the Treaty. The outcome is well known. In its decisions of April 28th 1998, the ECJ largely upheld the view of the two citizens from Luxembourg. Since then, a steady stream of cases on cross-border healthcare have been brought before the ECJ. These cases and the rulings of the ECJ have attracted considerable attention and have made clear the impact that the SEM has on health services of Member States.

Clearly, with Decker and Kohll, the volume of literature on the subject has increased with remarkable speed and has now reached almost impenetrable proportions. And the end of this growth is not in sight, since a number of new cases are pending with the ECJ (Wismar & Busse 1998; Mountford 2000; Palm et al. 2000; Wismar & Busse 2001; Wismar 2001).

The ECJ cases have put a number of fundamental issues on the agenda. Some authors have analysed the types of social benefits are in principle subject to European legislation (Füßer 1997). Another issue of real relevance is the future of the benefit-in-kind principle. The argument was put forward that the Kohll and Decker rulings may imply that the option for cost-reimbursement has to be provided at least as an alternative to the benefit-in-kind principle by the competent institution. This would entail a different patient-provider relation (Wille 1999). The ECJ rulings also raised questions concerning the elective in-patient sector, especially since free cross-border mobility of elective patients might result in high expenditure, with the consequent impact on existing budgets and the potential to undermine public capacity planning (Burger 2001). Clearly, this body of literature is not only concerned with the extend to what the free movement of people and services has to be applied to healthcare institutions but also to the repercussions on institutional settings, delivery, management and governance of health services (van der Mei 1998; van der Mei 1999). Related to the court cases there are accounts on the political perception of Kohll and Decker throughout the Member States (Gobrecht 1999).

2.7 Competition law and self-governing bodies

Another strand in the scientific and political debate on European integration and health services refers to competition law in the TEC. According to Article 81, all agreements between "undertakings" or their associations which may prevent, restrict or distort competition within the SEM are incompatible with European law. This article refers in particular to direct or indirect price fixing or any other trading conditions. Competition law applies to all undertakings no matter whether they are private or public (Eichenhofer 2001). And indeed, undertakings are not assessed by their formal or legal status but by the function they fulfil.

National health services are less affected by competition law since European competition law does not apply to state activities. But, in Social Health Insurance countries, many tasks are delegated from the Ministry or state institutions either to the self-governing bodies of physicians or to sickness funds. Their status as institutions under public law with a set of explicitly delegated powers does not, in principle, prevent them from becoming subject to European competition law. Not surprisingly, research – mainly by lawyers – is based in countries such as Belgium (e.g. Pieters & van den Bogaert 1997), Germany or the Netherlands.

There are various areas which are currently under debate. For example in Germany the reference price system in the pharmaceutical sector is being questioned. According to § 35 Social Code Book V, the federal associations of the sickness funds have the responsibility to set the prices of the reference price list. A pharmaceutical which exceeds this price ceiling is still available an may be prescribed, but any amount of money above this ceiling has to be paid out of pocket by the patient. It is up to the physician and the patient to make the decision whether a pharmaceutical which is below the price ceiling shall be prescribed. The current discussion focuses on the question as to whether price setting by the federal associations of the sickness funds is incompatible with European competition law since it is suggested that they fix prices and a form of cartel which is incompatible with Article 81 of the TEC (Giesen 2001). To be on the safe side, the regulations regarding the setting of reference prices were recently suspended for 2002 and 2003 in favour of governmental price-setting by ordinance. But the debate on the applicability of European competition law goes far beyond single mechanisms such as the pharmaceutical price regulation scheme. In Germany, it reaches the Federal Committee of Statutory Health Insurance Physicians and Sickness Funds which is performing a variety of highly relevant functions essential to the whole system architecture (Busse 2000). Even the collective contracts between sickness funds and physicians may come under the suspect of cartel building (Eichenhofer 2001). The situation is new insofar as the application of social legislation in the area of social security in Germany had priority over German competition law. But this is not the case for European law which is considered to have priority over domestic law and is instantly applicable (Knispel 2001).

2.8 Comparing prices, benefits and quality

It has been argued that with the introduction of the Euro in most Member States, cross-border price comparisons will be made by patients, purchasers and politicians. This might result in an intensified "shopping around" across Europe for best value healthcare (Kücking 1998). Yet, our knowledge on prices and contents of benefit packages in Member States is very limited. Nevertheless initial attempts to compare certain parts of benefit packages have been made (Kupsch et al. 2000). Other studies have focused on specific benefits and price comparisons (Kaufhold & Schneider 2000). Pharmaceutical pricing policies are another relevant issue in this debate (Mossialos 1998). Cross-border care also raises the question of quality. The ECJ has argued, in regard to Kohll and Decker, that cross-border care does not pose a threat to human health, since a similar standard of healthcare can be expected in all Member States. This opinion was based on the assumption that mutual recognition of diplomas and established minimum training requirements for health professions will guarantee this standard. But not all health professions are regulated by these directives, and it remains questionable if the assumption is valid (Nickless 2001). Undoubtedly, this strand of research has gained new relevance in the light of the ECJ court cases.

2.9 European integration, healthcare and policy development

The completion of the SEM, the Interreg programmes and the Maastricht Treaty have all raised awareness and interest in the political arena about the relationship between European integration and health and healthcare. This interest has certainly intensified with the Kohll/Decker rulings and more recently with the Peerbooms case. Border regions in particular attempted to respond proactively to the new developments by supporting cross-border health planning and delivery, for example in the German "Land" of North Rhine-Westphalia and its neighbouring regions in the EU (Sendler 1996; Ministry for Women Youth Family and Health of the State of North Rhine-Westphalia 2000). During the last German presidency of the EU the Minister of Health acknowledged the impact of European integration (Fischer 1999).

In the Social Health Insurance countries – Austria, Belgium, France, Germany, Luxembourg and the Netherlands – the self-governing bodies and their associations investigated this matter. There is, for example, a study on the Austrian social security system's compatibility with European economic regulations (Schulz-Weidner & Felix 1997). In the Netherlands, at the request of the Council of Health and Social Services, a report was commissioned to assess the scope, risk and chances of the SEM in healthcare (Belcher 1999). The resulting main report by the Council came to the conclusion that the Dutch health system is facing major challenges (RVZ 1999). In order to reach political conclusions, the SEM in healthcare for purchasers, providers and patients has also been analysed in Germany (Gesellschaft für Versicherungswissenschaft und -gestaltung 1996). The working committee of the federal associations of sickness fund in Germany has agreed on a common position in regard to the ECJ rulings (Arbeitsgemeinschaft der Spitzen-verbände der gesetzlichen Krankenkassen 2000). Various sickness funds in Germany have made attempts to develop positions (Klusen 2000; Lorff & Maier-Rigaud 2000).

Clearly, the impact of the SEM, European competition law and the EU health mandate on health services in the Member States is not only an academic affair, it is of relevance for the various actors in the domestic health policy arenas.

References

Abel-Smith B, Figueras J, Holland W, McKee M, Mossialos E. Choices in health policy – an agenda for the European Union. Aldershot-Brookfield-Singapore-Sydney: Dartmouth; 1995.

Altenstetter C. Health policy regimes and the single European market. J Health Polit Policy Law 1992;17(4):813-46.

Altenstetter C. Regulating healthcare technologies and medical supplies in the European Economic Area. Health Policy 1996;35(1):33-52.

Altenstetter C. Regulating and financing medical devices in the European Union. In: Leidl R, editor. Health care and its financing in the single European market. Amsterdam-Berlin-Oxford-Tokyo-Washington DC: IOS Press; 1998. p. 116-49.

Arbeitsgemeinschaft der Spitzenverbände der gesetzlichen Krankenkassen. Strategischer Umgang der GKV mit den aktuellen europarechtlichen Entwicklungen – Herausforderung Europa annehmen und gestalten [Strategy of the statutory health insurance in regard to current European legal developments - tackling the European challenge and shaping the future]. 2000.

Bastiani A. Die private Krankenversicherung in ausgewählten Ländern der Europäischen Union. Eine vergleichende Analyse vor und nach der Deregulierung [The private health insurance in selected Member States of the European Union. A comparative analysis before and after deregulation]. Karlsruhe: VWW; 1995.

Belcher P. The role of the European Union in Healthcare. Zoetermeer: Council for Health and Social Service (RVZ); 1999.

Bellach BM, Stein H, editors. The new public health policy of the European Union. Past experience, present needs, future perspectives. München: Urban und Vogel; 1999.

Berg W. Gesundheitsschutz als Aufgabe der EU: Entwicklung, Kompetenzen, Perspektiven [Health protection as a EU-task: developments, competencies and perspectives]. Baden-Baden: Nomos Verlagsgesellschaft; 1997.

Burger S. Europäischer Gerichtshof: freier Dienstleitungsverkehr auch für stationäre Leistungen – Beschränkungen sind möglich [European Court of Justice: free movement of services for in patient servcies - restrictions possible]. Die Betriebskrankenkasse 2001;89(8):356-8.

Busse R. Health care systems in transition – Germany. Written in collaboration with A. Riesberg and edited by A. Dixon. Copenhagen: European Observatory on Health Care Systems; 2000.

Calnan M, Palm W, Sohy F, Quaghebeur D. Cross-border use of health care. A survey of frontier workers' knowledge, attitutdes and use. Eur J Public Health 1997;7(3 Suppl.):26-32.

Calnan M, Palm W, Sohy F, Quaghebeur D. Implementing a policy for cross-border use of health care: a case study of frontier worker's knowledge, attitutes and use. In: Leidl R, editor. Health care and its financing in the single European market. Amsterdam-Berlin-Oxford-Tokyo-Washington DC: IOS Press; 1998. p. 306-11.

Coghlan T. Commission Report on the Integration of Health Protection Requirements - A response. eurohealth 1996;2(4):6-8.

Deppe HU. Perspektiven der Gesundheitspolitik: Bundesrepublik Deutschland und Europäische Gemeinschaft [Perspectives in health policy: The Federal Republic and the European Community]. Frankfurt/Main: VAS, Verlag für Akademische Schriften; 1990.

Deppe HU. Auswirkungen der europäischen Wirtschaftsintegration auf die Gesundheitspolitik in der Bundesrepublik Deutschland [Effects of European economic integration on the health policy of the Federal Republic of Germany]. In: Deppe HU, Friedrich H, Müller R, editors. Öffentliche Gesundheit = Public Health. Frankfurt/Main-New York: Campusverlag; 1991. p. 60-83.

Deppe HU, Lehnhard U. Die Gesundheitsssysteme in den Ländern der EG und der westeuropäische Integrationsprozeß – Ein Überblick unter besonderer Berücksichtigung der Bundesrepublik [Health systems in the Member States of the European Community and the West-European integration – An overview in special consideration of the Federal Republic of Germany]. In: Deppe HU, Lehnhard U. Westeuropäische Integration und Gesundheitspolitik [West European integration and health policy]. Marburg: Verlag Arbeit und Gesellschaft; 1990. p. 7-46.

Eichenhofer E. Der Bundesausschuss der Ärzte und Krankenkassen und das EU-Wettbewerbsrecht [National Committee of SHI-Physicians and Sickness funds and the EU-competition law]. G+G Wissenschaft 2001;1(2):14-8.

Fischer A. A new public health policy in the European Union. In: Bellach BM, Stein H, editors. The new public health policy of the European Union. Past experience, present needs, future perspectives. München: Urban und Vogel; 1999. p. 10-22.

France G. Cross-border flows of Italian patients within the European Union. An international trade approach. Eur J Public Health 1997;7(3 Suppl.):18-25.

Füßer K. Transfer sozialversicherungsrechtlicher Komplexleistungen ins Ausland – zur Öffnungsbereitschaft des aktuellen Sozialversicherungrechts aus der Sicht des europäischen Gemeinschaftsrechts [Transfer of social insurance complex benefits into foreign countries]. Arbeit und Sozialpolitik 1997;51(9/10):30-49.

Gerlinger T. Arbeitsschutz und europäische Integration: europäische Arbeitsschutzrichtlinien und nationalstaatliche Arbeitsschutzpolitik in Großbritannien und Deutschland [Health protection at the working place and European integration: European and national health protection policy at the working place in Great Britain and Germany]. Opladen: Leske und Budrich; 2000.

Gesellschaft für Versicherungswissenschaft und -gestaltung (GVG). Auswirkungen der Politik der Europäischen Union auf das Gesundheitswesen und die Gesundheitspolitik in der Bundesrepublik Deutschland. [Effects of the European Union's policy on health services and health policy of the Federal Republic of Germany] In: Gesellschaft für Versicherungswissenschaft und -gestaltung (GVG), editor. Einfluß der Europäischen Union auf das Gesundheitswesen in der Bundesrepublik Deutschland – Bestandsaufnahme und Perspektiven. Bonn: Irmgard Vollmer; 1996. p. 1-103

Gesellschaft für Versicherungswissenschaft und -gestaltung (GVG). Medizinische Leistungen im EU-Ausland [Medical benefits in other Member States of the EU]. Hamburg: Techniker Krankenkasse; 2001.

Giesen R. Das Kartellrecht der GKV-Leistungserbringung und die dafür gültige neue Rechtswegzuweisung [Cartel law of statutory health insurance service provision and the the newly assigned courts]. G+G Wissenschaft 2001;1(2):19-23.

Gobrecht J. National reactions to Kohll and Decker. eurohealth 1999;5(1):16-7.

Grünwald CA, Smit RLC. Zorg op Maat in der Euregio Maas-Rhein – Evaluierung eines Modellprojektes. Amstelveen: Ziekenfondsraad; 1999.

Ham C. The European Community and UK, health and health services. In: Harrison A, editor. Health Care UK 1991. London: King's Fund Institute; 1991.

Ham C, Berman P. Health policy in Europe: Many changes will result from new chapter on public health. Brit Med J 1992;304:855-6.

Heppell S. The new European system for regulating medicinal products. eurohealth 1996;2(4):28-9.

Hermans HEGM. Patient's rights in the European Union. Eur J Public Health 1997;7(3 Suppl.):11-7.

Hermans HEGM, Berman PC. Free movement of citizens in the EU: Consequences for health provision. Report for the Commission of the European Communities. Dublin: European Healthcare Management Association; 1996.

Hermans HEGM, Berman PC. Access to health care and health services in the European Union: regulation 1408/71 and the E111 process. In: Leidl R, editor. Health care and its financing in the single European market. Amsterdam-Berlin-Oxford-Tokyo-Washington DC: IOS Press; 1998. p. 324-43.

Hermesse J, Lewalle H, Palm W. Patient mobiltiy within the European Union. Eur J Public Health 1997;7(3 Suppl.):4-10.

Hofmann B, Kochs U. Freier Zugang zu Gesundheitsleistungen in Grenzgebieten – Grenzüberschreitendes Projekt in der Euregio Maas-Rhein [Free access to health services in border regions - cross border pilots in the Euregio Maas-Rhein]. Die Betriebskrankenkasse 1998;6(6):306-8.

Hunter W, Hübel M. Integration of health protection requirements into European Community policies. eurohealth 1996;2(4):4-5.

Jinks C, Ong BN, Paton C. Mobile medics? The mobility of doctors in the European Economic Area. Health Policy 2000;54(1):45-64.

Kaufhold R, Schneider M. Preisvergleich zahnärztlicher Leistungen im europäischen Kontext [Price comparison of dental benefits in the European context]. IDZ - Information Institut der deutschen Zahnärzte 2000;(1):1-33.

Keck J. The European Union Single Market in pharmaceuticals. eurohealth 1999;5(1):23-5.

Klusen N. Chancen und Risiken auf dem europäischen Gesundheitsmarkt. Rechte der gesetzlich Krankenversicherten in der Europäischen Union [Chances and risks in the European health market. Legal entitlements of the statutory health insurance insurees in the European Union]. Baden-Baden: Nomos Verlagsgesellschaft; 2000.

Knispel U. Zur Bedeutung des europäischen Wettbewerbsrechts für die gesetzliche Krankenversicherung [Relevance of the European competition law for the statutory health insurance]. G+G Wissenschaft 2001;1(2):7-13.

Kupsch S, Kern AO, Klas C, Kressin BKW, Vienonen M, Beske F. Health service provision on a microcosmic level: an international comparision; results of a WHO/IGSF Survey in 15 European Countries. Kiel: Institut für Gesundheits-System-Forschung; 2000.

Kücking M. Europa und die Zukunft der sozialen Sicherungssysteme [Europe and the future of social security systems]. Die Ersatzkasse 1998;78(5):214-6.

Kyriopoulos J, Gitona M. Cross-border health care in Greece: a macro- and micro-analysis of pre-authorised care. In: Leidl R, editor. Health care and its financing in the single European market. Amsterdam-Berlin-Oxford-Tokyo-Washington DC: IOS Press; 1998. p. 312-23.

Lehnhard U. EG-Binnenmarkt und Arzneimittelpolitik Arzneimittelpolitik [EU-internal market and pharmaceutical policies]. In: Deppe HU, Lehnhard U. Westeuropäische Integration und Gesundheitspolitik. Marburg: Verlag Arbeit und Gesellschaft; 1990. p. 63-104.

Leiner G, Schuppe M, editors. European Health Forum Gastein 2000: Information and Communication in Health. Bad Hofgastein: EHFG; 2001.

Lorff G, Maier-Rigaud G. Die europäische Krankenversicherung ist längst möglich – Weggestaltungen für die Zukunft [The European health insurance has been possible for a long time- perspectives for the future]. Zeitschrift für Sozialhilfe und Sozialgesetzbuch 2000;(9):393-8.

Lottman PEM, Wilt GJ. Projekt Grenzüberschreitende Behandlung in der Euregio Rhein/Waal. Patienten-behandlung ohne Grenzen für bestimmte Krankheitsbilder [Project on cross-border care in the Euregio Rhein/Waal. Treatment without borders for certain indications]. Nijmegen: Abteilung Medical Technology Assessment, Cluster biomedizinische Wissenschaften und nichtstationäre Heilkunde (BEG); 1999.

Mäder W. Gesundheitswesen im Binnenmarkt: Rechtsgrundlagen, strukturelle Rahmenbedingungen und Handlungsstrategien [Health systems and the internal market. Legal background, institutional frame-works and strategies for action]. In: Clever P, Schulte B, editors. Bürger Europas [Citizens of Europe]. Bonn: Dümmler; 1995. p. 117-33.

McKee M, Mossialos E, Belcher P. The influence of European Law on national health policy. J Eur Soc Policy 1996;6(4):263-86.

Ministry for Women Youth Family and Health of the State of North Rhine-Westphalia. Health Policy in Europe. Developments, Chances and Prospects from the Point of View of the State of North Rhine-Westphalia (NRW). Düsseldorf: Ministry for Women, Youth, Family and Health of the State of North Rhine-Westphalia; 2000.

Mossialos E. Pharmaceutical pricing, financing and cost containment in the European Union member states. In: Leidl R, editor. Health care and its financing in the single European market. Amsterdam-Berlin-Oxford-Tokyo-Washington DC: IOS Press; 1998. p. 85-115.

Mountford L. Health care without frontiers? The development of a European market in health services? London: Office of Health Economics; 2000.

Nickless J. A guarantee of similar standards of medical treatment across the EU: Were the European Court of Justice decisions in Kohll and Decker right? eurohealth 2001;7(1):16-8.

Palm W, Nickless J, Lewalle H, Coheur A. Implications of recent jurisprudence on the co-ordination of health care protection systems. General report produced for the Directorate-General for Employment and Social Affairs of the European Commission. Brussels: Association Internationale de la Mutualité (AIM); 2000.

Pieters D, van den Bogaert S. The consequences of European competition law for national health policies. Antwerp: MAKLU Uitgevers; 1997.

RVZ – Council for Public Health and Health Care. Europe and Health Care. Zoetermeer: RVZ; 1999.

Sachverständigenrat für die Konzertierte Aktion im Gesundheitswesen. Ausbau in Deutschland und Aufbruch nach Europa, Jahresgutachten 1992 [Extension in Germany and on the road towards Europe. Annual Report 1992]. Baden-Baden: Nomos Verlagsgesellschaft; 1992.

Sachverständigenrat für die Konzertierte Aktion im Gesundheitswesen. Gesundheitswesen in Deutschland: Kostenfaktor und Zukunftsbranche. Band I: Demographie, Morbidität, Wirtschaftlichkeitsreserven und Be-schäftigung; Sondergutachten 1996 [Health care system in Germany: cost factor and branch of the future. Vol. I: demography, morbidity, efficiency reserves and employment]. Baden-Baden: Nomos Verlagsgesellschaft; 1996.

Sachverständigenrat für die Konzertierte Aktion im Gesundheitswesen. Gesundheitswesen in Deutschland Kostenfaktor und Zukunftsbranche. Band II Fortschritt und Wachstumsmärkte, Finanzierung und Vergütung. Sondergutachten 1997 [Health care system in Germany: cost factor and branch of the future. Vol. II: Progress and growth markets, finance and remuneration. Special Report 1997]. Baden-Baden: Nomos Verlagsgesellschaft; 1998.

Schulz-Weidner W, Felix F. Die Konsequenzen der Europäischen Wirtschaftsverfassung für die Österreichische Sozialversicherung [The consequences of the European economic polity for the Austrian social insurance]. Soziale Sicherheit Fachzeitschrift der Österreichischen Sozialversicherung 1997;50(12):1121-60.

Schwanenflügel M von. Die Entwicklung der Kompetenzen der Europäischen Union im Gesundheitswesen [The development of European Union competences in the health sector]. Berlin: Erich Schmidt Verlag; 1996.

Sendler H. Bestandsaufnahme und Perspektiven der EU-Politik im Bereich des Gesundheitswesens aus Sicht eines Bundeslandes [Survey on and perspectives of the EU-Policy in the area of health services from a state's point of view]. In: Gesellschaft für Versicherungswissenschaft und -gestaltung, editor. Auswirkungen der Politik der Europäischen Union auf das Gesundheitswesen und die Gesundheitspolitik in der Bundesrepublik Deutschland – Bestandsaufnahmen und Perspektiven [Impact of European Union politics on health services and health policy in the Federal Republic of Germany - Status-quo and perspectives]. Bonn: Irmgard Vollmer; 1996. p. 51-8.

Starmans B, Leidl R, Rhodes G. A comparative study on cross-broder hospital care in the Euregio Meuse-Rhine. Eur J Public Health 1997;7(3 Suppl.):33-41.

Theofilatou MA. The emerging health agenda. The health policy of the european community. Doctoral Thesis Universiteit Maastricht; 2000.

van der Mei AP. Cross-border access to medical care within the European Union - Some reflections on the judgements in Decker and Kohll. Maastricht Journal of European and Comparative Law 1998;5(4):277-97.

van der Mei AP. The Kohll and Decker rulings: revolution or evolution? eurohealth 1999;5(1):14-6.

Verschueren H. The patient's position under EC law. In: Bellach BM, Stein H, editors. The new Public Health Policy of the European Union. Past experience, present needs, future perspectives. München: Urban und Vogel; 1999. p. 236-41.

Wille E. Das Sachleistungsprinzip in der GKV im Spannungsfeld der europäischen Integration [The benefit-in-kind principle of the statutory health insurance in tension with European integration]. Die Krankenversicherung 1999;51(10):292-6.

Wismar M. Warum Herr Peerboms aus dem Koma erwachte [Why Mr. Peerboms rose from coma]. Gesundheit und Gesellschaft 2000;3(4):22-3.

Wismar M. ECJ in the driving seat on health policy – but what's the destination? eurohealth 2001;7(3):5-6.

Wismar M, Busse R. Freedom of movement challenges European health care scenery. eurohealth 1998;4(2):13-5.

Wismar M, Busse R. Effects of the European Single Market integration on the German public health system. In: Bellach B-M, Stein H, editors. The new public health policy of the European Union. Past experience, present needs, future perspectives. München: Urban und Vogel; 1999a. p. 83-99.

Wismar M, Busse R. The impact of Single European Market regulations on health services of Member States. In: Bellach BM, Stein H, editors. The new public health policy of the European Union. Past experience, present needs, future perspectives. München: Urban und Vogel; 1999b. p. 241-5.

Wismar M, Busse R. Europa Ante Portas. Gesellschaftspolitische Kommentare 2001;42(10):14-8.

The European Union and Health Services
R. Busse et al. (Eds.)
IOS Press, 2002

31

The Single European Market and health services - the research design

Philip BERMAN, Reinhard BUSSE, Matthias WISMAR, Bie Nio ONG and
Calum PATON

Abstract. This chapter describes first the three phases of the project and their objectives. It then explains how the four freedoms of persons, goods, services and capital were broken down into 14 analytical categories (e.g. labour market for doctors and dentists, pharmaceutical market, consumer choice services). Furthermore, definitions on terms are given, e.g. that *impact* refers to the effect of SEM interventions upon domestic legislation and the administrative rules of national or regional institutions while *outcomes* are defined in terms of effects on health services or healthcare. The final sections give details about the methods and research strategies used in the three phases; particular emphasis is given to the scenarios developed in phase 3.

1. Purpose and structure of the project

The purpose of the project was to analyse the impact of the EU Internal Market – or Single European Market (SEM) – on the regulating, financing and delivery of health services in the Member States. While the Treaty Establishing the European Community (TEC) defines several areas of competence for the European Union with potential impact on healthcare and health services, this project is concerned only with the SEM, with its four freedoms i.e. the free movement of persons/ individuals; the free movement of goods; the free movement of services; and the free movement of capital. The project did not therefore deal with other areas such as competition law, agriculture, social protection, environmental policy etc. Neither did it deal with public health measures, research on health, or health policy under EU programmes (Figure 1).

The study was an international research project conducted in three phases, each aiming at achieving two main objectives:

Phase 1
- To identify SEM regulations and directives as well as respective European Court of Justice (ECJ) decisions which explicitly refer to health services and which therefore are classified as having a potential impact on the purchasing, supply and delivery of health services.
- To identify both the methods used as well as the actual extent to which these EU directives have been transposed into the laws and rules of the Member States, whether at national or regional level.

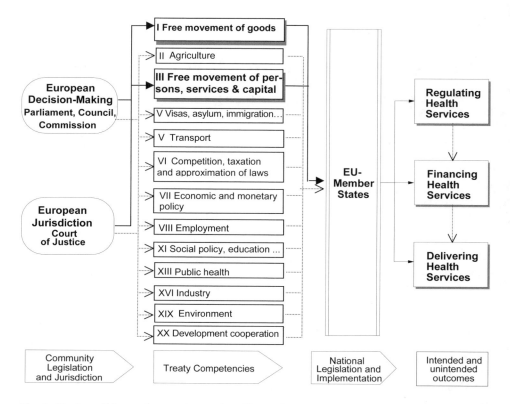

Fig. 1: Design of the study to estimate the effects of the Single European Market on the
     health services of the Member States

Phase 2
–   To analyse the factors involved in the extent to which EU regulations have been
     adopted.
–   To evaluate the impact of these national or regional laws and rules on the purchasing,
     supply and delivery of health services (i.e. to what extent has policy in Member States
     been changed?).

Phase 3
–   To identify outcomes, including both intended and unintended effects, of the SEM on
     Member States' health services and to develop futures scenarios exploring key issues
     identified in the earlier analysis and evaluation; and
–   To produce an overall report highlighting and analysing the key issues.
–   To explore whether duration of EU membership also has an influence on the impact of
     SEM interventions, four countries were selected for the project to represent the "four
     waves" of membership of the European Union. Germany represents the original
     membership group from 1952/58; the UK the first accession group of 1973; Spain the
     southern expansion in the 1980s; and Sweden the accession countries of 1995.

The design of the study (Figure 1) is intended to cast light on the individual research stages
and to illustrate the ways in which they are inter-related. The investigation firstly focused

on all legislative acts and court rulings issued by Community institutions ("European interventions"), in particular the elements of SEM legislation and court rulings which explicitly affect aspects of regulating, financing or delivering health services of the Member States. To explore the effects of the four freedoms on health services, relevant categories were defined for each of the four freedoms.

In Phase 1, the relevant European interventions – i.e. those referring both to health services and the SEM – were identified and categorised. In addition, the measures for their implementation and transposition in the Member States were identified and analysed.

In Phase 2, the outcomes of European interventions and their national transposition were considered to be of particular importance – such as mobility of medical manpower and the free movement of goods and services (or consumers of healthcare moving across national boundaries as part of consumer choice of goods and services). Each case study focuses on the issues that are of particular relevance to one country. For example, consumer choice has been based in Germany; medical manpower has been pursued primarily in the UK; public procurement in Spain; and pharmaceuticals in Sweden. Where appropriate, the case studies have incorporated brief information from the other three countries to provide a broader picture of the impact of EU regulations and policy.

In Phase 3, some of the topics were developed into *scenarios*. The scenarios seek to depict – at a very broad and general level – "alternative futures", based upon different assumptions about the behaviour of key actors and events. The scenarios are not full-blown, data-based scenarios but attempts to provide a basis for future policy by EU and Member State policymakers – by drawing attention to the possible consequences of different courses of action or inaction.

The chapters in this book present a selection of these case studies and scenarios.

2. Definitions

The term *intervention* includes both policy instruments (directives, regulations etc.) and the juridical instruments by the European Court of Justice.

In assessing the relevance of a single piece of legislation or jurisdiction, the terms *penetration power*, *outcomes* and *impact* are used. *Penetration power* refers to the degree a given intervention is binding on the national and regional level of Member States. For example the penetration power of a regulation is higher than that of a recommendation since the first is a binding legal instrument which the latter is not. Nevertheless, the *outcomes* of the same regulation could be smaller, if it aims at a very limited and detailed issue, while the recommendation may have a more relevant outcome, since the issues it refers to are of great importance to the health services of Member States.

A further distinction is made between the *impact* of SEM interventions and *outcomes* in terms of effects on health services or healthcare (Figure 2). *Impact* refers to the effect of SEM interventions upon domestic legislation and the administrative rules of national or regional institutions. Impact on Member States depends on a number of factors, including the extent to which directives are transposed, and the extent to which health system rules of Member States are changed. The same EU intervention may have different impact in different countries. For example, one country may already have all the data protection legislation required, while another country may have to introduce a considerable body of legislation.

Equally, countries may transpose legislation more or less effectively (or, in extreme cases, not at all). Full transposition can be explained in a number of ways: a political culture of enthusiasm for Europe ("being a good European"); an "automatic" process of transposition of regulations; or the perception that regulations offer national advantage.

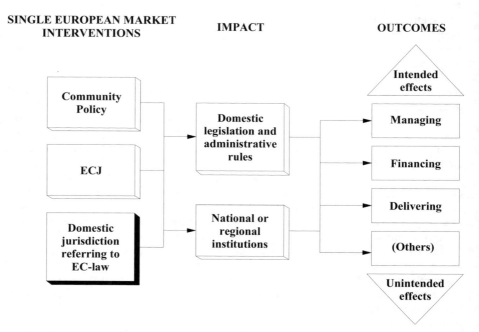

Fig. 2: Relation between interventions, impact and outcomes

The process of transposition differs from country to country – not least reflecting differences between unitary states (such as England); federal states such as Germany; and states such as Spain with varying regional autonomy. One must equally distinguish between formal transposition and implementation within the health sector. Equally one must distinguish between transposition and impact: it is possible to have full transposition but little impact and only partial transposition yet significant impact. Differences may be explained, for example, by the fact that the requirements of the European intervention a) were already covered by national or regional law, b) caused a modification of existing law, c) introduced a completely new set of national or regional law, d) were an opportunity to introduce national and regional law which goes beyond the requirements of the European intervention or e) were of considerable relevance for a national health service but not for a social health insurance system.

Outcomes refer to the effects of SEM interventions on health services and healthcare – in terms of management, finance, supply and delivery, i.e. they address the overall question what difference European integration makes for health services. Effects may be intended or unintended. The principal intended effect of each intervention, according to the selection criteria mentioned above, is to establish a SEM. Clearly, some of the interventions have more specific objectives but they will be described and analysed when appropriate. Unintended effects are those which do not comply with the SEM, which are indifferent towards it, or which have negative consequences for health services. The study paid particular attention to these effects and to the different perspectives of the EU and the Member States.

3. Formation of categories

To explore the effects of the four freedoms on health services, relevant categories were defined, taking both "supply" and "demand" factors into account (Figure 2). These needed to be sufficiently abstract to represent different health systems and sufficiently specific to enable the formation of meaningful categories.

For example, the free movement of individuals comprises both the free movement of doctors, nurses and other healthcare professionals as "suppliers" of health services as well as of persons undergoing short-term stays (business trips, tourism) or long-term stays in other countries who may "demand" health services during those stays.

In contrast, movement of consumers with the explicit intention to receive healthcare goods or services is classified under free movement of goods and services, respectively, to reflect the intentions of the respective SEM interventions. The other important demand-side categories regarding these two freedoms relate to public procurement, while regulations regarding the pharmaceuticals, medical products and health insurance market constitute the supply-side. As regards the free movement of capital, only one category, namely investments in hospitals, was addressed as a potentially relevant topic for health services.

The definitions of the categories were initially developed in an abstract form and agreed upon in a triangulation process among the participants of the project in order to obtain a consistent interpretation. They were refined in the light of the data that had been gathered.

In summary, Figure 3 presents a typology devised to explore relevant legislation and issues. This typology is not the only possible way to organise the study, but is a robust means of reflecting on the impact of the SEM on health services.

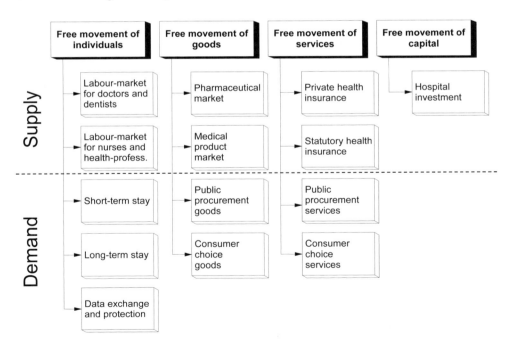

Fig. 3: The four freedoms and the categories defined to analyse the interface between SEM integration and health services

4. Research strategies and methods used in Phase 1

This study explored virgin territory as far as its empirical data were concerned. This meant that no existing databases or systems of categories could be utilised. European interventions had to satisfy two criteria in order to be included in the analysis:

1. the structures for regulating, financing or delivering medical care in the health service had to be clearly defined; and
2. the regulatory measure had to be clearly attributable to the SEM and thus to one of the "four freedoms".

At the European level, a research strategy consisting of several steps was applied in order to identify the relevant interventions:

–   perusing the academic literature;
–   perusing Commission documents;
–   searching the internal database of the ECJ;
–   systematically tracing back relevant references in documents already found.

These activities were accompanied by less systematic research which was either limited to certain subject areas or certain periods of time:

–   a manual search in the Official Journal of the European Community, concentrating on periods where we assumed we would find documents which were relevant;
–   searching the Internet database of the ECJ: http://europa.eu.int/cj/de/jurisp/index.htm (only contains decisions as from 17 June 1997);
–   searching according to search criteria on the Internet pages of the EU server: http://europa.eu.int/index.htm.

Finally, the material was arranged according to the defined categories and sent to experts in those areas who were asked about the comprehensiveness of the interventions found and invited to amend the lists. The numerous tips received from colleagues as to which documents could be relevant cannot be underestimated. The analysis of these data was largely quantitative. It addressed questions in regard to the number of interventions, the dynamic of interventions, the number by instrument, the number of interventions by category etc.

In order to fulfil objective 2 (measures introduced in Member States to implement the relevant EU regulations, whether at national or regional level) specific investigations were carried out in each of the four Member States to capitalise upon the particular databases, information sources and networks available in each. For this purpose, the legislative or administrative acts on the national and regional level were collected as far as possible and available.

The data were then analysed quantitatively and qualitatively by asking questions such as following: Are directives transposed or not at national level? How long does this take? What (if any) is the difference between the content and scope of European legislation and the regulations formulated at national, regional and/or local levels to implement it?

5. Research strategies and methods used in Phase 2

This second phase was intended to assess the actual outcome and to formulate explanations for any differences and variations. Therefore, the following questions were posed:

– Does an intervention have intended and/ or unintended effects, and if so, at what level and in which way?
– Where and how does an intervention influence outcomes (range, quantity and quality of services; or equitable distribution of access)?

Research strategies and methods varied depending on the topic. The methods included interviews, focus discussion groups, surveys, analysis of documents and published literature etc. In order to produce a robust interpretation of the research data, a review mechanism was put in place for the studies. To this end, national experts were asked to assess the validity of the research findings and to identify further or other effects and associated expectations.

6. Research strategies and methods used in Phase 3

This final phase aimed at setting out the consequences of *alternative scenarios* using the appropriate methodologies. The effect of changes in EU policy was traced and predicted, and likely outcomes at Members States level forecasted. Scenarios are compilations of trends into differing images of the future. As such they are a tool for considering how interacting sets of trends might lead to a range of conditions in the future (Bezold & Hancock 1993; Garrett 1999).

Scenarios can be developed in a number of ways and with varying degrees of detail. Most often a "base scenario" is formulated which is an extrapolation of current trends. This is then contrasted with a number of alternative scenarios that might represent a more optimistic and a more pessimistic extrapolation. The main underlying strand is that the scenarios must be plausible, yet at the same time they should challenge current thinking. This is an important function of scenarios i.e. pushing the boundaries of orthodoxy and stimulating creative approaches to issues and problems.

First, scenarios in health can be based on a contextual analysis and this type of scenario considers large social, political and economic environments within which health is situated. Often some sort of visioning exercise takes place in order to formulate a long-range scenario with transformative characteristics, and this will be contrasted with a set of alternatives. These sorts of scenarios depend on multi-disciplinary research and the analysis of wide-ranging empirical data.

The second type of scenario is focused upon answering a specific question, most commonly associated with treatments of diseases or interventions aimed at specific sub-populations. The Dutch Steering Group on Future Health Scenarios uses this type, and their scenarios have included diabetes, ageing and cancer. These scenarios are based upon complex research, including detailed analysis of large data sets on mortality and morbidity, health technology assessments, Delphi techniques or other consensus methods.

The third type of scenario is an analytical exercise whereby various kinds of theory (e.g. social, political, economic or organisational) are tested by modelling predictions. These predictions can then be tested to different degrees: observationally and naturalistically (Sheaff 1999) using empirical research methods, or through focused analytical discussions in expert groups.

The scenarios developed in this project can be grouped under the type 3 scenario, specifically the scenarios developed through expert discussions. The rationale behind this methodological choice has been primarily pragmatic: the resources (time and money) for the project were insufficient to conduct type 1 or type 2 scenarios. By carefully selecting national experts in the fields under investigation, it was possible to organise structured workshop discussions, using the country reports and other relevant documentation, were held in order to formulate base scenarios and alternatives.

References

Bezold C, Hancock T. An overview of the health futures field for the WHO Health Futures Consultation. In: Taket A, editor. Health Futures in support of health for all. Geneva: WHO; 1993.

Garrett MJ. Health Futures. A handbook for health professionals. Geneva: WHO; 1999.

Sheaff R. The development of English Primary Care Group governance. A scenario analysis. Int J Health Plann Manage 1999;14(4):257-68.

Part II

Single European Market legislation and jurisdiction

The European Union and Health Services
R. Busse et al. (Eds.)
IOS Press, 2002

Analysis of SEM legislation and jurisdiction

Matthias WISMAR and Reinhard BUSSE

Abstract. The creation of the European dimension in the health service started immediately after on the formation of the EEC. In total, a substantial number of 233 Single European Market interventions with at least potential effects on the health systems of the Member States could be identified. About two thirds originate from Community policy and one third from the European Court of Justice. These interventions are usually based on highly effective instruments, particularly directives and requests for preliminary rulings. The regulation density is particularly high as regards the free movement of persons and goods, especially in the area of pharmaceuticals. On the whole, the supply side is affected by more interventions than the demand side.

1. Europe is regulating – the scope of the regulatory measures

Over a period of more than 40 years (1958 to June 1998), 233 legal documents which met the inclusion criteria – i.e. referring both to health services and the SEM – were identified (Table 1). When allocating them to the categories defined for each of the four freedoms, it was necessary to make multiple citations. Comprehensive documents, in particular, such as Regulation 1408/71, had to be allocated to several categories. A total of 17 interventions were allocated several times.[1] Thus the total number of interventions with potential effects on the individual categories amounts to 260 data records.[2] An analysis revealed that the ECJ represented 35 % of interventions, clearly playing an important role in terms of the number of interventions.

Table 1: Single Market legislation and judicial decisions of the Community institutions with potential health service effects in the Member States 1958-30.6.1998

	Number of interventions identified	Total number of interventions allocated	Total number of interventions (%)
Community policy		168	65 %
ECJ		92	35 %
Total	233	260	100 %

---

[1] Regulation 1408/71 was allocated six times, Regulation 2001/83 five times, Regulation 1290/97 four times and Regulation 1390/81 three times. All other multiple cited interventions were allocated only twice.

[2] This second figure represents the total number of interventions for all calculations and statements unless otherwise stated.

2. The dynamism of the regulatory process

The total number of interventions already indicates that the interventions of Community institutions with potential effects on the health systems of the Member States are not just a recent phenomenon. The analysis of the time series (Figure 1) demonstrates that, from the very inception of European integration, Community institutions were at least co-regulating aspects relating to the regulation, financing or delivery of health services.

As early as in 1958, shortly after the formation of the EEC, "Regulation No. 3 on the Social Security of Migrant Workers" regulated the social security status of persons moving across national borders.

After sporadic interventions in the sixties, the beginning of the seventies saw regular regulation on the part of the Community institutions. Although this was subject to fluctuation, it is evident that there was an increase in the frequency of interventions until at least the mid-90s.

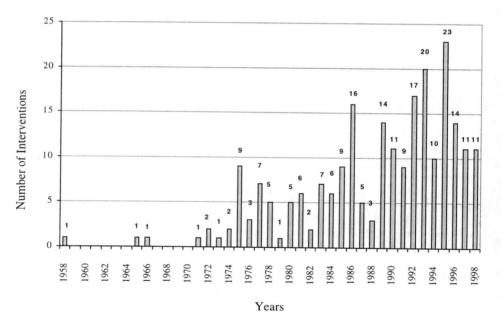

Fig. 1: Dynamism of SEM legislation and judicial decisions with potential health service effects in the Member States 1958 to 30.6.1998

3. Regulation according to categories

An initial assessment indicates the particular frequency of interventions for the interfaces of the free movement of persons and goods with the health system. In total they combine 248 interventions. This corresponds to 95 % of the total number of interventions found (Table 2). If the total number of interventions is broken down according to interventions on the supply side and interventions on the demand side, the regulation of the supply side prevails (Table 3).

Table 2: Allocation of the interventions according to the "four freedoms"

	The free movement of persons	The free movement of goods	The free movement of services	The free movement of capital	Total of the four freedoms
Number	128	120	12	0	260
Percentage	49 %	46 %	5 %	0 %	100 %

Table 3: Allocation of the interventions to supply side vs. demand side

	Supply side	Demand side	Total
Number	175	85	260
Percentage	67 %	33 %	100 %

While this allocation of interventions in relation both to the "four freedoms" and to the supply side and the demand side already reveals a certain imbalance, the picture can be further clarified by an analysis of the allocation of the interventions to the individual categories, i.e. "intervention density" which, in terms of quantity, focuses on the particularly active interfaces between Single Market integration and health services.

For the free movement of persons (Figure 2, white columns 1-5) it is evident that "short-term stay" and "Data exchange and protection", with 11 and 3 interventions respectively, have a considerably lower intervention density than the other categories.

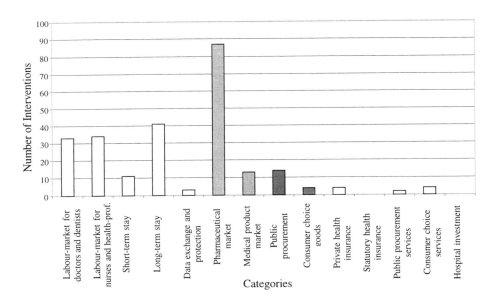

Fig. 2: Intervention density according to categories

A different picture results from the analysis of the categories for the free movement of goods (Figure 2, black columns 6-9): One category – "Pharmaceuticals market" – quite clearly predominates and, with 87 interventions, reaches the highest regulation density of all categories.

For the categories of the free movement of services (Figure 2, white columns 10-13) the regulation density is considerably lower in comparison with the previous freedoms, although more equally distributed. It is strikingly apparent that no intervention for "statutory health insurance" – in the sense of offering insurance – could be identified.

For the category "hospital investment" (Figure 2, column 14), which falls within the sphere of the free movement of capital, it was not possible to identify any intervention.

4. The "penetration power" of the instruments of the Community institutions

The previous stages of the analysis have shown that there is a large body of legislation and judicial decisions at the interface between Single Market integration and health services, that this is a dynamic development and that it is of particular quantitative significance for certain categories.

In order the gauge the qualitative significance, a further analysis examined the instruments with which the institutions of the EU intervene. This analysis provides information concerning the addressees, the effects, the contents and the form of the interventions. In this way conclusions can be reached concerning the potential significance of the instruments. This is referred to as "penetration power" (i.e. how effectively they penetrate national legislation and regulation).

Table 4: Instruments of Community policy

	Instrument				
	Regulation	Directive	Decision	Recommen-dations	Other resolutions
Addressees	All citizens of the European Community	All Member States	All or individual Member States	All Member States (and in rare cases individual Member States)	EC institutions and the administration
Effective-ness	Generally and directly effective	Binding objectives, but free selection of the means	Individual or specific regulation of the individual case	Statement which is not binding, but which is politically authoritative	Internally effective
Content	Of an abstract and general nature	Skeleton legislation	Individual Member States, administrative acts, all Member States, skeleton legislation	Random	Autonomous resolutions, organisational acts

Community policy has five instruments (Table 4) – regulations, directives, decisions, recommendations and other resolutions – of which the weakest instrument is "recommen-dations". Recommendations are generally addressed to all Member States and thus have a universal character, but they are not binding in any way. The instrument "Other resolutions" are binding, but are exclusively addressed to the institutions and the administration of the EC. These resolutions have no potential direct effect on health services. However if the institutions of the EU are reformed by resolutions in such a way that this results in institutions whose organisational objective has potential effects on the health systems of the Member States, these are included in our survey. "Decisions" have a universal character and are binding. However they regulate individual cases and not general matters. (For example, new pharmaceuticals approved by the European Agency for the Evaluation of Medicinal Products are licensed via a directive; this type of directives has, however, been omitted here in order to avoid distorting the numbers.)

The instruments which are particularly relevant and which have a binding, general and universal character are, without any doubt, "directives" and "regulations". A directive defines an objective which all Member States need to achieve. The means employed to achieve the objective are, however, a matter for the Member States. A regulation harmonises not only the political objectives, but also the means and can thus be regarded as the most powerful instrument in Community policy.

In the section of Community policy under investigation considerable use is made of powerful political instruments (Figure 3). Regulations and directives together account for 124 interventions, which corresponds to a proportion of almost 80 % of all interventions of Community policy. Directives alone account for 81 interventions – or 75 if double allocations are omitted. To put this number into perspective, the total number of SEM directives in force in May 1999 was 1405 (Single Market Score Board No. 7 [November 2000]), i.e. 5 % of them have at least potential effects on health services.

In addition to Community policy, the ECJ plays an important role in the field (see Table 1). Of the six instruments of the ECJ, four are only of minor significance for the area of health services (Table 5). Proceedings for annulment, proceedings for failure to act and actions for damages always relate to the actions of the Community institutions or to their failure to act and are not directly relevant to the Member States. The same applies to appeals heard by the ECJ, the so-called remedies.

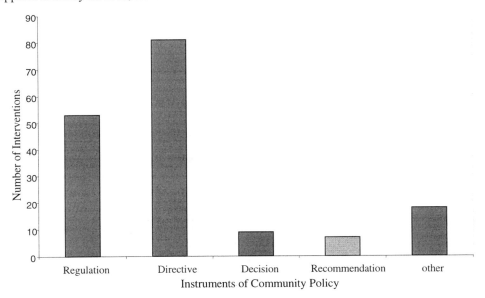

Fig. 3: Instruments of Community policy according to the number of interventions

The instruments of the ECJ which are relevant to the analysis are the request for a preliminary ruling and proceedings for failure to fulfil Treaty obligations. Both types of proceedings are engines of European integration. One is aimed at bringing about a harmonisation of interpretation and application of Community law and the other at enforcing its implementation in the Member States.

Table 5: Instruments of European jurisdiction

	Instruments					
	Proceedings for failure to fulfil Treaty obligations	Proceedings for annulment	Proceedings for failure to act	Actions of damages	Remedies	Requests for preliminary rulings
Objective	Examination as to whether Member States have complied with their obligations under the EC Treaty	Examination of the legality of the actions of Community institutions	Examination of the legality or the failure to act of a Community institution	Clarification of the Community's liability outside the Treaty obligations	Clarification of legal questions	Harmonisation of the interpretation and application of EC law
Defendant	Member State	Community institutions	Community institutions	Community institutions or their employees	Court of first instance	
Plaintiff	Commission; Member States (seldom)	Member States; Council; Commission; Parliament (under certain circumstances); individual persons affected	Court of Justice	All natural persons or legal entities	Parties to the proceedings	All courts can, and in the last instance must, request a preliminary ruling in as far as the matter concerns EC law
Sanctions	Payment of a lump sum or a fine	Declaration of annulment pertaining to legal acts of the Community or parts of such acts	Formal complaint			

The most common type of proceedings are requests for a preliminary ruling, which account for 73 % of all types of ECJ interventions with at least potential effects on health services (see Figure 4). This type of proceedings also has particular significance outside the health care area. The 1997 statistics on the rulings of the ECJ show that requests for preliminary rulings accounted for 66 % of all proceedings in which judgements were announced. This type of proceedings has the objective of bringing about a consistent interpretation and application of EC law throughout the whole of the Community. Only courts of the Member States may request a preliminary ruling from the ECJ. This will be the case if the outcome in a national case is largely dependent on Community law. The ECJ decides how European law should be interpreted with binding effect. The ruling on interpretation is returned to the national court which then has to apply the law as it has been interpreted by the ECJ. The request for a preliminary ruling is therefore a very important hinge between EC law and the national courts. This hinge function is intended to make national courts "guardians of Community law".

The much-discussed cases of Kohll and Decker were preliminary rulings. The idea that the ECJ, with its rulings on the Luxembourg disputes, judged merely on individual cases that have no import outside Luxembourg and are without general application cannot be sustained in view of the significance of Community law, the function of the ECJ, the effect of this type of proceedings and the close interrelationship between the ECJ and the national courts.

The second most common form of proceedings are proceedings for failure to fulfil Treaty obligations. This type of proceedings accounts for 21 % of all types of ECJ interventions identified. They enable the ECJ to ascertain whether the Member States are honouring their obligations under the Treaty. This type of proceedings can be brought by the Commission and also by the Member States. The ECJ pronounces its judgement at the end of a staged procedure. If the Commission is of the opinion that a Member State is in breach of its obligations under the Treaty, it first sends a formal notice and then a reasoned opinion (as laid out in Article 226 of the Treaty). Member States are required to respond to such infringement letters within a certain deadline. If the Member State allows the time limit for submitting such a statement to lapse or if the Commission regards such a statement as being inadequate, it may then initiate the next stage of the proceedings by bringing the case before the ECJ. The ECJ will then ascertain whether the Commission is justified in its view. If the Commission is of the opinion that the Member State has failed to comply with the ruling of the ECJ within a certain time limit, it will initiate the final stage of the proceedings. Now the ECJ has to find whether the Member State in question has failed to comply with its obligations. The ECJ may impose the payment of a lump sum or a fine.

With a total of 86 interventions (or a proportion of 93 % of all interventions on the part of the ECJ) proceedings for a preliminary ruling and proceedings for failure to fulfil Treaty obligations are the major instruments applied. For both cases one can safely assume a considerable penetration power.

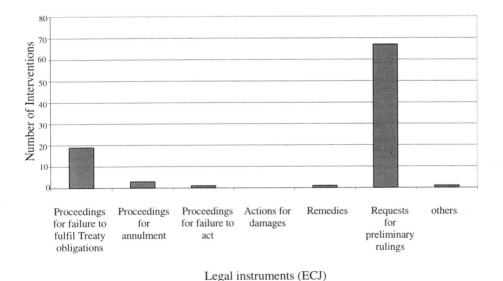

Legal instruments (ECJ)

Fig. 4: Instruments of the ECJ according to the number of interventions

5. Summary and conclusions

This chapter has taken a closer look at the fictional separation between the SEM on the one hand and health services on the other in terms of both quality and quantity. It has assessed the interventions of Community policy and the European Court of Justice (in relation to the four Single Market freedoms) with at least potential effects on the health systems of the Member States in terms of the number of interventions, their frequency and timing, and the regulation density for various health service categories. The results can be summarised as follows:

– The creation of the European dimension in the health service did not first come about with the ECJ rulings of April 1998, which attracted such wide public attention, but was commenced directly on the formation of the EEC.
– Since the seventies the frequency of interventions has become more dynamic and peaked in the first half of the nineties.
– In total, a substantial number of some 250 interventions with at least potential effects on the health systems of the Member States could be identified. About two thirds originate from Community policy and one third from the European Court of Justice.
– The interventions which have potential effects on the health systems of the Member States are usually based on highly effective instruments, particularly directives and requests for preliminary rulings.
– The regulation density is particularly high as regards the free movement of persons and goods. The interventions affect the EU-wide labour market for physicians, dentists and other occupations in the healthcare sector on the one hand, and short-term and long-term visits by tourists, employees etc. on the other. The intervention density as regards the free movement of goods can mainly be explained on the basis of the markets for pharmaceutical products. On the whole, the supply side is affected by more interventions than the demand side.

The European Union and Health Services
R. Busse et al. (Eds.)
IOS Press, 2002

Transposition of European directives into national legislation

Matthias WISMAR, Reinhard BUSSE, Calum PATON, Fernando SILIÓ VILLAMIL,
Nuria ROMO AVILÉS, Maria Angeles PRIETO RODRÍGUEZ,
Mona SUNDH and Barbro RENCK

Abstract. This chapter concentrates on the transposition of SEM directives as they
need to be formally implemented on the Member State level. In the case of the
Federal Republic of Germany with its 16 Länder, sometimes several dozens of transposition measures such as laws or ordinances are necessary for full transposition, a
process which often also takes considerable time. Similarily, the strong role of
Swedish counties in healthcare leads to several transposition measures per directive
while in Spain the number is lower. In comparison, a variety of transposition
patterns emerge.

1. Instruments and transpositions

According to the analysis in the previous chapter, on a European level there are four
principal instruments which have proved to be potentially powerful in their effect (Table 1).
Of these four instruments, only directives can be subjected to any meaningful and feasible
analysis of the incorporation of European legislation and court rulings into national
legislation and regulations ("transposition").

Table 1: Relevant instruments of legislation and judicial decisions of the Community
institutions and their mechanisms of implementation

	Community policy		**ECJ**	
Instrument	**Regulation**	**Directive**	**Proceedings for failure to fulfil Treaty obligations**	**Proceedings for a preliminary ruling**
Transposition	No transposition, no account needs to be given	Transposition; account needs to be given	ECJ examines transposition	"Transposition" is the decision of referring court
Result	No research possible	Research possible	Research is possible in principle but rare	Research is possible in principle but rare

The reason for this is that directives only specify the objectives, but not the measures themselves. Member States not only decide the appropriate measures to attain the objectives, but
also the legislative means which are appropriate to the circumstances. Member States are
under an obligation to ensure that directives are implemented in accordance with their objectives and to report to the Commission, within the prescribed time limits, that directives
have been transposed into national law. This means that directives leave "traces" in national
legislation. The measures that are selected in the various Member States, the means and the
time needed for implementation can be researched and analysed. As a reminder: A total of
75 SEM directives were identified which refer to health services.

In the case of regulations, on the other hand, there is a close interrelationship between the European and the national level. Regulations come directly into force – or within the prescribed time limits – and apply to all EU citizens. They do not need to be transposed into national law and leave hardly any traces that can be researched on the national level (except possible administrative orders).

Proceedings for failure to fulfil Treaty obligations are usually initiated if the transposition of a directive is not communicated in time, or is communicated incompletely, or if the Commission criticises the transposition as not being appropriate to the objectives. In principle, it is possible to find such proceedings. However, as the ECJ is now in a position to impose substantial lump sum payments and fines, most Member States make efforts to avoid such proceedings.

Preliminary ruling proceedings, which in terms of their quantitative and qualitative aspects represent a particularly effective type of proceedings in our investigation, take effect in two ways. First through the judgement of the relevant court which has clarified questions on the interpretation and application of Community law in the preliminary ruling proceedings. Here it can be expected that the court in question will abide by the interpretation. Second, the courts in subsequent judgements can refer to judgements that have already been pronounced. In principle it is possible to search for at least some of the subsequent judgements in databases. However, due to the disproportionate relationship between research effort and results, this was not done in this project. Although it is quite possible that a large number of the preliminary rulings that are relevant can be found in the databases concerned, they would also be cited if the judgement is of only marginal relevance or does not fulfil both criteria for inclusion. The qualitative analysis that would then be necessary would go beyond the scope of the research project, without necessarily enabling any additional insights.

2. Transposition in Germany

2.1 Methodological remarks

In theory, there should be two ways to analyse the transpositions of European directives, either through the body in Germany that is responsible for reporting back to the Commission or through the recipient of that information at the Commission. In practice both methods are only feasible to a limited extent.

On the German side there is a collection office which reports all transposition measures to the Commission. This collection point is at the Federal Ministry for Industry and Technology. From there contact is cultivated with the relevant liaison offices in the individual Ministries and with the Commission. Department 4 at the Federal Ministry for Health (consumer protection, veterinary medicine) collects all transpositions that the Ministry has initiated. This is handled in a similar way in the other Ministries. The Federal Ministry for Industry and Technology then reports the transpositions to the Commission.

Unfortunately, the database at the Federal Ministry for Industry and Technology proved to be unsuitable for the purposes of the study. First, the data it contains only goes back as far as 1980 and secondly it contains sensitive information which could give rise to problems under the data protection laws.[1]

---

[1] At this point the authors would like to offer their most grateful thanks to the officials of the Federal Ministry for Industry and Technology who were a great help to in every respect, despite the data protection rules.

An attempt to gain access to a database of the Commission containing the transpositions as reported by the Member States also failed – surprisingly, such a database apparently does not exist.[2]

As a way out of the dilemma, it was decided to examine the Juris database which was searched for legislation transposing European legislation on the national level. The Juris database proved useful as a way out of this situation. The Commission reports the implementation reports it receives to Juris. These are entered into the database and are available for a search. The interpretation of the database search commissioned, must be made subject to a number of reservations, however:

- If no report has been received regarding implementation, this can, but does not necessarily have to mean that the directive in question has not been implemented. It is possible that Germany has failed to report the implementation measure or that the Commission has not (yet) passed on the report.
- The report regarding the implementation measure is forwarded over a lengthy route: from the implementing office, via the collection office in the Ministry in question, via the contact point at the Ministry for Industry and Technology, then to the Commission and finally to Juris. Some of the information can get lost along the way (passive postal effect) and this makes it difficult to retrieve when conducting the search.
- In accordance with the federal structure, statutes are published in so many different publication media that it was hardly possible to obtain a clear picture of them and no search can be carried out for them, so that, in some cases, only the report concerning the source was available for analysis.

2.2 The implementation of directives in Germany

A total of 202 transpositions were identified implementing 54 European directives (Table 2), and thus there were no results for 21 out of the total of 75 directives identified during the first stage of the project.[3] As the majority of these directives were issued in the nineties it is quite likely that they are still either at the reporting or the implementation stage.

Table 2: The total number of transpositions in Germany

Total number of directives (without double allocations)	Directives for which no search could be made	Directives with transpositions	Transpositions for those 54 directives
75	21	54	202

If the 202 transpositions are allocated to the categories (Figure 1), it can be seen that once again in terms of quantity, the free movement of persons (columns 1-5) and the free movement of goods (columns 6-9) represent the main interfaces between health services and the SEM. However, the weighting of the intervention density for the individual categories differs from the weighting at both the European level and that found in Spain and Sweden. Thus "Public procurement goods" is regulated by more transpositions than the "Pharmaceuticals market" in Germany, even though the latter has more than twice as many EU directives.

---

[2] The authors would like to thank Mr Paul Belcher, Head of EHMA's Brussels Office for the research activities in Brussels.

[3] Directives 66/454, 73/240, 76/764, 77/65, 83/189, 83/570, 90/366, 92/25, 92/28, 93/4, 93/36, 93/37, 93/42, 93/93, 94/38, 95/43, 95/46, 96/6, 96/71 and 98/21.

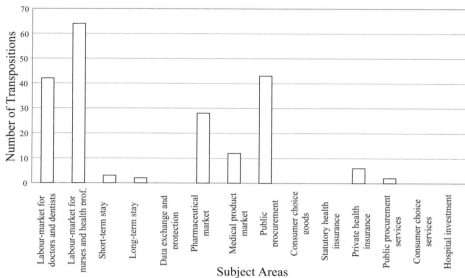

Fig. 1: Number of transpositions in Germany according to categories in the four freedoms

As there are on average almost four transpositions for each European directive; shifts between the subject areas can partly result from the very unbalanced allocation of the transpositions (Figure 2).

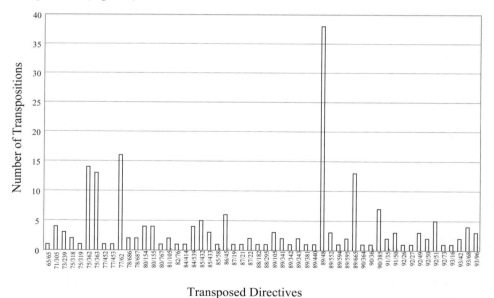

Fig. 2: Number of transpositions according to directives

As far as the implementation of European directives in Germany is concerned, the question of the regulatory strength and thus the type of instruments that are used for implementation must also be considered.

In the section of Community policy under investigation, European directives in Germany are mainly implemented by means of laws and decrees (Figure 3). These two instruments at the level of the Länder and the federal government together accounted for a total of 80 % of all transpositions. This means that the high penetration power of the instruments used, which could already be ascertained at the European level, continues on implementation in Germany.

Out of the 202 transpositions that were identified during the database search, 49 % were initiated at the federal level and 41 % at the level of the Länder. This relative balance of transpositions between the federal government and the Länder has to be interpreted careful-ly, though, because as soon as a transposition falls within the competence of the Länder, it is usually implemented by the majority of Länder using corresponding measures. The activities of the Länder are therefore counted several times. Thus, more directives at the interface between health services and the SEM are actually transposed at the federal level.

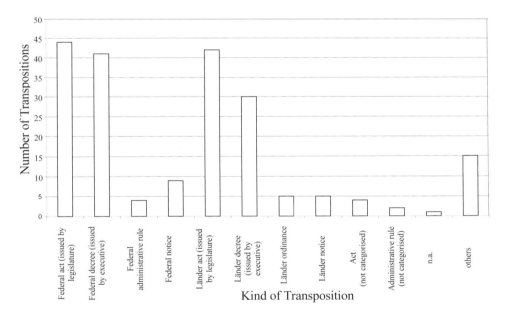

Fig. 3: Transposition measures according to instrument and level of politics

The time taken to transpose directives is of particular interest (Figure 4). Major delays or even the postponement of implementation would in effect suspend European legislation in Germany. While the danger is not the intentional failure to comply with the prescribed deadline for the implementation of the relevant European directive, there is, in a worst-case scenario, a danger of proceedings for failure to fulfil Treaty obligations if one Land does not transpose a directive, perhaps resulting in lump sum payments or punitive fines for Germany as a whole.

However it has proved difficult to determine the exact date of implementation. In Germany, a European directive can simultaneously be implemented through several trans-positions and by several agencies, such as the federal government and the Länder, so that the process can often be a lengthy one. There is also a methodical problem to be considered in interpreting the period required for implementation. Transpositions that have met with no objection over the years can suddenly be examined by the Commission as to whether the Member States implement the directive correctly. For this analysis, the European database was compared with the German one. Out of the 54 European directives for which German transpositions could be identified, 50 contained sufficient information concerning details such as implementation, the date of coming into force, the date that they were passed etc.

In some cases, a negative period of implementation can be noted in Figure 4. This is the case if existing German law complies with European directives that have recently come into force. When the measures were reported to the Commission therefore, the German authorities reported the laws or decrees that guarantee the implementation of the European directives, although some of these were enacted a long time ago. This is an interesting indicator for the fact that not all directives will actually impact upon national legislation.

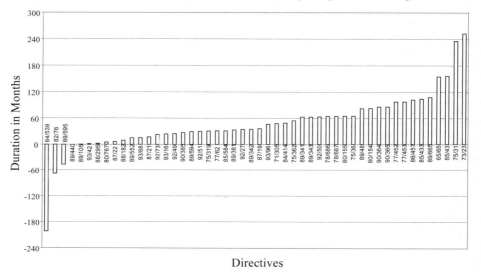

Fig. 4: Time required to implement directives in months

European directives which require no further implementation are, however, a marginal phenomenon. Roughly two fifths of all directives are implemented in Germany only after they have come into force AT a European level, i.e. after the set deadline. However, there are also outliers which required up to 20 years to be fully transposed.

Whether the transposition actually fulfils the requirements of the directive is another matter. For example, the first stage for initiating proceedings for failure to fulfil Treaty obligations in relation to the Third Directive concerning Indemnity Insurance (92/49/EEC) has been commenced with Germany as the defendant. The Commission was of the opinion that Germany, in putting the directive into effect, was in indirect breach of the provisions of this directive. This directive was intended to guarantee the free movement of services for private health insurance. Insurance companies that are domiciled in the Member States of the EU were to have access to the entire SEM. However, a clause was incorporated into the German Social Code Book V (SGB V) which made the eligibility of private health insurance for a premium subsidy by employers dependent on the separation of branches of industry. This meant that private health insurance companies could only offer their services in the field of health care, but not in other branches (SGB V, Article 257, paragraph 5). But this excluded a number of potential competitors from the German market for private health insurance. In all probability, however, the conflict will be settled amicably. The offending clause is not of central importance.

2.3 Conclusions

The implementation of European legislation in Germany can generally be said to lack transparency. Although the Federal Ministry for Industry and Technology collects the transpositions for the implementation of directives so that they can be reported to the Commission, the data kept by the Commission, just like the data in the Juris database, suffers from the many different types of implementation and the many different implementation agencies involved. Although most directives are implemented at the federal level, there is an increasing number of acts and decrees on the level of the Länder, as it is often also necessary for directives to be implemented at this level. Whether and when implementation has actually occurred is often very difficult - and sometimes impossible - to ascertain under present circumstances. As regards the chronological dimension of transposition of directives into German law, it has been shown that it has usually taken about three years until final transposition was reported. In individual cases, however, it took more than ten years and Directive 65/65 has still not been transposed into German law to the satisfaction of the Commission. The traditionally weak German transposition record has improved however during the study, a fact which might not yet be reflected in the transpositions identified: While in November 1997, it was - together with Belgium – ranked second last failing to transpose 8.5 % of all SEM Directives, that rate had fallen to 2.4 % in May 1999 and 3.1 % in November 2000 – placing Germany at number 5 and 9, respectively (Single Market Score Board No. 7).

3. European Union law and British law

This brief section outlines the procedure for translating European law into British law. First, the UK is not a federal country – although a devolved parliament for Scotland and a devolved assembly for Wales may alter things somewhat. Second, Britain has a record of automatic implementation of EU law. This does not square with the perception of Britain as a "European laggard", but the paradox is that the UK "moans a lot and then obeys" whereas other countries may appear to be "good Europeans" but are then less likely to implement EU laws automatically. (Of course it is useful for British politicians – as for any politicians – to moan about Europe in order to "pass the buck" to Europe for laws which they are' at the end of the day, reasonably happy to translate into British law!) As recently as in November 1997, the UK was fourth after Denmark, the Netherlands and Finland in its transposition of SEM directives record Due to increased efforts in Sweden and Spain and the relatively slow transposition progress in the UK, its position had however decreased to the sixth place by November 2000 (Single Market Score Board No. 1 and No. 7).

It is the responsibility of Member States to "do as necessary" to translate directives into national law. One question (in the UK as elsewhere) is whether the transposition of the Directive requires a new law, a modification of existing law, or overturning of a law? In the UK, in normal circumstances, a strong executive and a compliant parliament with an overall majority of the government means that parliament acts as a rubber stamp. Most contentious issues have been dealt with at the level of the Council of Ministers (or, less likely, the Commission) and once the directive has been framed, the transposition in the UK is an automatic matter. There are, clearly some sensitive issues, but these normally resolved by the permanent representatives in Brussels prior to the framing of directives. One example was the Directive concerning working hours – exemptions for junior doctors was heavily pushed by Britain.

European law is traditionally transposed into British law in late night sessions which are ill-attended. There is, of course, the well-known anecdote of Mrs Thatcher's Government signing more centralising European legislation than any other British Government in history. The conclusion for Britain is that the transposition of EU directives into British law is not really a matter of interest.

4. The transposition of SEM directives in Spain

4.1 Implementation of EU legislation in Spain

The right to healthcare protection, which is recognised by the Constitution, is looked after at varying levels of public administration. According to the Spanish Constitution, Article 149.1.16, the State has sole responsibility healthcare issues across the Spanish borders, access and entitlements to as well as general co-ordination of healthcare, along with the legislation on pharmaceutical products. The regional governments are widely responsible regarding healthcare, above all in the management and planning of health services, along with further developing legislation within the rules set by the national level. Local councils also have responsibilities in this area, though subsequent to the General Law on Healthcare their resources are included within that of the region. Thus, the range of the norms transposed differs according to the body in charge and whether it is of a fundamental nature or not.

Another factor to be taken into account is the configuration of the national health system in Spain in which, unlike other Member States, and excluding certain regions such as Catalonia or Navarra, the provision of health services is a public service and healthcare is mainly carried out in the public sector.

Alongside transposition control, there needs to be application control. This is one of the major problems posed from a legal point of view, since a norm may be technically transposed but, afterwards, the various practices of the operators or Member States make it inapplicable.

4.2 Methods and results

Spanish ordinances that are affected by and also stem from previously identified legislation were located by means of a systematic search using IBERLEX-UE, a legislative database that provides the national transposition of Community directives.

The number of Spanish transpositions increased gradually over the years and 65 % of the identified 32 Spanish transpositions, mainly in the area of legislation, were passed during the years 1992 to 1994. This rhythm of transposition dropped from 1995 onwards.

As with SEM directives, Spanish legislation on transpositions concentrates on the transposition of directives that regulate the free movement of persons and goods (Table 3). In transpositions concerning the free movement of persons, the most predominant area is that which regulates the job market for nurses and other health professionals (57 % of those found). Legislation transposition regarding the regulation of the pharmaceutical market is predominant among those transpositions identified within the free movement of goods (66 % of those identified).

Table 3: Transpositions in Spain and Sweden – free movement of persons and goods

Free movement of persons

	Labour market doctors	Labour market nurses	Short-term stay	Long-term stay	Data protection
SEM directives	21		3	3	2
Transpositions in Spain	3	8	1	2	0
Transpositions in Sweden	49		16	10	9

Free movement of goods

	Pharmaceutical market	Medical devices market	Public procurement goods	Consumer choice goods
SEM directives	23	10	8	0
Transpositions in Spain	12	3	3	0
Transpositions in Sweden	83	22	29	0

5. The transposition of SEM directives in Sweden

5.1 Implementation of EU legislation in Sweden

As with other Member States in the EU, Sweden is obliged to implement and follow EU law. This obligation is, among other ways, communicated by the principle of loyalty according to Article 5 of the EC Treaty. The principle means that, for example, Sweden is obliged to take all actions that can be regarded as appropriate to ensure that the obligations are fulfilled under the treaty or other Community measures.

The Swedish government is responsible for Sweden implementing and abiding by EU legislation and is thus responsible for ensuring that the authorities instructions agree with the requirements stated in EU legislation. It is not required that EU legal acts are implemented in Member States by means of formal laws. The Member States can implement EU legal acts by means of national statutes based on their own legal systems. In Sweden the legal acts are implemented in accordance with the distribution of norm-establishing powers between the parliament, the government and the administrative authorities. The way an EU legal act is implemented in Sweden depends on how the issue has previously been dealt with within Swedish legislation.

The implementation process starts with a proposal for new Swedish act or regulation being studied and worked out by order of the Government. Subsequently the Government can present a bill for a new law, which will then be dealt with by the parliament. The implementation of EU legal acts in Sweden often means that the Government works out regulations and/or that authorities issue instructions. Coordination between the Government and the authorities is required in the latter regard. The authorities are therefore obliged to inform the ministry in question of the implementation of EU legal acts with instructions. The ministries inform the EU Commission of the Swedish implementation of the EU legal act and subsequently the Commission scrutinises the statute text (Agency for Administrative Development 1998).

Swedish authorities can implement EU directives in various ways. The main rule is that the text of the directive should be rewritten into a public authority instruction, but it could also be reproduced verbatim. A third alternative is that an instruction could refer to the text of the directive.

The Agency for Administrative Development (1998) has conducted a study on the adaptation of Swedish regulations to the EU body of regulations, which shows that authorities in several cases have introduced regulations in EU-related directions that are more far-reaching than the requirements in the underlying EU legal acts. The same study shows that authorities, generally speaking, meet the EU legal requirements when implementing EU directives and completing EU regulations and instructions but that there is usually no control or follow-up of the authorities' instruction work. The lack of control is explained by the fact that public authorities' instructions due to EU legal acts mostly concern detailed, specific matters that require special competence. The Cabinet Office and the Ministries lack such competence.

5.2 Methods and results

For the Swedish transposition data, the National Board of Trade in Sweden has provided information. The database on the Official Journal of Community Legislation in Force and Others Acts of the Community Institutions (Volume I, Analytical Register) has also been used in the analysis. In addition, the Internet has also been used as a research tool and searches of relevant web sites have been made.

Regarding the free movement of individuals in the health sector, the overwhelming number of Swedish transpositions concern the labour market for doctors, nurses and other health personal. It further shows that the relatively few SEM directives within the category of short-term stay have necessitated quite a number of transpositions. Possibly even more surprising is the number of transpositions in the category of data protection.

Regarding the free movement of goods and services in the health sector, the overwhelming number of transpositions (62 %) are concerned with the pharmaceutical market, i.e. a situation similar to that in Spain but different to that in Germany. Further, it can be seen that there are also a number of transpositions within the categories of medical devices and public procurement of goods and services.

5.3 Conclusions

In the results scoreboard "Single Market Scoreboard No. 7" issued by the EU, it is maintained that "transpositions of Internal Market directives has considerably improved in most Member States. Denmark, Finland and Sweden have successfully kept their transposition deficit to below 1.5 %. ... The 'fragmentation factor', the percentage of directives not yet implemented across all Member States remains high (12.8 %). One in eight Internal Market directives has not been transposed in every Member State. ... Three years since the first launch of the Scoreboard it has become clear that administrations can achieve a significant reduction in the implementation deficit of Internal Market legislation only if intense administrative activity is coupled with political support at the highest levels. Internal Market legislation involves important reforms that can only be successfully implemented if there is adequate political backing. ... Denmark, Sweden, Finland and Spain have done best in coming to grip with the transpositions process, and though they face some delays, they are well on course for eliminating their transpositions backlog." According to these statistics, Sweden ranked second in the EU when it came to implementing SEM directives in November 2000 – a drastic improvement in comparison to November 1997 when it ranked only eighth.

In Sweden it is commonly thought that the country is relatively conscientious concerning the transposition of those directives from the EU to national law. However, tendencies towards over-regulation have also been identified. Directives are usually implemented within the EU time-frame and reports are made to the Commission after the directives have been implemented. Perhaps this efficiency can be traced to the fact that Sweden is a relatively new member of the EU.

References

European Commission. Commission Staff Working Paper. Single Market Scoreboard No. 7; November 2000.

Statskontoret [Agency for Administrative Development]. EG-regler och svensk regelkvalitet. Åtgärder för att förbättra det svenska arbetet med att reformera och förenkla regler, 1998:27. Lägesrapport [EC regulations and Swedish regulation quality. Measures to improve the Swedish work to reform and simplify regulations. Situation report]. Statskontoret [Agency for Administrative Development]; 1998.

Part III

Free movement of persons

The European Union and Health Services
R. Busse et al. (Eds.)
IOS Press, 2002

The mobility of doctors and nurses –
a United Kingdom case study

Clare JINKS, Bie Nio ONG and Calum PATON

Abstract. This chapter presents a description and analysis of the labour market for doctors and nurses in the European Economic Area (EEA). We first discuss the policy context of labour mobility, followed by a detailed case study of one of the participating Member States, the United Kingdom. After the discussion of the main site comparisons with the three other partners in the BioMed Concerted Action, Germany, Sweden and Spain, will be drawn. The conclusions outline the main policy implications and the contours for possible future work.

While the intention of this study was to examine the labour market for doctors and nurses, we have been hampered by the paucity of reliable data on nurses. Where possible we will refer to nurses, but of necessity, more data and in-depth analysis on the situation regarding doctors is presented.

1. The policy context of the labour mobility of healthcare professionals

As one of the largest employers in Europe, health services, clearly, have the potential to be affected by the impact of labour mobility on the demand for and supply of doctors nurses, and other health professionals. Health service workforce planners in Europe have traditionally overlooked this potential impact. Integrated workforce planning that adopts a European dimension is an undervalued but increasingly important process.

In the UK, for example, adopting a European dimension to workforce planning is important not least in terms of the Government's Comprehensive Spending Review (Department of Health 1998) and the announcement of an increase of 7,000 more doctors, 15,000 nurses and 6,000 more nurse training places for the National Health Service (NHS). This announcement must be considered in parallel with identified pressures that the British health service has recently faced (Buchan 1998; Friend 1998; Jinks et al. 1998; Lambert and Goldacre 1998; Lyall 1997; Snell 1998). These pressures include, for example:

- major domestic nurse and doctor recruitment and retention problems
- a change in gender balance to the UK Physician workforce. This has led to a rise in the number of UK physicians seeking part time employment
- a trend towards early retirement
- specific concerns about recruitment difficulties for general practice

In the past, the above pressures have been moderated by the supply of doctors from both overseas and the EEA. For example, EEA qualified doctors contribute significantly to the Senior House Officer cadre (SHO). Recent figures show that ten percent of SHOs in England and Wales are from the EEA (Jinks et al. 1998). The potential impact of labour mobility thus becomes apparent when new registration figures from the General Medical

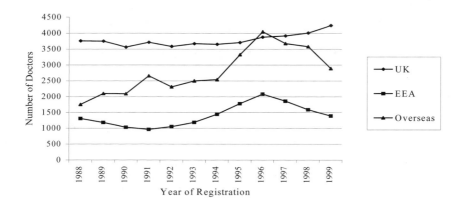

Fig. 1: New full GMC registrations of EEA, UK and Overseas doctors[1] (1988-1999)
(Source: GMC Notes on the Medical Register 2000)

Council (GMC) are examined. These figures indicate that the number of new full registrations of doctors from other EEA Member States are in decline. See Figure 1 above.

Figure 1 suggests that European junior doctors are now less likely to come to the UK to train. This decision could be affected by employment opportunities in their host country. Indeed, a recent study undertaken by the Permanent Working Group (PWG) of European junior hospital doctors (PWG 1996) has indicated that medical unemployment in mainland Europe will continue to fall well into the early part of this century. This trend has clear implications for policy makers both in the UK and in the rest of Europe and, thus, presents important research questions: to what extent are people moving; what are the factors that facilitate or prohibit mobility; and, what are the implications of mobility for health services?

To address the questions identified above, a case study on the movement of doctors into the UK has been undertaken. Originally, the remit of the project was to investigate doctors, nurses and other health professionals. It soon became clear that comprehensive and reliable data was only available on EEA doctors. This case study has, therefore, primarily focused on the movement of medical professionals.

The aims of the case study were to:

–   Describe the EU legislative framework for the free movement of individuals and it's impact on labour mobility.
–   Enumerate the number of physicians from other EEA Member States working in the UK.
–   Identify the number of physicians from other EEA Member States in one health region of the UK (North West Region).
–   Investigate the reasons for mobility; and, the training opportunities and experiences of EEA doctors in the UK (and barriers to training, if they exist).

---

[1] Overseas doctors include all doctors except those from the UK and the EEA.

During the case study, a combination of research methods have been employed. The policy framework and national and regional data have been derived through literature review and "desk study". Quantitative methods were used to survey EEA doctors practicing in one health region. Finally, a small sample of doctors and clinical tutors were interviewed to discuss in more depth the reasons for and experiences of working in UK.

2. The European policy framework for free movement of UK doctors and nurses

The Treaty of Rome lays the foundations for the free movement of labour within Europe. Key articles that facilitate freedom of movement are illustrated in Table 1:

Table 1: Articles from the Treaty of Rome (Mobility of Labour)

Article Number	Description
48	Freedom of Movement for Workers
52	Freedom of Establishment in another Country
59	Freedom to Provide Services
07	Prohibition of discrimination based on Nationality
57	Mutual Recognition of diplomas, certificates and other evidence of formal qualifications

The above policy framework facilitates the free movement of doctors and nurses across the EU as there is mutual recognition of qualifications. Furthermore, language ability does not have to be proven. Doctors who wish to work in the UK need to register with the General medical Council, while nurses UK need to be registered with the United Kingdom Central Council.

European directives (75/362/EEC and 75/363/EEC), passed in 1975, aimed to facilitate the entry of doctors into Member States other than the ones in which they trained. They specified that immigration rules do not apply to a national of the EEA, (or the family member of a national), who is entitled to an automatic right of residency in the UK under EC Law; and, that all professional qualifications were equally acceptable across the community. Directive 75/362/EEC and 75/363/EEC have since been consolidated in a third directive, 93/16/EEC (The Doctor's Directive). This came into effect in January 1993.

The key features of 93/16/EEC, are illustrated below:

1. In accord with citizenship and completion of training, doctors are entitled to register in other Member States.
2. Member States must recognize as specialists doctors who meet the above criteria. Specifically, Member States must recognise as specialists doctors who hold a recognised specialist certificate (equivalent to Certificate of Completion of Specialist Training in the UK) have trained in a specialty that is listed in the Doctor's Directive and recognised in the country to which they wish to move
3. The implementation of vocational training programmes must last at least two years for general practice.
4. The establishment of Competent Authorities. These bodies have two main functions. Firstly, to supervise training within each Member State and to issue certificates to doctors who complete training satisfactorily. Secondly, to issue or verify certificates and diplomas under 93/16/EEC for doctors entering the Member State. Host states are required by the directive to recognise certificates and diplomas issued by other Member

States. In the UK, competent authorities include the General Medical Council (GMC), The Joint Committee on Postgraduate Training for General Practice (JCPTGP) and the recently formed Specialist Training Authority of the Royal Colleges (STA)

Under the EU regulations, recognition of nursing and medical qualifications does not depend on the individual's ability to demonstrate linguistic competency in the language of the country they are moving to. The Treaty of Rome precludes discrimination on the basis of language, and unlike professionals from overseas (non-UK and non-EEA), EEA nationals do not have to pass the language test administered by the Professional and Linguistic Assessment Board (P.L.A.B.).

One example of how EU policy on the freedom of movement has had a direct impact in the UK can be seen from recent changes to postgraduate and specialist medical training. In the early 1990s, the European Commission questioned the way in which the UK issues certificates to its own specialists and the way it recognised specialist medical qualifications issued in other countries.

This disparity in training between EU countries has been summarised by Lowry (1996) as follows: the duration of specialist training in most specialties in the UK has always been longer than the minimum laid down in 93/16/EEC. Until 1996, the GMC issued a certificate of specialist training (CST) to doctors whose training met the minimum requirements of the directive. The CST was accepted by other countries as evidence of specialist status although it did not confer such rights on doctors in Britain. British doctors could obtain a CST and practice as specialists elsewhere in Europe at a stage in their training far short of that required for an appointment as a consultant in the NHS. Many European doctors, particularly from countries with high medical unemployment, came to Britain to obtain training leading to CST which enabled them to return home and work as specialists. Effectively, this meant that Britain was operating a two tier system, with a lower standard of training for those who wanted to work elsewhere as specialists than those staying in Britain.

In 1992, the British Government responded to pressure from the EU by establishing a working party to consider how Britain could be brought into line with the EU directives. The working party made a number of important recommendations, (the Calman proposals), including, for example: the introduction of a Certificate of Completion of Specialist training (CCST). This is awarded to a doctor when the relevant medical Royal Colleges considers that training has been satisfactorily completed to a level of competence compatible with independent practice and eligibility for consideration for appointment to a consultant post. Another important recommendation was the unification of registrar and senior registrar grades to a new grade of Specialist Registrar.

In response to the proposals and subsequent NHS Executive guidance, new arrangements for postgraduate specialist training, certification and specialist registration came into force on 12th January 1996. The legal basis for these changes is the European Medical Specialists Order 1995 (as amended by the European Specialist Medical Qualifications Amendment regulations 1997 on 31 December 1997). This implements the UK's obligations to training of medical specialists and the mutual recognition of qualifications. For the first time, fulfillment of the requirements became mandatory. The Order established the "Specialist Training Authority of the medical Royal Colleges" (STA). This competent authority, in conjunction with the GMC, issues certificates on satisfactory completion of Specialist training (CCST) and is legally responsible for ensuring adherence to training requirements stipulated in 93/16/EEC. Individual Colleges and Faculties publish appropriate syllabuses, handbooks, conduct appropriate tests etc. However the STA has responsibility for ensuring that Colleges' relevant publications and activities comply with the requirements of the European Medical Directive.

A better indication of the numbers of EEA doctors actually working in the UK can be obtained by examining data from the annual NHS Executive Medical and Dental Census. Figure 3 illustrates figures for EEA doctors practising in England between 1996 and 1997. Figure 4 offers comparative data on UK doctors.

Figure 3 supports data from the GMC that the numbers of EEA doctors coming to the UK are in decline (a total decline in England by 227 between 1996 and 1997). A shift in the profile of doctors between grades is also evident.

For example, there has been a rise in the number of EEA doctors at Consultant or Specialist/Senior Registrar grade; and, a decline in the number at Registrar grade.
This pattern is replicated in Figure 4 for UK doctors and is not unexpected. It has emerged as a result of the Calman recommendations and the unification of registrar and senior registrar grades described earlier. Importantly, Figure 3 illuminates a decline in the number of EEA doctors at Senior House Officer (SHO) and House Officer (HO)[2] grades. Traditionally, EEA doctors embark on training programmes in the NHS at SHO grade. This is where the greatest decline in the number of EEA doctors practising in the UK is seen – a decline in number of 207. The number of UK SHOs has, however, increased. Figure 4 indicates that between 1996-7 there has been an increase in the number of UK SHOs practising in England by 330.

Figure 5 illustrates the number of EEA doctors working in one health region in England, the North West Region. These figures are again derived from the NHS Medical and Dental workforce census. Again, an increase in the number of EEA doctors at Specialist/senior registrar grade and a decline in the number at SHO and HO grade can be seen.

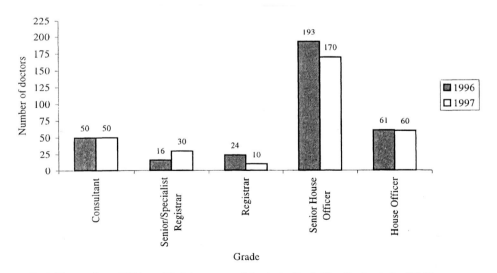

Fig 5: The number of EEA qualified doctors practising in the North West Region in the UK (Source: Department of Health. Medical and Dental Workforce Census 1996/7)

---

[2] House Officer is the most junior hospital doctor grade after graduation, and Senior House Officer is the next grade.

3.2 National data: nurses

The mobility of nurses can, at present, only be traced at a national level. No systematic data collection takes place at regional or local level and even if NHS Trusts[3] record country of origin, there is no consistency across different organisations. Thus, we only present national level data here.

Table 2 demonstrates the rise in EU nurses in 1996, with a more modest increase in 1997 and then the levelling off of this trend. In contrast, the rise of nurses from other countries, notably South Africa, Australia, Philippines and the West Indies has been considerable. Buchan (2000) argues that this differential rise is due to the importance of communication with patients, giving advantage to staff from English-speaking countries.

Table 2: Initial registration of nurses and midwives

Year	EU countries	Other countries	Overseas total
94/95	798	1,654	2,452
95/96	763	1,999	2,762
96/97	1,141	2,633	3,744
97/98	1,439	2,861	4,300
98/99	1,412	3,568	4,980
99/00	1,416	5,945	7,361

Source: UKCC press release, 14/6/00

A more detailed breakdown of practitioners registered with the UK Central Council for Nursing, Midwifery and Health Visiting (UKCC) as to the EU country of origin is provided through an analysis of trends in the number of European nurses and midwives coming to the UK. For example, in 1999/2000, 4.93 per cent of the total number of admissions to the UKCC's professional register were from practitioners qualified in other EU countries. Figure 6 illustrates how admissions of practitioners from EU countries compare with admissions from elsewhere (1996-2000).

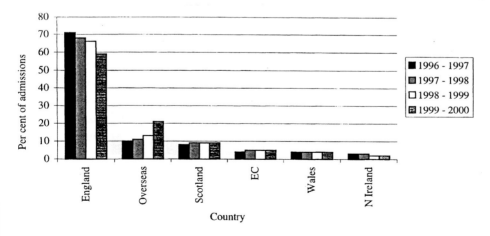

Fig. 6: Nurses registered with the UKCC, 1996-2000 (Source: Statistical analysis of the UKCC's professional registers 1997-2000)

---

[3] NHS Trusts are the statutory authorities responsible for running hospitals in the UK.

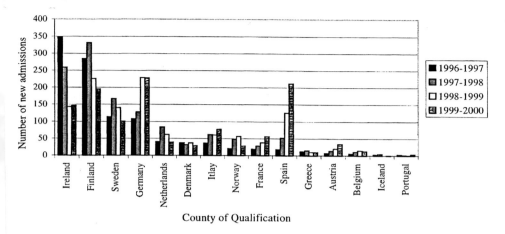

Fig. 7: New admissions to the UKCC via EC arrangements by country of qualification, 1996-2000 (Source: Statistical analysis of the UKCC's professional registers 1997-2000)

The number of admissions of EU practitioners to the UKCC professional register rose for the first time between 1997 and 1998. The greatest number of new admissions in this period were from practitioners who had qualified in Sweden and Finland. The number of admissions of EU practitioners to the register rose recently from 1,165 between 1998/99 to 1,416 between 1999/2000. Admissions of practitioners from Sweden and Finland have fallen, whilst admissions of practitioners from Spain have risen. Figure 7 illustrates admissions to the register between 1996 and 2000 by country of qualification.

It is important to bear in mind when looking at the figures that registration with the UKCC does not necessarily mean that the nurse in question is working within the health system. Conversely, nurses might work in the UK as auxiliaries during a period of adaptation before being accepted onto the UKCC register (Buchan 2000).

The Department of Health issued guidance at the end of 1999 stating that 'all NHS employers [should] ensure that they do not actively recruit from developing countries who are experiencing nursing shortages of their own'. This was reiterated in the NHS Plan (DoH 2000) and in a statement by Lord Hunt in August 2000. In the autumn of the same year a bi-lateral agreement was reached with Spain aimed at bringing 5000 Spanish nurses to the UK (already reflected in the 2000 figures). It is doubtful whether the intended numbers will be reached in practice as Spanish nurses enjoy better salaries and working conditions than British nurses (Silio, personal communication), although there is an oversupply of nurses in Spain.

Broad trends in terms of deployment are available with Inner London attracting 31.3 % of overseas trained nurses and England 3.5 %. However, a detailed breakdown by country of origin, country of training and geographical location of workplace is not available. This would require a survey by individual NHS Trust, and even then, many Trusts do not hold this type of information (in a personal communication with a North West Regional Human Resource Director we were told that they could not see the need to collect this data).

4. Survey of EEA doctors in one region in the UK: impact and comparative analysis

In order to investigate labour mobility in the region's EEA doctor population, a questionnaire was sent to all EEA doctors that could be identified. The primary aims of the survey were to:

- Identify EEA doctors in the area covered by the Manchester Deanery[4]
- Investigate the reasons for labour mobility and, therefore, for coming to the UK
- Investigate the process of registering to practice in the UK and actually practising in the UK.
- Investigate the experiences of training in the UK and satisfaction with training progress.
- Identify EEA doctors' career intentions.
- Identify a sample of doctors for interview.

The Region's Postgraduate Dean's medical staff database was used to identify a sample frame of EEA doctors. A total of 167 EEA doctors were identified (110 SHOs, 48 SpRs and 9 GP Registrars).

Each EEA doctor was sent a short postal questionnaire. Pre-paid return envelopes were provided. A reminder (including a second pre-paid envelope) was administered after four weeks. There were 17 exclusions due to "addressee unknown". An adjusted response rate of 53 % was therefore achieved: 56 SHOs, 5 GP registrars and 17 Specialist registrars.

4.1 Reasons for mobility

The main reason for labour mobility reported by doctors who responded to the survey is related to labour market conditions in EEA doctors' home country. Figure 8 illustrates the

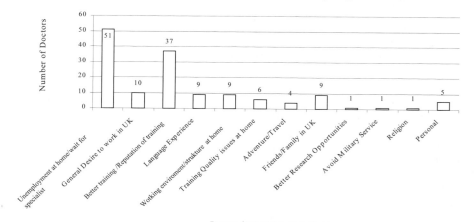

Fig. 8: Reasons for leaving country of qualification

---

[4] The Deanery is the geographical area covered by the postgraduate dean responsible for medical education. The progress of students working as junior doctors in hospitals/primary care in that area can be closely monitored by the Deanery.

reasons why doctors decided to leave their country of qualification. Medical unemployment or lack of specialist training posts were most frequently given as the reason for leaving the host country and coming to the UK. A higher standard of training in the UK was also a commonly cited reason.

4.2 The experience of labour mobility

When asked how easy or difficult it was to obtain permission from UK authorities to train or practice in the UK, an overwhelming majority of respondents, (89 % in total), found it was very easy or easy. A smaller number, jut over half, found it easy or very easy to obtain an actual training position once in the UK (total 51 %). A very small number of EEA doctors who responded to the survey found obtaining permission to train in the UK to be a difficult process (1 %). However, the number of those respondents who found it difficult or very difficult to obtain an actual training position was much larger (14 %).

Of those doctors who expressed difficulty in obtaining a training position, 37 % were Greek, 18 % German, 18 % from the Netherlands and 9 % each from Ireland, Poland and Spain.

When asked whether satisfied with their current training programme the majority of answers were favourable. However, 9 % stated that they were dissatisfied and 20 % were neither satisfied nor dissatisfied. The group of dissatisfied doctors consisted of Dutch and German nationals.

When asked whether they felt that patients accepted them just as they would accept a UK doctor, the overwhelming majority (90 %) of respondents felt that they were accepted on an equal basis. Only 8 % felt that they were not accepted by patients as UK doctors would be.

When asked whether they felt UK doctors accepted them as they would accept other UK doctors, the number who responded "no" was much higher than above (18/79 or 23 per cent). 59/79 (75 per cent) of respondents felt accepted just as a UK doctor would be accepted.

4.3 Career intentions

EEA doctors were asked about their career intentions and; whether, or not, they intended to remain in the UK. These findings are of particular interest. Only a quarter of those who responded intend to remain long term in the UK with over a half intending to leave in the short and medium term. The data highlight the considerable uncertainty among EEA doctors who responded to the survey. 16 per cent of SHOs and 17 percent of SpRs are currently undecided as to whether or not to remain in the UK. Furthermore, the majority of SHOs stated that they intend to remain only in the medium and short term (32 per cent and 26 per cent respectively) rather than in the longer term (21 per cent). Those who intend to leave in the short term will do so, for example, "after obtaining Membership of the Royal College of Physicians (MRCP) qualification."

More SpRs than SHOs stated that they intend to remain here in the long term and qualified this statement with, for example, "until retirement" and "indefinitely". Twenty three per cent of SpRs also indicated that they intend to stay only in the short term: and, on completion of specialist training they intend to leave the UK. It is possible to assess the intentions of EEA doctors to stay in the UK by country of qualification: For example, it is interesting to note that Greek doctors, in particular, intend to remain for short periods in the UK (1 month), with an even number of German doctors intending to stay for short and long periods. Only 2 of 12 Irish SpRs anticipate long term stay.

5. Interviews with clinical tutors and EEA doctors: a comparative analysis

The role of clinical tutors is important in the selection and monitoring of junior doctors, and thus, EEA doctors fall within their remit. Seven clinical tutors from the NW region were selected, representing the full range of hospital settings (general and teaching hospitals) and geographical locations. The purpose of the semi-structured interviews was to explore the specific issues relating to EEA doctors in comparison to both UK and overseas doctors. The interviews took a chronological format and also considered experience with EEA doctors against both EU regulations and the doctors' impact on the UK health care system. Interviews were either conducted face-to-face (tape recorded and then fully transcribed), or via telephone format on prepared schedules. The interviews lasted between 30-60 minutes.

From the EEA doctor survey a stratified sample was drawn consisting of twelve 12 doctors reflecting the composition of the overall sample in terms of grade and nationality. The purpose of the follow-up telephone interviews was to explore the issues covered in the sample in more depth in order to get a better understanding of the perspectives and experiences of EEA doctors. All doctors were asked to provide times, which suited them to be interviewed. Notes were taken during the interviews on prepared schedules and after the interviews they were transcribed. The interviews lasted between 30-45 minutes.

All the interviews were analysed using the QSR NUD*IST computer package. The open-ended answers from the survey reported above were also introduced into NUD*IST and formed an important additional data set. The main comparative categories for the doctors' group were grade and nationality. Comparisons were also drawn between the responses from clinical tutors and doctors. All the transcripts were coded according to the questions and additional categories were derived from the evolving analysis, reported in the discussion below.

5.1 Reasons for coming to the UK

The reason that many of the EEA doctors come to the UK is related to the labour market in their own countries. In particular, Germany and the Netherlands have an oversupply of doctors coupled with a limited opportunity for training posts in hospital and general practice. In the case of male Dutch doctors, they had, until recently, the additional problem of conscription which delayed their final graduation with 12-18 months.

The German doctors not only mentioned unemployment, but also the narrow range of options available whereby "once you have chosen your specialty you are committed". In comparison with the UK they expressed satisfaction with the opportunity to rotate here and to get a feel for different specialties. A second reason for leaving their home country cited by German doctors was the nature of the medical system, which was perceived to be strongly hierarchical. Two doctors explicitly stated that junior doctors are "treated badly" by senior staff and thus they did not enjoy the working environment.

Other factors attracting EEA doctors to the UK included the reputation of the training and teaching which was perceived as of good quality. Language also played a role in that most EEA doctors were proficient in English. Word-of-mouth was quoted by the majority of doctors who had heard from friends about work in the UK and sometimes were actively encouraged by those friends to join them.

The southern-European doctors discussed their desire to train abroad and they felt that information about opportunities in the UK was more readily available, either through agencies or through friends. One of the Spanish doctors mentioned that she did not progress in Spain partly because of the over-provision of doctors, but also because she needed contacts. Or as she put it:

"I am the first doctor in my family and we do not have access to the medical networks."

Summarised in terms of supply factors, EEA doctors come to the UK because the job situation in their own country is tight with an over-supply of doctors limiting the choice of options and career progression – together with hierarchical systems in some countries. Factors specific to the UK are the reputation of the UK training and that English is taught in most European countries as the second language.

5.2 The application process

Two main routes into the application process were mentioned. First, through friends who alerted EEA doctors to advertisements/vacancies and second, through specialised employment agencies. The latter route was seen as the more comprehensive and easy, because the individual was guided through all the stages of the application to the acceptance of a job offer. This was considered particularly useful in relation to validation of qualifications by the GMC, which included the proper translation of documents. Timing was an important advantage of using agencies as one German doctor explained:

"In Germany it is expensive to subscribe to the British Medical Journal (BMJ) and it is better if you know someone who lives in England who can alert you to a job. There is a real problem because, if you wait for them to contact you, you have often missed the closing date deadlines. So, in fact, it is much easier to let the locum agency sort it out."

One doctor mentioned that UK consultants came to visit Germany for an active recruitment drive and he was interviewed for a job in Frankfurt. Another German doctor was interviewed over the telephone and he only had to present his evidence of qualifications to the agency, and not to the NHS Trust employing him. This process was confirmed by one of the clinical tutors who said that he had done telephone interviews. However, he saw that as an exception rather than a rule. At the same time he realised that EEA doctors could be at a disadvantage when

"they are in their home country and they send their c.v. through the post. It is unlikely that they can attend for interview."

The clinical tutors emphasised that EEA doctors have equal rights and opportunities to the UK graduates, and that they are appointed on merit. However, in practice the clinical tutors realise that it is not always an entirely fair process because EEA doctors cannot always attend interviews and can be subject to implicit bias (which will be discussed later in this report).

Most doctors felt that getting a job has become more difficult, and particularly for registered training posts. They mentioned the increasing number of people applying, but were unclear why that has altered over the last few years. One of the Spanish doctors said that he had sent over 25 applications before he got his first interview, but that resulted immediately in a job offer. Perhaps this suggests a prejudice, or unwillingness to recruit from such sources until wholly necessary – in which case, however, such applicants measure up well. Such anecdotal "evidence" could benefit from further investigation.

The clinical tutors argued that it was relatively easy for EEA doctors to acquire training posts, depending on the specialty. At the SHO level they did not see great difficulties, especially in the shortage specialties. One of the clinical tutors mentioned that there is sometimes implicit prejudice:

> "People naturally look towards appointing a UK graduate. There is a matching scheme in operation where graduates are automatically allocated to training places and the European graduates have to somehow fit into that."

Thus, while formally there are equal opportunities, EEA doctors can be "streamed" into certain directions as structural circumstances are interpreted in a particular way by the people appointing junior doctors.

5.3 Induction and conditions of service

All the EEA doctors interviewed were invited to participate in a general induction programme in their employing organisation. Most hospitals had an information booklet with all the necessary information. This proved to be an important source as some doctors said that they could not attend the actual verbal introduction as they were "on call". None of the doctors had received an induction specifically tailored to the needs of EEA doctors. In a number of cases this appeared to have led to crucial information being missed. A Spanish doctor explained the lack of proper information has hampered his progress:

> "I am three years down the line now and I know that I have not done things that at the time I should have. Nobody has told me things that I needed to do to progress my career. Some Trusts are only interested in getting you to service. You need more information and direction on what training you have to do and over what period you should expect to have done it."

This doctor had not known about the central role of "the logbook"[5] and has wasted considerable time as a result. The same happened to a Dutch doctor who was asked for his logbook when he wanted to change jobs. Only then – after having worked for a year in the UK – did he realise its importance.

Understanding of policies such as "the New Deal"[6] was sketchy. This was also a problem amongst UK graduates but more pronounced in the case of non-UK graduates who felt advantage had been taken of them. A number of doctors reported that they worked much more than the 56 hours, but did not know how to remedy the situation. Similarly, the amount of teaching that they could expect was a source of confusion, and one of the doctors said that he received no specific guidance for EEA doctors and that "you find out by yourself — slowly!" This problem was acknowledged by one of the clinical tutors who was concerned that EEA doctors did not always know all the opportunities available to them.

The clinical tutors admitted that there is no separate policy for dealing with the induction of EEA doctors and that they are treated the same as other junior doctors. One explanation given was the following:

> "We do not have a separate policy. This does not mean we don't want to. If we have a greater volume of EEA doctors, and on a regular basis, then perhaps we

---

[5] The logbook is a personal record for doctors in training, describing clearly the scope of their activities and skills, and this is ratified by their trainer.

[6] The New Deal represents an agreement in 1996 between the UK Government and organisations representing the medical profession that junior doctors should not work more than 56 hours per week. They can be on duty for 72 hours per week but, of that, 16 hours should be on call.

will need to have one, or some sort of system that provides a special induction. That is not the case at the moment."

The same clinical tutor made reference to the Mersey Postgraduate Dean who commissioned a video introducing non-UK graduates to the NHS. This could prove an important resource for people who have to cope with the complex mix of adapting to a different country and culture, and operating within a different health care system and training structure.

5.4 Career opportunities

In theory the career opportunities for EEA doctors are the same as for UK graduates. In practice the picture is more complex. On the one hand there are doctors who testify that they are satisfied and feel that there is equality of opportunity. They state that they are treated the same as the UK graduates and that they feel well integrated and accepted. On the other hand, a number of doctors expressed doubts as to whether an implicit hierarchy is in operation, which goes as follows:

> "First, British doctors, then EEA doctors and then Indian doctors. It all appears to depend on skin colour."

This issue appears to be bound up with notions about British culture and education, because EEA doctors feel that there is a certain "superiority", which is expressed in various ways. Moreover, EEA doctors sometimes felt that the experience they had built up in their own country was misunderstood and not considered equivalent. This "de-valuation" of their knowledge and experience meant that they often had to go back a few steps, and thus slow down their career.

When comparing the EEA doctors' perspectives with the opinions of the clinical tutors a number of interesting issues arise. At the formal level mutual recognition of previous training exists, but in practice the clinical tutors describe concerns that they themselves and their colleagues within the health service have about equivalence. This is clearly expressed by one of the clinical tutors:

> "In practice we are sceptical and cautious about people's qualifications. I don't have a good understanding of their capabilities just on the strength of the letters after their name. I don't have enough information about their medical school and its standards. It's more at the macro level, and specific information would be more useful to know what the standards are."

To some extent the clinical tutors share the perspective of the EEA doctors when they say that

> "we don't have sufficient understanding of what their training means and how you can compare their training with UK training."

However, in the absence of an agreed framework for assessing equivalence it is easy to adopt stereotypical approaches based upon previous – and often ad hoc – experiences:

> "Rightly or wrongly when assessing the training received by EEA doctors and in employing them you tend to be influenced by which country they are from."

This was clearly demonstrated in the remarks made by clinical tutors such as "Spanish graduates have theoretical book knowledge" or "the Spanish have by far the worst reputation". On the other hand "there hasn't been a bad German or Dutch doctor" and "they are better with language". The comparison between northern and southern European doctors was captured by the metaphor "above or below the olive line". Whilst there might be objective differences, the generalisations built upon anecdotal evidence could prejudice against individual doctors and thus counter equal opportunities in career development.

The clinical tutors argued that EEA doctors had the same opportunities as UK graduates, and that they were encouraged to work towards CCST. At the same time there were contradictions concerning the deployment of EEA doctors. First, doubts were voiced as to whether equality of opportunity existed in practice across the board. One of the tutors said that

"they tend to fill the spots that haven't been filled by UK graduates."

Second, one clinical tutor explained that some hospitals see the EEA workforce as a "transient resource" and

"there has never been the incentive on either part to treat vacancies filled by European doctors as anything other than short term vacancies."

Taken those tendencies together it is easy to consider investment in career development of EEA doctors as a waste of resources. In this sense the comments from the EEA doctors and the clinical tutors point towards a problem of perception about the role of EEA doctors and their aspirations. They all express the wish to take advantage of the same career opportunities as UK doctors, yet do not all feel that these are available to them. This can lead to an under-investment in professional development with possible negative consequences for individual EEA doctors and the quality of the service provided by them.

Two other issues warrant mention: for EEA doctors there is no requirement to provide evidence of proficiency in English (unlike overseas doctors who have to do a PLAB test). This means that some EEA doctors can practice in the UK with insufficient mastery of the language which is problematic in various areas of their work e.g. report writing and communication with patients. This has a detrimental effect on their career opportunities as they are not able to function to their maximum potential – and they will also be hampered in demonstrating their clinical competence – and thus they encounter barriers in progressing up the ladder.

The second issue was the lack of systematic support for EEA doctors. None of the respondents interviewed (clinical tutors and EEA doctors) mentioned the existence of a formal mechanism. Some of the clinical tutors explained that EEA doctors fitted into the normal junior doctor support structures, and that informal support was sometimes available. However, there was no explicit recognition of special needs of this cohort of doctors. A few EEA doctors mentioned feelings of isolation and lack of exchange of ideas about career options, but none knew whether targeted support existed. Given that EEA doctors do not always receive the right amount of information at induction this support is important if they are not to pursue "blind alleys".

5.5 Career intentions

The long-term career intentions of the EEA doctors differed between individuals and no clear pattern could be ascertained in terms of nationality. The factors which determined whether individuals wanted to pursue a career in the UK or at home were a combination of personal considerations such as marriage and family, structural considerations such as changing employment patterns and professional choices such as moving into new territories such as practicing in developing countries.

Specific issues warrant further discussion. First, there was considerable confusion whether qualifications such as CCST obtained in the UK would be recognised in the home country. Most German and Greek doctors were confident that their UK CCST was recognised, while the Dutch, French and Spanish doctors appeared uncertain. This is somewhat surprising given that these doctors have embarked on training programmes and invested time and resources in something with an unclear long-term pay-off.

Second, most of the German doctors want to stay in the UK, not only because of the poor job prospects in Germany but primarily because they feel that they have been trained for the UK context and therefore their career is geared towards the needs of the British health service. One doctor expressed it thus:

"I have done my full post-graduate training in the UK, I think and work as a British doctor."

Furthermore, certain specialist qualifications are not recognised (such as Membership of the Royal College of Obstetricians and Gynaecologists (MRCOG)) and doctors who have completed such training feel that it would be wasted time if they went back:

"I would have to do another year in Germany and the German own exams before settling as a specialist."

Clinical tutors have the impression that 50 % of EEA doctors stay and 50 % go back home. One of the clinical tutors surveyed the EEA doctors in his own Trust who all wanted to complete their training in the UK. He found that the people who wanted to return to their home country did so for family reasons, but only returned to their own countries if they managed to secure a comparable position there. This impression was backed up by the observation of another clinical tutor who said that most EEA doctors come for specific training and then return home. However, it is difficult to disentangle individual motivation from professional and structural reasons, and predictions about long-term career patterns are not possible from this study.

In view of recent policy statements about extending the UK medical workforce by 7,000 doctors (Department of Health, 14th July, 1998) recruitment from outside the UK will probably be continuing, but the relative proportions of EEA doctors and other doctors (including the former Eastern block, South African and Commonwealth) cannot be stated with accuracy.

5.6 Patients' acceptance of EEA doctors

An important area explored in both the survey and the interviews was how EEA doctors thought that patients perceived them. The majority of doctors said that they had experienced little or no difficulties with acceptance by patients. The reasons given can be categorised as follows: first, Britain is increasingly seen as a multi-cultural society and patients are used to being attended by professionals from different nationalities. Second, almost all the EEA doctors are white (or shades of white) and this makes acceptance easier. Third, most doctors feel that any possible barriers can be overcome by a professional attitude.

Despite this optimistic assessment caveats were mentioned on a few occasions. For example, acceptance depends on the experience and education of the patient. In the case of patients who have not had exposure to foreign doctors "there could be a language and/or attitude barrier". Many doctors mentioned that speaking the language well was considered important, as well as coping with the various English accents.

The clinical tutors confirmed the experience of the EEA doctors and provided the same reasons for the positive acceptance by patients. Perhaps they emphasised the professional attitude even more than the EEA doctors themselves:

> "I don't think the patients mind who their doctor is as long as they come across well and communicate well [...] I can only remember a handful of incidents since I have been a clinical tutor. I think I can ascribe to the idea – which has been shown in research – that the initial prejudice that could arise with a doctor is completely dispelled within a few minutes by that doctor's personal approach. If the doctor communicates well and is obviously competent to talk with the patient or the parent, I am sure the patient does not mind where the doctor comes from."

On the whole very few problems were reported in this study and any incidents were dealt with as exceptions rather than the rule.

5.7 Acceptance by professional peers

The picture emerging about acceptance by peers is less homogeneous, and positive and negative reactions are balancing each other out. The interviews "put flesh" on the bones of the survey data reported above. While most EEA doctors say that they are accepted by their peers, they do mention the conditions which made this acceptance easier, including the fact that being a national from an EEA country generally meant having a white skin. A Spanish doctor felt that he was accepted only in so far he was not competing against UK doctors, and one of the clinical tutors felt that EEA doctors were especially welcome in areas suffering from staff shortages.

The negative aspects have been partly discussed above in relation to the perceived British superiority concerning their own educational system and standards. EEA doctors expressed dismay at their previous training being considered as inferior, or in the words of a German doctor "there is a tendency to mistrust anything other than the British way of training and practice".

They also felt that there was little knowledge of non-UK systems and a lack of interest in finding out because

> "they are not interested in what happens in medicine anywhere else than Britain."

A Greek doctor linked the staff shortages in medicine to the negative attitude he has encountered as follows:

> "They are probably annoyed by the increasing number of foreign doctors working in the UK."

The most recent trends show that demand for NHS training places by overseas doctors is outstripping supply and this is becoming a concern within professional circles. This issue, alongside wider workforce planning issues will be discussed in the "outcomes" section below.

6. Comparisons with Germany, Sweden and Spain

6.1 Regulatory frameworks

Around 1970 Germany's health care system was modernised and resulted – besides a huge hospital expansion and modernisation programme – in the opening of new medical schools (e.g. Medizinische Hochschule Hannover). In addition, the right of the medical faculties to limit the number of students was challenged. Accordingly, universities had to admit as many students as they could teach (not necessarily reflecting their own preferences or what the Health Ministry deemed necessary). As higher education was a responsibility of the Länder (states), they had to agree a "state-contract" in order to regulate capacity nation-wide. In 1972 the first state-contract was introduced which mandated the teaching of a certain number of students per faculty member (or patients for students in their clinical years). As a result, the number of medical students rose from 26,000 in 1960/61 to 43,400 in 1975/76 and further to 68,800 in 1980/81 (West Germany only, excluding dental students).

Almost coincidentally with the introduction of cost-containment policies, the political debate on the adequate number of doctors assumed a dramatic over-supply of physicians for the near future. "Doctors are sweeping the health sector" was the dominant metaphor of the political debate. The assumed oversupply was expected to be responsible for a sharp rise in future expenditure (Döhler 1990; Alber & Bernadi-Schenkluhn 1992). Although there was neither clear scientific evidence as to what constitutes the adequate number of doctors, nor was the hypotheses sufficiently tested that more doctors will necessarily increase expenditure, nevertheless a new policy was introduced aimed at reducing the number of physicians. In order to regulate the number of physicians two sets of policies were introduced:

- First, policies aimed at reducing the number of medical students which is difficult due to constitutional rights as explained above. As downsizing medical schools met with opposition from the universities, increasing the number of teaching hours and decreasing the number of students per teacher was the only possible – but limited – way. Another policy was intended to make medical education unattractive – through the introduction of a "Arzt im Praktikum", representing a very low salaried period for young doctors in hospitals. After the number of medical students peaked in 1988/89, it is slowly but steadily dropping (in the unified Germany): from 95,200 in 1990/91 to 82,700 in 1998/99 (Bundesministerium für Gesundheit 1999).
- Second, legislation was introduced to limit the number of office-based physicians. According to §§ 99-105 of the Social Code Book V, "needs-based" plans have to be developed to regulate the number of social health insurance (SHI) – affiliated office-based physicians. Originally, the intention was to guarantee that shortage specialties would also be available in rural areas. Since the 1980s, however, the focus has been on avoiding over-supply. From 1993 onwards, the Social Code Book regulates matters so that new practices may not be opened in areas where supply exceeds 110 % of the average number for the particular specialty. Accordingly, the Federal Committee of Physicians and Sickness Funds has developed guidelines that define these limits. The

guidelines classify all planning areas into one of 10 groups – ranging from large metropolitan cities to rural counties – and define the "need" per group as the actual number of physicians working in counties of that group in 1990 (divided by the population). Accordingly, "over-supply" is defined as 110 % of that figure (Busse 2000). This limits possibilities for new practices but still leaves – mostly rural – areas open. Moreover, since 1999, physicians older than the age of 67 have to give up their practice (affecting around 2,500 doctors or 2 % of the total in 1998 – the oldest being 92!).

A fundamental principle of the health care system in Sweden is that it is a public sector responsibility to provide and finance health and medical services for the entire population. Two characteristics of the Swedish system are its decentralised structure and it being based upon democratic principles.

Sweden comprises 21 county councils and regions. The county councils and the regions decide on the allocation of resources to the health services and are responsible for the overall planning of the services offered. It is also the county councils and the regions who own and run the hospitals, health centres and other institutions, even if these institutions are supplemented by private organisations. In certain cases these organisations have contracts with the county councils or the regions. The county councils and the regions are also responsible for the recruitment of doctors and nurses.

In Spain the regulation of student number in medical faculties operates through a "numerus clausus". However, the "numerus clausus" has been applied on an irregular basis, and coupled with the creation of new medical faculties, this has resulted in the admission of some 20,000 new students over the last decade. This figure is now decreasing, and it is stated that the number of students admitted to Spanish faculties of medicine should not in any case exceed the existing admission figures (Ministry of Health and Consumption 1998). The proposed decrease would reduce the number of students to 4,000 per year, with a student/population quotient (1/10,000) being equivalent to the admission average in European Union countries. Yet, the rate of doctors per inhabitant remains higher than that in neighbouring countries.

Current legislation requires that all medical graduates who wish to become specialists or generalists participate in the same training scheme, the MIR (Medico Interno Residente). This scheme is based on supervised professional and practical training which consists of two key elements: a training programme and a system of teaching accreditation. The number of accredited teaching centres has risen from 96 in 1987 to 227 in 1999. The number of teaching units have increased from 1543 to 2376 during the same time period.

6.2 The production of doctors and workforce profile

The number of new physicians in Germany has fluctuated over the last decades. After World War II, the "production" of new physicians was very limited since medical faculties had the right to curb the number of students. A further hurdle for new physicians consisted of the fact that possibilities for opening up a (new) practice were severely limited as the ratio of physicians to sickness fund insured was fixed at 1/600. However, according to a ruling from the constitutional court of 23rd March 1960, the freedom to choose a profession – guaranteed in article 12 of the "Grundgesetz" (constitution) – is not only a formal freedom but entails the right to settle in the ambulatory sector and the obligation of sickness funds to contract with any physician who wishes to do so.

The number of physicians working is still growing, although more physicians work in the hospital sector than in the ambulatory sector. The number of physicians grew from 244,238 in 1991 to 287,032 in 1998.

The percentage of foreign physicians among all practising physicians has remained constant at slightly below 5 % over the last few years at 13,836 in 1998. Equally, the number of physicians from other EU countries has remained constant over that period, at around 28 % of all foreign or 1.3 % of all physicians. Actually, even the numbers by country are remarkably stable – reflecting the fact that most of the foreign physicians come to Germany for long periods (or even stay, as it may be assumed for most foreigners in private practice (around 25 %). A specific phenomenon in Germany is the high (and still increasing) number of physicians from Iran.

Although often claimed differently (see the remarks by German junior doctors in the UK), unemployment is comparatively low among physicians and dentists. In January 2000 11,082 physicians and dentist were registered unemployed, which is a drop compared to January 1999 by 5.7 % (Bundesanstalt für Arbeit).

In Germany a side issue with relevance to this project is the fact that – besides their post-graduate training as defined by the medical chambers – physicians as well as dentists had to take part in a mandatory introductory course about managing a practice before being able to apply to open their own practice. This additional requirement was considered to violate the freedom of movement for physicians (78/686 EEC) and after the Commission had taken steps against Germany in the summer of 1998, the requirement was dropped through the Act to Strengthen Solidarity in Social Health Insurance late in 1998. It is doubtful, however, that the previous requirement constituted a real hurdle for foreign physicians

The only EU country with a noticeable (but with +20 % still small) increase in numbers of doctors working in Germany is Austria after its joining the EU, possibly reflecting a modest effect of the freedom of movement for physicians. Only 4 EU countries are among the top ten countries with doctors working in Germany in 1998: Greece (at no. 3), the Netherlands (8), Italy (9) and Austria (10).

In Sweden doctor density is high with about one doctor per 300 inhabitants. Currently there are about 2,800 more doctors compared to 5 years ago, which means that supply is relatively good. However, the need for doctors has increased, mainly for two reasons. Firstly, patients and the general public express increasingly greater health care demands and want a wider range and more responsive services. Secondly, new methods of treatment have been developed resulting in increased need for care in certain areas (e.g. within orthopaedic and ophthalmic surgery). Metropolitan areas (Stockholm, Skåne, Västra Götaland, and Uppsala) are well served with doctors, which is not primarily due to career and research opportunities but rather appears to be related to the availability of social, recreational and cultural activities.

Cardiology is the most popular speciality. The supply of cardiologists and of ophthalmologists is good, but there is a shortage of general practitioners. This shortage is set to increase and will be first noticed in "intermediate" county councils such as Västernorrland, Dalarna, Halland, Jönköping, Värmland and Kalmar. In response, several county councils have started to recruit doctors and general practitioners from Poland, Russia and similar countries. These doctors are given a crash course in the Swedish language before starting to practice.

Emigration of fully qualified doctors to other countries (i.e. doctors who are registered abroad) is relatively small, around 3-4 % of two sample batches of registered doctors (doctors registered in 1989 and 1995 respectively). It is, however, popular to take temporary employment in Norway during compensatory leave for on-call duty and during holidays.

Spain has a surplus of doctors. However, the post-graduate medical training system which has expanded as a result of the rise in accredited training centres (see above) cannot accommodate the large numbers of new graduates that have to be incorporated in the

Spanish NHS. A total number of 6145 accredited places are currently available, and consequently the training system is saturated causing a large gap between the number of students and the number of places on offer. Thus, the training system as linked to the NHS demonstrates a major weakness, namely a marked lack of elasticity. This could severely hamper the process of rapid absorption of excess training demand originating in the 1980s, and remaining unresolved.

Analysing the rates of doctors in active service, and the number of new graduates in neighbouring countries leads to the conclusion that it is necessary to continue the policy of reducing the number of medical graduates. No robust figures exist about the breakdown by specialties and regions.

6.3 The production of nurses

The nursing crisis was an issue in Germany for a considerable period. The reasons were that the turnover of nurses in the hospital sector was very high, due to low salaries, night shifts, family breaks, difficult working conditions and poor career prospects. There were several attempts to fill shortages with nurses from Asia and especially from Yugoslavia. Nevertheless, the nursing crisis remained endemic until the mid 90s.

Under the full cost cover principle, manpower planning for nurses in the hospital sector was guided by the so-called "Anhaltszahlen", an indicator which specified how many minutes of care a nurse would have to spend on average per patient/day. From this indicator the number of nurses for a particular hospital was calculated. It was an important guide for the negotiations on per-diems between the individual hospital and the sickness funds. The indicator was revised several times due both to technological change in the hospital sector and to the working time reduction which took place from 1958 to 1990 which reduced the weekly working time from 48 to 38.5 hours.

With the introduction of prospective financing and hospital budgets, the indicator lost its relevance, since effective manpower planning was now (in theory) in the hands of the hospital management, allowing the best use of allocated financial resources to be made.

But as a reaction to the ongoing debate on the nursing crises the federal government decided in 1993 to introduce an interesting instrument, namely "nursing time standards". Through this instrument, a daily documentation of nursing activities placed every patient in one of nine categories with a standardized amount of necessary nursing time between 52 and 215 minutes per day. The total amount of minutes per ward and per hospital could be calculated into the necessary nursing staff for the unit. Nursing time standards were introduced to end the period of (perceived) nursing shortages. It was expected that new jobs would be created – and this did, indeed, occur. However, the regulation was suspended in 1996 and abolished in 1997 for the official reason that the standard had led to almost 21,000 new nursing positions between 1993 and 1995 when the policy makers had anticipated only 13,000. It was also argued that it did not leave sufficient room for managerial decisions. Since then the nursing crisis is no longer on the political agenda.

It is unclear, whether the Schools of Health Service "Schulen des Gesundheitswesens" have trained sufficient number of nurses. Currently, hospitals appear to down-size or close Schools to save money, with some schools merging. In some Länder (states) the permission to run a School is handled more restrictive (this not yet reflected in the numbers of graduates, however).

Since nurses are not legally considered to be a profession, they do not need to register and hence no good data on nurses are available. The only reliable data relate to those working in hospitals. In 1991 there were 389,500 hospital based nurses and in 1998 419,300.

In Sweden nurses are the biggest group of employees in the health sector, and make up 29 per cent of the work force. In 1998 there were 129,581 registered nurses in Sweden (Hälso- och sjukvårdsstatistisk årsbok 1998) but not all of them actually work as nurses. The figures for 1997 show that 70,059 nurses were employed in the county councils and 95,897 nurses were employed in the municipalities. There is a shortage of nurses and this is expected to increase in the future. This phenomenon has started in the 80's and 90's when the County Councils gave notice to a lot of health services personnel. The result of this policy is the current high average age of employed nurses in Sweden, with the average age in 1998 being 43 years.

The Swedish Federation of County Councils published a report in 1998 illuminating the future requirement of staff and education in the health sector for the years 2005-2015. They calculated that in the future there will be a need for about 7,000 nurses each year in the councils, the municipalities and regions. Of this overall figure the Swedish Federation of County Councils estimated that about 2,300 could be recruited internally. They foresaw a number of ways: more nurses, who are already employed, could work increased hours; through changing the organisation of work by keeping a reserve army of substitutes. External recruitment could be helped by making it easier for nurses with a foreign education to enter the labour market. The remaining 4,700 nurses had to be produced through education and training. At present, there are about 3,450 places in nurse education and in the future an increase of 1,600 more places is required. However, the Swedish Federation of County Councils has decided that increase in 750 education places is more realistic. The national Swedish Labour Market Board has given more money for nursing education.

In a report from the Swedish Federation of County Councils in April 2000 two thirds of the county councils estimated that they have a large need for recruitment of nurses with further education. One third of the county councils reported that they need to recruit nurses with further education. Only one county council thought that they had a balanced number of nurses with further education. This report highlighted that the main shortages are within intensive care units, anesthetics, midwifery, oncology and child health nursing.

One explanation of shortages in specialty areas is because of the age structure with cohorts of employees retiring at the same time. At the same time the municipalities need to employ more nurses in order to meet increasing health care demand, particularly for general nurses, geriatric and psychiatric nursing and district nursing. Additional pressure is exerted through the changes in nursing work with trained nurses having to take on tasks previously carried out by enrolled nurses. A further explanation is an increase in the mobility. Statistics from Statistics Sweden (1998) shows that, in 1996, 570 nurses emigrated from Sweden. According to The National Board of Health and Welfare around 150 nurses from other countries each year gain a Swedish certification as a nurse, thus there an overall deficit in nurses.

It has not been possible to ascertain reliable figures from Spain and thus no comparison is made with the nursing situation there.

7. Outcomes

EU regulation with regard to free movement of labour has resulted in easy registration for EEA doctors with UK authorities to train and practice in the UK. Obtaining registration with the GMC was not considered difficult, but finding an actual training position could sometimes be more problematic. There is evidence in our study that a relationship with how prior qualifications are interpreted exists. Whilst qualifications are formally recognised by the GMC, and NHS Trusts do generally not demand proof of qualifications, the recognition *in practice* is less straightforward. The local medical establishments appear to perceive non-UK qualifications in paradoxical ways: on the one hand formal recognition is espoused, but on the other hand a lack of confidence in community-wide standards of basic medical and postgraduate education becomes apparent when judging individual candidates. This leads to inconsistent assessment of candidates' suitability for training posts, with distinction made between educational qualifications from Northern versus Southern European countries. The effect of these localised, unsystematic judgements is a potential inequality of training opportunity for certain EEA doctors.

The second issue relates to information concerning the training structure. The European Commission's Green Paper on Transnational Mobility (European Commission 1996) and the subsequent EU action plan on Free Movement of Workers that was adopted in 1997 emphasise this, because insufficient information in the Member States can create obstacles to mobility. At a local level this could be adapted to the needs of EEA doctors through information sharing strategies, including regional booklets, Internet based material, induction videos and so on. At a more personal, level support networks for EEA doctors could be helpful in breaking isolation, sharing information and experiences and possibly providing guidance to local medical establishments about educational qualifications gained in EEA countries.

At the time of writing this report, the Department of Health has issued a consultation document "A health service of all talents" (DoH 2000a) outlining a radical reform of workforce planning in the health service. The current complex system of medical manpower planning with its 'top-down' approach does not sit comfortably alongside the planning system for nurses and professions allied to medicine which is 'bottom-up' service-led (Davies 2000). The proposals are to develop an integrated planning system encompassing the whole workforce, and this is to take place against the backdrop of the NHS Plan (DoH 2000b) promising to increase the number of doctors by 9,500 and nurses by 20,000 by the year 2004. At the same time, the 12-year limit to implement the EU working time directive and the reduction in the number of training places available as a result of the alignment of medical training with European criteria pose considerable problems that the new system has to address urgently. The drive in the UK to develop local solutions, whilst at the same time to deliver national targets will be a delicate balance to achieve. Moreover, when taking into account the transnational context of the European Union which generates its own political, educational and service trends, it will be difficult to predict the exact outcomes of the national and international changes in the labour force. The shortages in all cadres of health personnel has meant that the UK is increasingly seeking to recruit from other countries, but pressure from developing countries, notably South Africa, have meant at least a public cautionary stance that recruitment will "have to be done on an ethical basis in countries with a surplus of staff" (Lord Hunt, Junior health minister, August 2000).

In general terms, it is clear that the EU directives have influenced the UK health service in that the free movement of labour allows the mutual acceptance of qualifications and thus the uptake of training places for medical personnel. The reputation of British training and the status of English as the dominant international language results in Britain being primarily an importer of personnel. However, the attraction of the UK appears to be lessening for EEA doctors while doctors from other English speaking countries (esp. South Africa and Asia) are on the increase.

When comparing to the three other countries, Germany appears to attract doctors from specific EU countries such as Austria and Greece, and is increasingly becoming attractive to personnel from Central and Eastern Europe. Whether this is due to EU Directives or geographical proximity is difficult to say. In Spain and Sweden the issue of inward mobility of doctors is less apparent, but the outward migration on either a temporary or permanent basis is more significant. The EU Directive has facilitated movements, but not destabilised the national system.

8. Conclusion and policy implications

EU-wide policies and directives are in place and have been transposed in most countries, but the key question now lies in their implementation at country-level. The UK case study has illuminated the tension between formal and "real life" recognition of medical qualifications, and the lack of guidance throughout the training period for EEA doctors in the UK. It is vital that the implementation discrepancy between formal and informal recognition and access to information are tackled if equal access to medical training is desired as envisaged in the Medical Directive 93/16/EEC.

Related to this is the question of the quality of medical and nursing training. Even though formal recognition exists, there is uncertainty as to the comparability of actual skills and competencies. The differences in national curricula are difficult to ascertain because they depend on a multitude of factors: clinical knowledge and content of educational programmes, training context, cultural expectations, roles and responsibilities in different health care systems and so on. Judgements as to what constitutes appropriate quality are problematic and contingent upon specific structural and cultural conditions. An argument could be made for the development of a minimum competency framework to be adopted across the EU.

The (implicit) assertion underlying the EU legislative framework is that labour mobility is "a good thing". Clearly, in an economically and socially homogeneous Europe, which is a super-national political entity, such mobility is likely to be considered as a basic human freedom. This study highlights the positive aspects of mobility which are both at the individual level in terms of widening experiences and opportunities, and at the institutional level where organisations are enriched through a wider range of cultural and educational inputs.

Yet, in a Europe "at the crossroads", there may be unpredictable effects upon individual countries. If, for example, doctors are in shortage Europe-wide or in certain economically better-off countries, then free mobility may lead to shortages in economically poorer countries. The migration of doctors from Greece to the UK would be a case in point. The situation could be the other way round: surpluses in better-off countries could aid poorer countries, or countries with shortages, or both. The recent (only temporary) surplus of German doctors is a case in point.

What is clear, however, is that national manpower planning in the public sector may often be inadequate to achieve its goals in the context of unpredictable international mobility. As a result, there may be a politically difficult choice to be made between developing a European manpower planning strategy for substantially publicly funded provision (e.g. of doctors); the maintenance or even increase in regulatory restrictions on mobility to prevent national strategies from being undermined; and the increasing privatisation of public planning (e.g. leaving the supply of doctors to the private market with individuals investing in their own training). The last is likely to be unattractive and inequitable – for poorer individuals and also poorer countries. The second option goes against the grain of developing EU policy. Yet, the first option is an attack upon subsidiarity within the EU as currently understood.

This overview on four EU countries has only begun to investigate these matters. Yet, the pervasiveness of "informal" barriers to implementation of free mobility perhaps suggests that – in the absence of clear European policy compatible with Member States' own policy and reality – Member States will use informal policy, or barriers, to render national and EU directives superficially compatible.

References

Alber J, Bernadi-Schenkluhn B. Westeuropäische Gesundheitssysteme im Vergleich: Bundesrepublik Deutschland, Schweiz, Frankreich, Italien, Großbritannien [West European health systems in comparison: West Germany, Switzerland, France, Italy, United Kingdom]. Frankfurt a. M.: Campus Verlag; 1992.

Blomqvist K, Lindberg L.Uppföljning av personalbehovet inom landstingen, regionerna och Gotlands sjukvård [The follow-up about the need for staff within the County Councils, the regions and the Health care in Gotland]. Stockholm: Landstingsförbundet [The Federation of the County Councils]; 2000.

Buchan J, Seccombe I, Ball J. The international mobility of nurses, a UK perspective. Institute of Manpower Studies; 1992.

Buchan J. Your country needs you. Health Serv J 1998; 16th July: 22-5.

Buchan J. Pressure is on. Health Serv J 2000; 7th December: 26-7.

Bundesministerium für Gesundheit. Daten des Gesundheitswesen. Ausgabe 1999 [Health care data - edition 1999]. Baden-Baden: Nomos Verlagsgesellschaft; 1999.

Busse R. Health care systems in transition – Germany. Copenhagen. European Observatory on Health Care Systems; 2000.

Davies J. The devil is in the detail. Health Serv J 2000; 1st June: 18-21.

Department of Health. Comprehensive Spending Review. Press Release; 14th July 1998: 294.

Department of Health. A health service of all talents. London: DoH; 2000a.

Department of Health. The NHS Plan. London: DoH; 2000b.

Department of Health. NHS Hospital, Public Health Medicine and Community Health Services. Medical and Dental Workforce Census, England - Detailed Results: 30th September 1996/7.

Döhler M. Gesundheitspolitik nach der "Wende": Policy Netzwerke und ordnungspolitischer Strategie-wechsel in Großbritannien, den USA und der Bundesrepublik Deutschland. Berlin: Edition Sigma; 1990.

European Commission. Education, training, research. The obstacles to transnational mobility. Brussels: COM(96)462 final; 1996.

Friend B. Quick march. Health Serv J 1998; 3rd December: 26-7.

Hurwitz L. The Free Circulation of Physicians within the European Community. Aldershot: Avebury; 1990.

Jinks C, Ong BN, Paton C. Catching the drift. Health Serv J 1998; 17th September: 24-6.

Lambert TW, Goldacre MJ. Career destinations seven years on among doctors who qualified in the UK in 1988: Postal questionnaire survey. BMJ 1998;317:1429-31.

Landstingsförbundet [The Swedish Federation of County Councils].Vården: en framtidsbransch, personalens kapacitet [Nursing: a branch for the future, the capacity of the staff]. Stockholm; 1998.

Lowry S. Certify a specialist. BMJ 1996; Career Focus: 2-3.

Lyall J. Doctors' orders. Health Serv J 1997; 5th June: 12.

McKee M. Workshop discussion report. In: Normand C, Vaughan P, editors. Europe without Frontiers. Implications for Health. Chichester: John Wiley and Sons; 1993. p. 105-110.

Ministry of Health and Consumption. Report on Spanish citizens' health. Madrid; 1998.

Permanent Working Group of European Junior Hospital Doctors (PWG). Medical Manpower in Europe by the year 2000. From Surplus to Deficit. Copenhagen: PWG; 1996.

Socialstyrelsen [The national board of health and welfare]. Hälso- och sjukvårdsstatistisk årsbok 1998 [Yearbook of Health and Medical care 1998]. Stockholm 1998.

The European Union and Health Services
R. Busse et al. (Eds.)
IOS Press, 2002

Scenarios on the future mobility of doctors and nurses

Calum PATON and Bie Nio ONG

Abstract. Based on the results of two expert workshops, this chapter presents possible developments of the mobility of doctors and nurses in an enlarged EU under four scenarios: 1. The SEM and labour mobility are strengthened. 2. Health services are removed from the SEM. 3. Human resource planning is undertaken on a EU-wide scale. 4. The pragmatic status quo continues. The latter situation is considered the most likely but unstable nonetheless as certain countries continue to rely on importing health professionals. The first scenario is considered the most likely alternative, with possibly increasing negative consequences for candidate countries if doctors and nurses emigrate.

1. Introduction

Within the context of the Single European Market, there is at present uncertainty about future employment patterns and mobility of doctors in the European Union. At the political level – certainly in Member States and possibly at EU level – it is unclear whether mobility should be regarded as something that is desirable or whether it should merely be tolerated. Is mobility a symbolic expression of European unity or is it the "solution" to a human resources problem? Are these problems – such as shortages of doctors and nurses – the same in all EU countries? If some countries have shortages and others have surpluses, will these needs be met by market forces in an equitable manner which preserves solidarity within healthcare systems? Is quality an issue which has implications for mobility or is it used as a smokescreen for protectionist measures? How does the different organisation of medical and nursing specialties affect mobility? Do the sectoral directives (concerning the health professions) need to be preserved?

Medical education is mostly public in the countries of the EU, but this could change in the long-term as the result of unintended consequences of the single market policy. How will European mobility and employment policy affect national plans for medical education and national terms and conditions of employment? How will doctors' organisations react? How will medical education be changed, if at all?

Patterns of mobility may be unrelated to the SEM. Most migration into the UK by doctors is not from the European Union but is based upon historical, political and economic links with developing countries. Is the same true of other European countries?

The enlargement of the European Union may also have important consequences for the mobility of doctors. The former communist countries of Central and Eastern Europe have, in some cases, highly-educated yet poorly paid doctors. Will mobility lead to shortages of key personnel in those countries? Will it lead richer countries to under-invest in educating their own doctors (and nurses and other professions?) on the grounds that it is cheaper or easier to import them?

Scenarios can be based on a number of steps:

1. selecting the policy outcomes of interest (for the EU, Member States and doctors)
2. identifying the key actors (EU policy-making bodies; national governments; and medical regulatory bodies)
3. tracing alternative possible decisions and actions by key actors and alternative possible "external events", in the light of the political, professional and managerial environments and any relevant theory which may help to predict behaviour or events
4. suggesting the relative likelihood of such alternatives
5. predicting what effects the most likely decisions and actions will have on the policy outcomes identified above. This creates the "base" scenario and alternative scenarios that can then be traced by taking combinations of less likely decisions, actions and events.

In this study, steps 4 and 5 are not formally undertaken – since insufficient data are available. The hypothetical "base scenario" and alternative scenarios have therefore been merged. Future research is recommended to develop more detailed scenarios so that policy, both at EU level and within Member States, can be appropriately refined in accordance with the values underpinning healthcare systems as well as the SEM.

2. Methods

An initial reconnaissance of the issues was undertaken. Two expert workshops were then held – one consisting of UK experts and the other involving international experts from the four countries participating in the project. Each workshop was furnished with background information concerning the UK case study on mobility of doctors, statistical data on movement of nurses and a framework for the scenarios to be discussed. The outcome of the expert discussions and relevant literature forms the basis for the following scenarios.

2.1 Scenario A: Strengthening the SEM and labour mobility

This scenario is predicated upon a drive by the EU Council, the Commission, and Member States to strengthen the SEM in order to establish large industrial and economic sectors in Europe as a major economic force in the world i.e. encouraging supra-national business and economic concentration rather than competition. It assumes that the concerns of health policy, such as equity and solidarity, may have to be sacrificed to economic concerns.

At the EU level, strengthening the SEM makes mobility of doctors and nurses easier, and the mutual recognition of qualifications allows free movement of individuals across borders and health systems. The impact at national level is, however, not as straightforward: Member States do not want to invest in the education of doctors and nurses who are going to emigrate. Economically poorer countries, such as the candidate countries, may either suffer such emigration or may attempt to "sell" medical and nursing education on the international market, then educating domestic doctors and nurses at marginal cost.

Some Member States will see the SEM as a means of solving human resource shortages and will actively recruit staff from other countries. The UK is an example of such a policy, with recruitment of non-UK doctors and nurses (from Europe, English speaking countries and former colonies). Even where there are currently no shortages, some countries encourage non-nationals to apply for jobs because they anticipate shortages of health professionals. Conversely, there are countries that "over produce" doctors and nurses and which resolve these embarrassing surpluses by stimulating emigration of their health professionals.

Medical and nursing organisations might come under some pressure to expand the number of doctors and nurses because of commitments made by politicians. This is the situation in the UK, where the NHS Plan has promised substantial investments in staff: 7500 additional consultants, 2000 more GPs, 20,000 extra nurses and 6500 more therapists. An interim "solution" is to seek to attract 'staff from elsewhere in Europe, North America or Australia. Staff are currently being recruited from developing countries, but this is increasingly regarded as ethically questionable except where the countries in question are deliberately "exporting" professionals.

The quality of professional staff moving between EU Member States is a matter of concern both to employers and professional organisations. In some countries, the best people find jobs at home and only the lower quality people emigrate, while in other countries the best professionals may move, leaving the host country with the lowest quality (e.g. accession countries). Interestingly, Spain and the UK have recently agreed (November 2000) that 6000 Spanish nurses will work in the UK. Given that Spanish terms and conditions for nurses are generally better than in the UK, it is as yet unclear whether it is the ambitious nurses, wishing to learn English and to extend their experience who have accepted the offer, or whether those nurses who have had less successful careers in Spain have moved to the UK. There is the danger that unacceptable cultural resistance to foreign doctors and nurses will be supported by genuine concerns about quality. This leads to attempts to subvert European policy.

Two further perverse trends can be envisaged within this scenario. First, "imported" staff are assigned to fill temporary and/or non-career posts, rather than positions which will enhance their career prospects. Second, the UK case study demonstrates that, as a result of restructuring medical education, the number of training posts (Specialist Registrar) has been severely restricted, and implicit preference has been is given to UK doctors, which means that European doctors find it extremely difficult to obtain proper training and post-graduate qualifications. The only exceptions have been where there are shortages such as anaesthetists, urologists, and paediatric intensive care nurses.

Strengthening labour mobility through the SEM may therefore lead to inequity in both the quantity and quality of medical and nursing human resources.

2.2 Scenario B: Removing health from the SEM

This scenario is less likely to become reality but should be considered. The belief that national governments wish to achieve self-sufficiency and determine the quality of their medical and nursing workforce is the basis for this scenario. The EU plays a marginal role, leaving mobility to bi-lateral or multi-lateral arrangements between Member States. Governments will formulate their own manpower planning requirements and will work with professional organisations to define both quantity and quality of staff.

There is some scepticism about the effectiveness of national human resources planning with its long history of regular waves of either over or under production of doctors and nurses. In certain countries, over production of one group (e.g. nurses) is linked to under production of another (e.g. doctors). However, despite its imperfections, national human resource planning is clearly necessary.

Supply and demand of doctors and nurses is clearly linked to the complementary skills of the two professions. In the UK nurses are increasingly taking over medical tasks and developing an extended nursing role. However, with the increasing shortage of nurses many nurses do not have time to carry out their full and enhanced range of nursing tasks. Resolving these problems within the context of a policy of self-sufficiency is not easy, and there will continue to be demands to import doctors and nurses to overcome shortages. However, this may occur globally rather than specifically in the context of the European Union. Member States are likely to recruit staff wherever and whenever it is in their self-interest. Even if health is excluded from the SEM – which it is difficult to envisage – it is not clear what that would mean in practice for the free movement of doctors and nurses, since self-sufficiency (in the UK) is unlikely to become a reality, and the UK will continue to need foreign doctors and nurses.

The medical profession will wish to avoid a surplus of doctors, as this weakens economic, and political power. At the same time, it seeks to avoid large shortages as this results in unacceptably large workloads. Medical organisations are likely to support a "slight shortage" that can be managed through limited immigration.

A Europe-wide consequence of this "national self-sufficiency approach" is that the concept of subsidiarity in relation to health care is reinforced, possibly undermining the convergence of other policies which are affected by health policy. Furthermore, a return to national human resources planning in health would result in "closed" systems, by re-establishing "border controls" for those health professionals, thus undermining the entire principle of the free movement of labour. The foundations of the SEM could therefore be under threat, as one of the four freedoms would be compromised. In reality, it will be extremely difficult to stop individuals from moving between Member States in pursuit of new experiences and/or better career opportunities.

2.3 Scenario C: EU-wide public planning

This scenario is also unlikely but again is worth considering for its heuristic value. In order to overcome the inequities caused by the SEM (Scenario A) or by the return to national planning (Scenario B), an EU-wide public planning process might be considered. This would ensure the preservation of a social model for public services. The argument is that the SEM does not give priority to the European social model and that the four freedoms need to be placed within a wider framework that counteract the factors causing inappropriate flows of health professionals between EU countries. The main issues concern quantity and quality of medical and nursing resources. Poorer countries cannot afford to import health professionals, and they therefore have to produce a surplus, since they are in danger of losing personnel as a result of the attraction of richer countries. If the best people leave, the quality of the remaining service provision will suffer, and the vicious circle of low quality – high quantity is will be perpetuated.

This important question of quality/quantity could be addressed by EU-wide planning. This would involve a number of parallel strategies: first, the balance of different professional groups is carefully calibrated with "over-and-under-supply" being addressed both within individual Member States and between Member States. Second, the varying roles played by professionals with similar names in different countries need to be explicitly addressed in the planning process so that needs for different types of professionals, with different combinations of skills, can be accommodated in Member States. Third, harmonisation of education and training has to be developed through the formulation of an EU-wide competency framework. This is required in addition to the mutual recognition of qualifications as professional skill and knowledge varies within apparently similar certification. German nurses, for example, have a more restricted role and range of competencies than UK nurses.

Public health resource planning at the EU level would almost certainly require EU-wide coordinated investment in medical and nursing education to ensure an appropriate of doctors and nurses in Europe. A sophisticated system will also be required to track and regulate the numbers and location of medical and nursing jobs, the numbers admitted to medical and nursing training, as well as the process to identify distribution problems (e.g. under or over supply in specific areas). Any legal or policy barriers to implementing such an overarching approach have to be recognised and addressed.

A major issue both at EU and national levels is whether human resource planning is capable of delivering robust and sustainable outcomes. At the EU level, such planning would require reliable information on numbers of staff trained and employed, national health care needs and service structures, salary bargaining machinery etc. Changes in any of these factors in any of the EU Member States could unbalance EU-wide planning. Since such changes are highly probable, it is unlikely that EU-wide planning could ever be effective.

Would Member States be willing to contribute the resources, through taxation, to create such a system rather than taking national action and retaining national political control?

2.4 Scenario D: the pragmatic status quo

The basis for this scenario is the realisation that achieving a consensus on labour mobility across Europe is difficult, and that national interests will continue to be too varied for such a consensus both at the level of policy and implementation. This scenario is also based upon the assumption that mobility of health professionals is of limited importance, perhaps of greatest value in the "Euregios", and that an activist role by the EU to "run health services" is neither desirable nor likely, given the principle of subsidiarity and recent ECJ decisions.

As described in Scenario A, the mobility of doctors and nurses is determined by a number of factors that do not necessarily operate in concert. There are, however, both advantages and disadvantages in maintaining this unregulated movement across borders.

The principal advantage is that Member States retain control over human resource planning while they can also rely on labour mobility to redress over and under supply of doctors and nurses. The pragmatic status quo offers scope either for bi- and multi-lateral staff exchange agreements, or for EU-wide short-term labour mobility arrangements. The most important disadvantage of unregulated movement of professionals is the loss of control over the quality of personnel, resulting from differences in training and professional roles. Governments and medical/nursing organisations might wish to resolve this problem by agreeing a minimum set of competencies to be recognised across throughout the EU.

Retaining the status quo would allow the SEM and its four freedoms to operate – at least in principle – in relation to health care. However, implicit national control can be re-asserted by aligning curriculum development to national priorities (e.g. the NHS Plan in the UK) and a close monitoring of deployment of staff.

3. Assessing the scenarios

Following expert discussions, Scenario D was considered to be the most plausible scenario. Member States would retain control of health services and would attempt to achieve self-sufficiency in the provision of human resources. Some countries (e.g. UK) will, however, continue to rely on imported doctors and nurses. Recent ECJ decisions, though, may make the "status quo" unstable. It is therefore necessary that the EU proactively manages change, raising the profile of health policy at European level.

The most likely alternative scenario is that the EU seeks to strengthen the SEM (Scenario A), focusing on the pursuit of mobility at the expense of equity and/or quality. The reaction could be that national governments will try to influence the EU or use legal channels (European Court of Justice) to exempt certain aspects of health care from SEM directives (a move towards scenario B). It is, of course, very unlikely that such an exception would be made for health care.

In the long term the challenge is to ensure that the SEM and national health care policies are compatible. The four scenarios illustrate different ways to resolve the contradiction: letting the SEM (mobility and market) dominate; exempting healthcare from the SEM on a more systematic basis by stressing subsidiarity; exempting healthcare from the laisser-faire aspects of the SEM by public planning at EU level; or "managing the SEM" by ensuring that the SEM's benefits are maximised and damage minimised in terms of access and equity.

The European Union and Health Services
R. Busse et al. (Eds.)
IOS Press, 2002

The mobility of citizens –
a case study and scenario on the health
services of the Costa del Sol

Nuria ROMO AVILÉS, Fernando SILIÓ VILLAMIL and
Maria Angeles PRIETO RODRIGUEZ

Abstract. The objective of this chapter is to analyse the effects of health care provided to European patients in health centres in the Costa del Sol area, especially given the situation that many "tourists" live for six months or longer in the area but take advantage of the E111 form, which was originally designed for emergency assistance during short-term stays. While the documented number of such documented patients is rather low, their care nevertheless pose challenges, not the least economical which result from the fact that income due to this activity is not given to the district but kept in Madrid. Three scenarios outline and evaluate possible future developments, either improving or worsening the situation for the tourists, for the health service or for both.

1. Introduction

Within the framework of the free movement of citizens within the EU, Spain could be described as a recipient country for persons from the rest of Europe. The Costa del Sol in the province of Málaga is one of the major tourist resorts in Spain. The fact that Spain belongs to the European Community means that European tourists and citizens staying on the Costa del Sol have the right to access certain health services when vacationing or living temporarily in the area.

The description and analysis of the current situation has provided a starting point from which to propose alternative scenarios, by analysing the response of the services and the professionals working in the area to possible future changes. The health care provided to foreign patients has an impact on health services in terms of economic management, personnel management, the organisation of services, the daily practice of the medical professionals and client welfare services.

2. Methodology

First, a description is given of the impact of health care demand by European patients on Costa del Sol services during 1999. This assumes that demand remained constant during this period and did not change its influence on the health services. Using this description of the current status, three situations that could be considered future alternatives will be projected:

– Scenario A: The distribution of finances in the Spanish health system will be changed in such a way that the income resulting from treating European patients will no longer go to a central institution in Madrid but will be passed on to the district and its personnel.

– Scenario B: There will be financial pressures from the health system on the Province of Malaga so that the expenditures on health, and specifically on medical prescriptions, for European patients will be reduced.
– Scenario C: The number of tourists attended on the Costa del Sol doubles in one year but the current administrative rules remain unchanged.

In order to assess the current situation, different research methodologies for the key areas of analysis have been used, namely:

– Economic management: Description and analysis of the impact that tourist demand has on the economic management of the health centres.
– Personnel management and service organisation: Description and analysis of the impact that tourist demand has on personnel management and organisation in the health centres.
– Health care professionals' opinion and practice: Description and analysis of the impact that tourist demand has on medical practice models and the opinion of professionals as regards treating this type of patient.
– Client Welfare Services (CWSs) and customer advice: Description and analysis of the impact that tourist demand has on Client Welfare Services in health centres.

The main research techniques employed were interviews and discussion groups. To be more precise, interviews were carried out with four of the top people in the health district (two Basic Zone Directors, one Hospital Assistant Manager and one Hospital Head of Client Management) and held three discussion groups with health care professionals from the First Aid Centre and the Hospital.

3. Background: the Health Care Zone

3.1 Characteristics of the foreign population

The Costa del Sol health care zone is located in the autonomous region of Andalusia (Spain). Andalusia is one of the Spanish regions, together with Madrid, Catalonia and the island regions, with the highest proportion of permanent foreign residents. As can be seen in Table 1, in 1998 almost 96,000 foreigners lived in the region, out of a total of 7.24 million. The resulting percentage of 1.3 % is, however, still lower than the average for Spain of 1.8 %. The data available reveal a "specific type of foreigner", mainly Europeans, who decide to live permanently in Andalusia.

The focus of this chapter is, however, on European citizens who are only resident for a short period of time in Spain. No quantitative information was available on what might be called "floating" Europeans; in other words, those who spend only a short time in the region as tourists and are not registered by official data.

In an interview, a person in charge of health care in the hospital explained that, according to estimates by the health care professionals, there are 700,000 non-Spanish residents living on the coast in the summer and 400,000 in the winter. Official data from the census reflect 230,000. In other words, there is an unaccounted group in between those in the official registers as residents and those who only spend some time in the area and then move on.

Table 1: Number of foreigners with permanent residence in Spain and total number of inhabitants, by region (1998)

Spanish Region	Total number of inhabitants	Number of foreign residents	Foreign residents as %
Andalusia	7,236,459	95,970	1.3 %
Aragón	1,183,234	11,877	1.0 %
Asturias (Principality of)	1,081,834	8,682	0.8 %
Balearic Isles	796,483	40,399	5.1 %
Canary Isles	1,630,015	68,848	4.2 %
Cantabria	527,137	3,910	0.7 %
Castilla-La Mancha	1,716,152	11,374	0.6 %
Castilla y León	2,484,603	20,113	0.8 %
Catalonia	6,1470,610	148,803	2.4 %
Com. Valenciana	4,023,441	69,972	1.7 %
Extremadura	1,069,419	9,063	0.8 %
Galicia	2,724,544	21,140	0.8 %
Madrid (Com. de)	5,091,330	148,070	2.9 %
Murcia (Región de)	1,115,068	15,731	1.4 %
Navarra (C, Foral de)	530,819	6,385	1.2 %
Basque Country	2,098,628	16,995	0.8 %
Rioja (La)	263,644	3,253	1.2 %
Ceuta	72,117	1,196	1.7 %
Melilla	60,108	1,054	1.8 %
Not attributable		16,812	
TOTAL	39,852,651	719,647	1.8 %

Source: Based on data by INE (National Institute of Statistics).

Likewise, there are also other characteristics of this population for which there is no quantitative information. For example, there are people who not only come to the area in summer, but live here for up to six or eight months a year. This population requests health services in the area as if they were residents, even though they are counted as tourists.

The variability of the fluctuating population of the Costa del Sol affects the management and planning of the health care services. The senior people interviewed expressed the need to have health care mechanisms in place in order to attend to this non-quantified fluctuating population.

3.2 Health care provider characteristics

The Costa del Sol Hospital is located in Marbella (Malaga). It has 197 beds, and it is a teaching hospital with high-technology equipment. Regarding primary health care, the Costa del Sol district has its base in Mijas (Malaga). It is made up of two basic health zones, each of which has eight health centres.

3.3 Private or co-ordinated health care services for foreigners

When a European citizen comes to the Costa del Sol as a tourist (rather than as a permanent resident) and needs health care, that person will normally use the EU form E111 (if covered by Social Security in his/her the country of origin). The E111 this form will give the citizen temporary coverage to those benefits covered by the Spanish health care system. E111 holders have the right to all kinds of health care in Spain (emergencies, programmed health care, home visits, nursing care, pharmaceutical prescriptions, complementary tests, etc.). In other words, they are provided with the same health care as anyone with Social Security health care coverage who requests or needs such health care (SSCC 6/89 circular).

When contacting a health care provider, E111 holders should present the form to demonstrate that they are covered by a Social Security institution in their country of origin. In the Costa del Sol District, many E111 holders are treated and given a wide variety of health care services (emergencies, programmed health care, home visits, nursing care, pharmaceutical prescriptions, complementary tests, etc.).

In accordance with the Community Regulation 1408/71, the E111 form covers two potential situations:

- The worker's right to receive the immediate medical attention he/she may need during a temporary stay in another EU Member State (art. 22.1a).
- The pensioner's right, and that of his family, to receive health care during a temporary stay in another EU Member State, irrespective of whether said assistance be of immediate necessity (art. 31). In consequence, the health care requested must be provided whenever, from a medical point of view, it is considered appropriate and necessary and when any delay is inadvisable from the patient's point of view.

Medical and pharmaceutical provision covered by the E111 form includes:

- The health care that workers and/or members of their family may immediately need during a temporary stay in another EU Member State.
- With regard to pensioners and/or family members, the necessary healthcare depending on their state of health, including specific, regulated treatment.

As for the bureaucratic steps to be taken when a European citizen is in Spain, it has to be borne in mind that in general people do not have to pay for health care received. Once the E111 form has been presented, the cost of the health care provided is calculated using a price list and documented on the H1 form (a document that allows the district to declare health care provided to European citizens). These forms are sent to the INSS (the National Social Security Institute – the Spanish body that charges its counterparts in the EU Member States). Once a citizen lives permanently in Spain, he/she will receive the same pensioner documentation as a Spanish citizen and, from that moment on, will have exactly the same rights.

4. Current situation

4.1 Number of patients from other EU countries (tourists) treated in 1999

Primary care: In 1999, the Costa del Sol Primary Health Care District treated 6,890 European patients, according to data based on processed H1s. This health care provision provided the INSS with income of 30,823,082 pesetas[1] (185,681 Euro).

Hospital care: The data provided by the hospital show the number of patients treated via the emergency unit. In 1999, of the total number of 90,834 patients treated in this unit, 4,316 were foreigners (4.75 %). In the outpatient unit, of a total number of 8,041 patients seen, 242 were foreigners (3 %). With regard to the number of patients hospitalised, of a total number of 12,226 registered in the hospital, 328 were foreigners (2.6 %).

4.2 Volume of foreign patients treated per centre and medical service

As an indirect indicator of the number of Europeans treated in the Costa del Sol Primary Health Care District, data regarding the number of H1s processed were used.

The number of H1s processed in the district in 1998 was 5,483. If the district's activity is calculated in terms of the total number of general medicine, paediatric, nursing and emergency consultations, the district treated 2,450,574 medical cases in that year. Foreign patients make up 0.22 % of the overall activity in the district. In 1999, there was a slight increase in the number of H1s processed in the Costa del Sol District, totalling 6,890 or 0.27 % of the district's overall activity (see Table 2).

Table 2: H1 processing and activity of the Costa del Sol District, 1998 & 1999

Year	H1s processed	District activity	Tourists as % of activity
1998	5,483	2,450,574	0.22 %
1999	6,890	2,582,782	0.27 %

The hospital in this zone has data referring to the number of foreigners treated in the emergency and outpatient units. In the hospital, according to the data provided by the information technology unit, out of a total of 90,834 people treated in the emergency unit in 1999, 4,316 were foreigners, a large increase from 297 in 1994 (Table 3). These "foreign" emergencies do not solely refer to Europeans. A total of 123,140 people were treated in the outpatient unit, of which 8,041 were foreigners (6.5 % of the total).

Table 3: Development of foreign emergency in-patients at Costa del Sol Hospital in absolute and relative terms, 1994-1999

Year	Total emergencies	Foreigners (number)	Foreigners (%)
1994	40,331	297	0.74
1995	57,964	718	1.24
1996	72,523	1,496	2.06
1997	80,036	3,526	4.41
1998	85,367	3,961	4.64
1999	90,834	4,316	4.75

Source: emergency unit database, Evaluation Unit, Costa del Sol Hospital

---

[1] One should bear in mind that this amount charged does not have a direct repercussion on the district or on its health care professionals, since it is charged on a national level by the Social Security.

4.3 Expenditure derived from treating European patients

The activity due to treating European patients has a cost for the district. As a basis, the idea was used that there is an average cost for each medical action, obtained by adding up personnel, supplies and pharmaceutical expenditure and dividing by the general medicine, nursing and emergency consultations made in the primary health care district. These calculations give an indication of health care costs (see Table 4).

Table 4: Economic implications for the Costa del Sol District, based on the H1s

Year	H1s processed	H1 income	Cost to the district	Difference (= profit)
1998	5,483	138,544	92,385	46,159
1999	6,890	185,681	133,109	52,571

In summary, the documented activity involving foreign patient health care in the district is not particularly significant (0.22 % for 1998 and 0.27 % for 1999) when compared with overall activity. At the same time, this information indicates that treating this population provides economic income. Since this income is not collected directly by the district, it only contributes to the national income of the INSS (National Social Security Institute).

4.4 Type of activities carried out on foreign patients

In this part of Spain, one can differentiate between two types of health services requested by the European population:

- Emergency services when on holiday in the area.
- Other health care services requested by a "floating" population which is difficult to quantify, living for long periods in the area and who principally need to renew pharmaceutical prescriptions issued in their countries of origin.

Generally, the health care professionals interviewed did not establish any differences between the pathologies of the foreigners who vacation in the area and those of the Spanish population. The only element that characterises these European citizens is that they are mainly elderly and, therefore, suffer from age-associated illnesses. However, these pathologies are the same as those of the elderly Spanish population living in the region.

In the discussion groups and interviews carried out in the area, a particular element which was highlighted was the fact that the foreign patients request medication that health care professionals consider to be excessive, along with unnecessary complementary tests. Frequently, this medication has been prescribed by doctors in their countries of origin. The Spanish health care professionals often do not share their diagnoses and some of those interviewed have expressed their uneasiness with this situation.

With regard to inclusion in health programmes[2], the reasoning among the health care professionals interviewed was rather varied. The interviewees' answers pointed towards the idea that inclusion or not in health programmes is something that corresponds to medical

---

[2] Health programmes are programmes that follow the health of the patient in the time as, for example, "women's programme".

questions and that the health care professionals should decide accordingly in each individual case.

4.5 Attitude of the health care professionals towards the increase in demand and the type of patient

Some of the health care professionals interviewed did not doubt that the European patient has every right to be treated in another EU country. They did, however, have their doubts as regards the economic profitability on a national level; in other words, the financial benefit for the Spanish health system as a whole.

During the discussion groups, a certain lack of trust as regards the foreigner was detected. The foreigner was seen as "crafty", trying to get more out of the system than appropriate. At the same time, the health care professionals expressed the view that European patients using the Spanish health services are "in search of added health care" due, in part, to the fact that the medication is free and the services provided are high-quality.

The health personnel believed that it is good for Spain that the Spanish health workers "treat the foreigners well". It is as if the health services were seen as another element to be included in the tourist package offered to Europeans visiting the area.

Together with the stereotypes of the "foreigner" and the "Spaniard" that appeared in the discussion groups and interviews, there was also mention of specific characteristics of the foreign population that affect their use the health services and, thus, the needs stemming from their situation. It must not be forgotten that, to a large extent, this is an elderly population without family nearby.

Foreigners, including Europeans, who are staying on the Costa del Sol, need longer and more attentive care from health care professionals, due to linguistic and cultural difficulties. These characteristics make the diagnosis more complicated for the doctor. Occasionally, the professionals interviewed noticed specific characteristics of foreigners and pointed them out. For example, this includes the building of a different doctor-patient relationship, based on a greater interest in knowing more about the pathology or gratitude for the treatment received.

Both in the hospital and in the district, some of the health care professionals interviewed recognised that they have achieved job satisfaction from treating foreign patients. For them, it is both positive and gratifying for foreign citizens to recognise that the Spanish health services provide quality treatment. The main problem in the daily relationship with this type of patients is the language barrier, which impedes the smooth running of daily work. In the hospital, this problem was overcome by employing multilingual staff. These patients also pose other problems, such as loneliness and particular personal circumstances stemming from the fact that they are generally an elderly population.

4.6 Organisational changes due to increased demand

The Costa del Sol District has created, in some of its basic zones, specific surgeries to attend to the needs of displaced persons, including Europeans who are in the area.

When the heads of the Costa del Sol hospital were asked whether the services could possibly be modified, they mentioned extending the list of available services, for which a calculation of needs would be necessary, taking into account the population which spends a short period of time in the region.

The hospital management considered that a problem exists with regard to the "floating" population, as it is not registered and, therefore, is not included when adapting the services to needs. Realistic estimations of the population requiring health care would allow better planning of the services for the future. Although there is no specific data on the proportion of this population treated in the hospital, the demands already justify increasing the services, according to the opinion of the hospital management.

4.7 Modifying available services

In the primary health care district: Treating foreign patients visiting the area generates extra work that affects the personnel in the primary health care district. During the interviews, the primary health care professionals explained how treating the foreign population requires extra effort for which they are not compensated. For this reason, they lack incentives and motivation. In certain primary health care centres, staff is increased at the time of year when there is a greater number of foreigners in the area. Having to attend to these types of "in transit" patients generates a work overload. This overload affects both the medical staff and the other staff in the centres, such as administrative staff, who are saturated at certain times of the year.

In the hospital: The health care professionals interviewed in the hospital have included the provision of health care for the extra population that enters the area as a norm in their working day. They are prepared for this task and consider it just another responsibility in their daily routine. Any possible problems have already been envisaged and planned for. The language barrier, however, is mentioned again as one of the aspects that makes their work more difficult.

4.8 Customer advice initiatives

The linguistic and cultural difficulties are the similar in the primary health care district and in the hospital. In the case of the hospital, the need to attend to foreign patients led to the hiring of multilingual specialised staff, both in the areas of administration and health care. The fact that this staff is specialised means that treating these patients is seen as not being too problematic.

According to the information provided in the interviews with health care professionals, it has been necessary to introduce a translation service during medical appointments. The foreign population has organised themselves in this task and often help each other out with this service free of charge.

5. Scenarios: possibilities for the future

5.1 Scenario A: The distribution of finances in the Spanish health system will be changed in such a way that the income resulting from attending European patients will be passed on to the district and its personnel.

This situation is based on the fact that the economic repercussions from treating European patients occurs indirectly in the health system. There are no direct financial benefits on the health centres in our study. This income is even collected by the Ministry of Labour, which has no direct link with the health system.

The first result of this situation could be a better identification of the European patients and the type of treatment given in the Costa del Sol health centres. If the economic repercussion on the district is indirect, attempts to attract income will be much less than if the income were to go directly to the health care personnel responsible for attracting it.

This possibility is based on the idea that productivity improvements are felt by the health care professionals personally and so, if their income were to rise with each European patient treated, the primary health care district's economic management would improve.

It must not be forgotten that the repercussion on the quality of the attention provided would not be solely influenced by the increase in economic incentives. Other factors also have an influence on quality, such as language and other cultural barriers.

If income generated by foreigners were to go fully to the district, part of this potential income would be used to improve the administrative infrastructure, overloaded by having to attend to European patients.

Scenario A has been proposed using the reality of the health services in Spain. Another possibility would be to look at systems in other European countries and, for example, have patients pay to receive medical treatment. This situation would probably reduce the current situation of misuse pointed out by health care professionals.

5.2 Scenario B: There will be financial pressures from the health system on the Province of Malaga so that the expenditures on health, and specifically on medical prescriptions, for European patients will be reduced.

This scenario is related to Scenario A in that if the economic benefits had a direct repercussion for the Andalusian Health Service, the regulations would be better applied. If the process were correctly carried out, residents would obtain a Social Security number and this would provide income for the primary health care district.

With regard to patients, the type of patient living on the Costa del Sol for "long periods" is usually "complicated" from a clinical point of view. They are generally elderly, with multiple pathologies that have generally been badly studied and with little follow-up. This means that they are patients whose treatment requires a high pharmaceutical expenditure. (In the discussion groups it was mentioned that two "displaced persons" *surgeries* – in other words, those created specifically to attend to the foreign population – generate an annual pharmaceutical expenditure which is equivalent to that of five surgeries attending solely to Spanish patients.)

Two possible repercussions for this scenario would be:

- If the pressure to reduce medical prescription expenditure were to fall directly on the health care professionals, this would lead to generalised dissatisfaction.
- If the pressure were to fall on the client misusing the system, health personnel would be satisfied.

Currently, doctors do not consider it to be their obligation to negotiate with the patients whether to prescribe medication or not for economic reasons. If the medication is justified from a clinical point of view, the doctors' opinion is usually that they should prescribe it. For the doctors, the norm should be clarified and supported by the higher echelons of the health service. If doctors have no support from above and have to make the decision themselves, they may decline to make such choices.

Pressure from the health system on personnel without clear regulations to back up the health staff so that they can work safely would cause negative effects on the system and would be difficult to implement.

In this case, clear regulations on the processing of documents E111 or the Social Security card) are needed, which would provide the doctor with support when refusing to prescribe a certain treatment.

This type of measure would have no impact on the tourist sector. People would continue to come to vacation in Spain. They would simply make sure their situation is in order, using the right documents and not misusing the E111 for all types of medical assistance. Currently, they ignore the administrative rules since they do not see a problem and they can obtain medical assistance whenever they need it.

5.3 Scenario C: The number of tourists treated on the Costa del Sol doubles in a single year but the current administrative rules remain unchanged.

If the number of tourists treated in a year were to double, a process of adaptation in the health services would have to be implemented. The balance sheet would probably be negative:

–   More health care professionals would need to be hired.
–   Pharmaceutical objectives would not be met.
–   An attempt would be made to justify treatment expenditure.

The primary health care district has the autonomy to cope with this kind of situation. On a small scale, a similar situation occurs every August. The feeling of those in charge is that they are already working virtually up to the limit of their possibilities. Currently there is no situation of chaos but there is very little room to manoeuvre with regard to personnel and the structure of the health services.

The primary health care district would require an increase in its resources to cope with a situation like this. An equilibrium is needed among resources, the list of services and the population treated. An increase in the number of people treated with no corresponding increase in resources would lead to a breakdown in services.

Under this scenario, it must be borne in mind that the Costa del Sol is an area with a population that is already on the increase. This general increase in numbers is accompanied by an adaptation of the services, in terms of structure, personnel etc., which is too slow. The situation causes problems with waiting lists.

The increase in the European population requesting health care in the area would cause a drop in service quality and, for example, longer waiting lists.

The data available on new residential construction in the area is an indirect indicator of the forecast for population increase up to the year 2015. (The data at the disposal of the heads of the primary health care district indicate that, in 1998, six times more houses per 1000 inhabitants were built in the province of Malaga than in the city of Seville. In absolute terms, the increase is higher than that for Madrid, i.e. a province of approximately one million inhabitants built more houses than the Comunidad de Madrid, with almost six million inhabitants.)

The effects on the medical profession would follow along the same lines. Increased demand implies treating more patients. These patients come with the added difficulty of language. Treating a higher number of people would require a greater effort by the health care professionals. This scenario highlights the need to have reliable data on the population in the area, in order to avoid situations of alarm in the health services.

6. Conclusions

6.1 Conclusions regarding economic management

The European population staying for varying periods of time on the Costa del Sol (Malaga) requests a series of health services in Spain. The hospital services in the area have planned ahead bearing in mind this part of the population and, therefore, have less need to change. Primary health care professionals have highlighted a saturation in service demand by European patients that is difficult to deal with. The planning of services in the centres is varied: in some cases, the European citizens are included in the same surgeries as Spanish patients and, in others, specific surgeries have been set up. It can be concluded that, at present, medical attention is carried out without service planning; in other words, demand is dealt with as it occurs.

The services requested by the European population are normally twofold: emergency services when they are vacationing in the area; or health services for a "floating" population, which is difficult to calculate, living for relatively long periods in the area and who mainly need to renew prescriptions for medication received in their countries of origin.

The administrative process that should be followed by European citizens residing temporarily in the area causes confusion and doubts among the health care professionals. In general, during the discussion groups and interviews, the problems regarding this administrative process have been highlighted, above all in relation to the E111 form.

Some of the senior people interviewed have referred to "strategies" followed in their respective services in order to rationalise the medical attention provided to this type of patient. For example, sometimes the administrative process is slowed down in order to delay the provision of medical attention.

The data analysed in this scenario indicate that there is a high proportion of foreigners that is not reflected in the H1 processing. Those that are accounted for through the H1s generate income for the district over and above expenditure.

Thus, this cost calculation may not reflect the true situation. One possible hypothesis that can be drawn from this data and which would need studying in greater detail is that, since the economic benefits from H1 processing do not have a direct impact on the district, given that the income is collected by the INSS (a body controlled by the Ministry of Labour and not the Health Service), less of them are actually processed in comparison to the number of patients actually treated.

6.2 Conclusions regarding personnel management and service organisation

In general, this scenario has revealed a series of problems related to planning in the centres. For example, currently there are difficulties including Europeans in health programmes, and also for Spanish and European doctors to make the same diagnoses.
In the discussion groups and the interviews, the health care professionals expressed the need to create a specific list of services to attend to the temporary population in the area. This need is more urgent in the primary health care district than in the hospital.

The costs associated with the European citizens are compensated for, according to Spanish health care professionals, by the income and advantages from tourism, one of the prime areas of wealth of the region. Those interviewed expressed the idea that the health services should be included in the tourist planning for the area.

6.3 Conclusions regarding health care professionals' opinion and practice

Foreigners who live temporarily on the Costa del Sol do not suffer from different pathologies to those of the Spaniards. One has to distinguish between people who are vacationing and who go to the health centres for an emergency, and the health services requested by the elderly retired population who live temporarily in the area and suffer from pathologies related to their age. For the latter, the Spanish health care professionals have expressed the need for them to have social services at their disposal, since many of them lack the social support of family or friends.

The image that the Spanish health care professionals have of the typical European, and which is analysed in this scenario, is one of a certain craftiness as regards the temporary residents, since they try to obtain the maximum benefits they can from the Spanish health system. The fact that the medication is available to all and is free of charge means that, at times, the Europeans enjoy easier access to it than in their home countries. For example, in different discussion groups and interviews, the case of Scandinavian citizens was mentioned, as they obtain free medication for the whole year from the Spanish system without ever having been diagnosed by Spanish doctors.

The demand for medical attention by European citizens has grown constantly since 1994. The data obtained show the need to carry out studies that would enable a reliable calculation of the population requiring health services in the area. This, in turn, would allow better planning of these health services.

6.4 Conclusions regarding the future scenarios

Among the future possibilities, scenarios A and C will probably become a reality in the Andalusian Health Service. The Andalusian Health Service is trying to implement a series of economic incentives for health care professionals dealing with patients. The particular characteristics of the people who live temporarily on the Costa del Sol mean that they have pensioner Social Security cards which will provide better incentives for those doctors who give medical assistance.

Scenario A would lead to an improvement in the system, with a sounder calculation and understanding of the Europeans visiting the area. This, in turn, would lead to various improvements, as shown in figure 1.

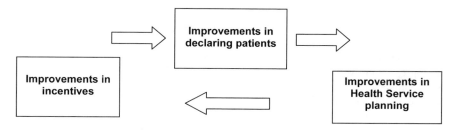

Fig. 1: Possible circle of improvements under scenario A

Scenario C, in a more modest version, is plausible in coming years, since all indicators point towards a growth trend in the tourist population entering the area. Scenarios A and C would inter-relate in order to achieve higher quality services.

The European Union and Health Services
R. Busse et al. (Eds.)
IOS Press, 2002

The impact of the SEM on data exchange and protection in the Swedish health system

Barbro RENCK and Mona SUNDH

Abstract. The Data Security Directive 95/46/EC required transposition into national legislation by October 1998. In the 1980s, Sweden, in the process of accession to the EU, postponed the amendment of existing domestic data protection legislation in order to build on the European law which was then being developed. The objectives of the Data Security Directive were difficult to meet, mainly because the balance between data protection of individuals and society's legitimate data requirements for administration, research and transparency were not fully in line with the Swedish approach, which is in general less restrictive. Due to the very recent transposition it is too early to assess intended and unintended outcomes conclusive. Yet, it is already clear that the new legislation is more complicated and difficult to interpret. On the operational level, authorities have to carry out new roles and responsibilities. Those bodies keeping and processing data are more involved in data protection matters. Collaboration between centre and regions in regard to data security is intensifying, and medical researchers using medical records will face increased difficulties. Almost all of these elements have resulted in an increased bureaucracy.

1. Introduction

All data protection legislation in Europe is built on the foundations laid down by the Council of Europe Convention for the protection of individuals with regard to automatic processing of personal data (Treaty 108 of 1981). The development of a Single European Market (SEM) and of the "information society" both increase cross-border flows of personal data between EU Member States. This chapter attempts to describe and analyse the impact of legislation and rulings introduced to implement the Data Security Directive 95/46/EC in relation to healthcare in Sweden.

2. Background and purpose

In recent years Swedish health services have undergone great changes. Shrinking financial frameworks, stricter budget control, guaranteed medical care and free choice of medical care are things which have resulted in a structural transformation of medical care (Spri 1996). Simultaneously, greater emphasis is put on improved efficiency and delivery of better, quality-assured products and services. This change has increased the need for electronic data communication both internally and externally, for example between authorities responsible for different kinds of medical care. The increased mobility of individuals and the development of the EU also require faster and better transfer of information.

Healthcare is an information-intensive operation. A large amount of information is handled; information which is usually very sensitive. An increased use of computers for processing data gives access to stored information. However, in the public sector, information technology (IT) has so far been used to a relatively small extent. When used, it has primarily been in administrative fields. Normally, the solutions have not been harmonised (HSS 1996). However, IT has not only purely administrative applications, but is used for storage, search and electronic transfer of information between different units (HSS 1999).

Computer support for handling patient information will become an aid for an increasing number of different professions. It is of the utmost importance that the use of computers does not threaten patients' confidence in the way submitted information is handled. Report 22 of the HSS (1998) deals with basic requirements concerning information security when distributing information within the health and medical services. The purpose of the requirements is to secure access, personal privacy, protection against alteration and traceability:

- *access*: to guarantee that the information is accessible when and where it is required
- *personal privacy*: to guarantee that there can be no unauthorised access or reading
- *protection against alteration*: to guarantee that transferred information has not been deliberately or unintentionally altered
- *traceability*: to guarantee the origin of the information, i.e. that it originates from the person who seems to be the author and that all activities for the transfer of information can be traced and linked to a responsible person.

Health informatics deals with the use of information and the application of information technology for treatment, training and research in the health and medical services (Pettersson & Rydmark 1996). Health informatics is interdisciplinary and can be defined as the science of collection, processing and use of information within the health and medical services. Health informatics covers the whole field of healthcare, i.e. hospital-based care, primary care, municipal medical care and care by doctors in private practice. When information systems for different activities within the health and medical services are developed, the developer has to base his work on concept models which show the significant concepts and phenomena of the area and their relationships. Examples of information systems within health and medical services which deal with concepts are computerised medical records, patient administration systems, laboratory systems, support for individual planning of care, monitoring systems for intensive care and diagnosis-supporting systems, e.g. digital X-ray systems, ECG-machines (HSS 1996).

Within health informatics, standardisation is in progress to enable us to make more extended and effective use of IT. This work has been going on since 1991 both inside and outside Sweden. The principal aim of this standardisation is to solve communication problems within health and medical services to allow an exchange of patient-related data between existing as well as future information systems. Results are beginning to show. Standards now allow the transfer of information between, for example, medical records systems and laboratory systems without special solutions for each manufacturer (HSS 1999).

Standardisation in Sweden is managed by the Swedish Health Care Standards Institution (HSS) and is conducted through committees and working groups, which cooperate with the corresponding international groups. HSS represents Sweden both in the international (ISO) and the European (CEN) standardisation work.

The use of IT within the public sector is, to a great extent, governed by various kinds of legislation. Most of it is so-called technology neutral. At the constitutional level there is the press law, to which the Official Secrets Act is linked. The Swedish principle of public access to official records is integrated in the press law. The principle of public access to official records, which is unique to Sweden, grants the citizens the right of access to the records of central and local authorities. The laws relating to public archives and administration also monitor information security. For healthcare there are specific laws, e.g. the Health and Medical Services Act, the Medical Records Act and - from 1998 - the Medical Registers Act. In October 1998 the Data Act was replaced by the new Personal Data Act based on EU Directive 95/46/EC.

The purpose of this research was to investigate the impact of legislation and rulings introduced to implement the data exchange and protection issues required to facilitate the free movement of EU citizens in relation to healthcare. Research was undertaken in four ways.

First, an analysis was done on the transposition of Directive 95/46/EC into Swedish legislation. Second, an examination was completed of how the central authorities and organisations concerned have worked with implementation issues relating to data exchange and protection within the health and medical services in county councils/regions. Third, the impact of legislation and rulings relating to data protection within healthcare in one county council, the County Council of Värmland, was analysed in detail. Fourth, the experience of the "personal data proxy" (see Section 5.6 for definition) with data security for health services after acceptance of the EU directive was assessed.

3. Methods and material

A combination of research methods has been applied. Amongst them is the technique of network or snowball sampling to get a clearer picture in regard to prospective developments - the sampling of subjects based on referrals from other subjects already in the sample. This approach is used when individuals with specific knowledge in a field are difficult to identify by ordinary means (Polit & Hungler 1987). Data were collected on a national and regional level by means of telephone interviews, personal interviews and a focus group interview. Representatives of the Swedish Federation of County Councils, the Ministry of Justice, the Data Inspection Board, the Swedish Health Care Standards Institution and those responsible for IT within the County Council of Värmland were interviewed.

In a focus group interview, which lasted one and a half hours, two Data Inspection Board officials were interviewed. The focus group interview has been completed through several telephone interviews. With a civil servant at the Ministry of Justice a telephone interview was carried out. At the Swedish Health Care Standards Institution two people were interviewed, one of whom was project leader in the field of health informatics. An IT strategist employed on a project basis was interviewed as a representative for the Federation of Swedish County Councils. A semi-structured interview guide was used for the interviews, which were recorded on tape and typed. Notes were made during the telephone interviews.

In a case study, the IT security of the health and medical services has been specially studied in one county council, the County Council of Värmland. Four people working with IT and security matters and/or with knowledge about legislation were interviewed. As a complementary activity, a telephone interview with a personal data proxy in one of the two regions was carried out.

In order to be able to more clearly describe how central authorities, organisations and county councils deal with IT matters, information has been obtained by means of brochures, information material, reports, fact sheets and newsletters. In addition, a search for relevant websites was undertaken in the Internet. The interviews were analysed manually. All the transcriptions were coded according to the interview questions but also in relation to other sources of information.

In the chapter, the results obtained through the interviews and other sources of information will be presented together. When appropriate, quotations from the interviews, which sometimes give a more detailed picture of an occurrence or opinion, have been included in the text.

4. The European Data Security Directive

The key directive of data protection is the European Directive 95/46/EC of 24th October 1995 concerning the protection of individuals with regard to the processing of personal data and the free movement of such data. The purpose of this directive is to create a common high level of protection privacy in order to allow the free movement of personal data between the Member States. Within the framework stated in the directive, Member States may specify more exactly the conditions when the processing of personal data may be carried out. These specifications may not, however, obstruct the free movement of personal data within the union (Regeringens proposition 1997/98:44).

According to the EU, the establishment of the SEM pre-supposes not only that personal data can be freely transferred from one Member State to another but also that the basic rights of individuals are protected. In particular, the individual's right to protection of their private information with regards to processing will be monitored. This directive concerns the processing of personal data which is done completely or partly in an automated way, whether the personal data are part of a register or not. However, the directive includes non-automated processing of personal data if they are part of or are intended to be part of a register.

The directive is a part of the European Community's actions designed to allow for the flow of personal data between different economic, administrative and social organizations on the SEM, reflecting the harmonisation of the rules for processing of personal data with a high level of protection within the European Community.

The directive have some other functions as well, including the right of the public to know what confidentiality and security controls are place within an organisation. Two other issues are important for the healthcare – access to health records by patients and freedom of information.

The preamble of the directive emphasises that the Member States will be allowed scope for action in connection with the implementation of the directive and that the states should strive to improve the protection granted by their current legislation; the measures chosen should aim at guaranteeing a high level of protection within the Community. Within the framework of this scope for action, there may thus be differences in the implementation of the directive. In accordance with Article 29 in the directive, a committee was formed at Community level with a spokesperson for every national supervisory board as well as a spokesperson for the European Union Council. The committee will advise the European Union Council and contribute towards the development of a uniform application of national rules that have been accepted in order to implement the directive.

When working on Directive 95/46/EC, Sweden acted powerfully to achieve solutions to ensure that the directive would not be in contrast to the Swedish principle of public access to official records and other constitutional regulations (Regeringens proposition 1997/98:44). In item 72 in the introduction, it is stated that the directive makes it possible to respect the Swedish principle of public access regarding access to public documents in connection with the acceptance of the provisions.

5. Impact on domestic legislation, national bodies and organisations

European legislation does not necessarily bear an immediate impact on the legislation of Member States. If, for example, new European legislation is already covered by domestic legislation, then changes are unnecessary. Obviously, Member States' unwillingness to transpose European legislation, or parts of it, would also result in no changes. This, however, would be challenged by the Commission. These two "no impact" scenarios have not taken place in Sweden. On the contrary, Sweden has used the opportunity of European legislation to overhaul the legal system of data protection in its health system. Yet, already in the process of transposition, it became evident that the Swedish approach to data protection differs from the approach proposed in the European directive.

The impact of the Data Security Directive had, in turn, an impact on national organisations. First, the new legal framework of data protection in Swedish healthcare changed and extended the role of the Data Inspection Board, which is the national authority responsible for data protection matters. Second, all those bodies and organisations processing or keeping data have greater responsibilities in data protection including the optional creation of a data protection proxy. Third, with the data protection laws of Member States, the Swedish Healthcare Standards Institution has gained a new strategic role in terms of representing Swedish interests in the creation of standards which will be introduced EU-wide and to adapt these standards in swiftly in the expanding IT-sector in Swedish healthcare.

5.1 The transposition of the European Data Security Directive

The Swedish government is responsible for Sweden implementing and abiding by EU legislation and is thus responsible for ensuring that the authorities' instructions agree with the requirements stated in EU legislation. The authorities are therefore obliged to inform the ministry in question of the implementation of EU legal acts with instructions. The way an EU legal act is implemented in Sweden depends on how the issue has previously been dealt with within Swedish legislation. Table 1 specifies the laws, regulations and instructions transposing Directive 95/46/EC into Swedish legislation.

Table 1: Transposition of Directive 95/46/EC into the Swedish legislation

Source	Title
SFS 1998:204	Personal Data Act
SFS 1998:544	Medical Register Act (special legislation)
SFS 1998:1191	Personal Data Ordinance
SFS 1998:1192	Ordinance with instructions to the Data Inspection Board
DIFS 1998:2	The Data Inspection Board's instructions regarding the obligation to report the processing of personal data to the Data Inspection Board
DIFS 1998:3	The Data Inspection Board's instructions regarding exceptions to the ban on the processing of personal data concerning criminal offences, etc, by anyone other than the authorities concerned

Responsible ministry: Ministry of Justice

5.2 Legislative procedure

The government charged the parliamentary Data Act Committee with the task of completing a total revision of the Personal Data Act and analysing how the EU Directive on personal data should be introduced into Swedish legislation. In accordance with legislative procedure and the introduction of the Personal Data Act, the government decided to allow the law to follow the text and structure of the directive with the exception of the regulations concerning transferral of personal data to countries outside the EU, stated in Articles 25 and 26. The provisions in the articles in the EU directive were viewed as complicated. The Data Act Committee's assessment was that legislation should not be introduced if it included more complicated rules than necessary with respect to the EU directive. The committee suggested a provision against the transfer of personal data to a country outside the EU as well as concrete exceptions from the restriction for those situations stipulated in article 26.1 a) – e) in the directive. A special provision regarding personal data, which is transferred for use in a country that has adopted the Council of Europe Convention, was also proposed in connection with Swedish obligations according to the convention.

The provisions in the EU directive allow transfer of personal data during treatment to an outside country if an adequate level of protection can be provided. The Personal Data Act (§§ 33 and 34) stipulated the restriction of transfer of personal data to an outside country with certain exceptions. Consequently, this entailed a stricter wording. The Swedish government, in accordance with the new legislation, wants to retain the tenor of the older Data Act in which it was allowed to transfer personal data to states that have accepted the Council of Europe Convention on Data Protection. The directive did not take into consideration the rapidly evolving information technology, which also has an impact on this restriction in Swedish legislation (Regeringens proposition 1999/2000:11).

The Swedish Parliament approved the government proposition for new personal data legislation (Personal Data Act). Along with the enactment of the Personal Data Act in October 1998, the legislation's rules regarding transfer of personal data to outside countries were met with criticism. The rules were thought to imply an unwanted limitation of the possibility to employ modern information technology, email for example. The legislation was difficult to apply in accordance with the Swedish principle of public access. The government proposed an alteration in the legislation soon after the Personal Data Act was enacted. Transfer to outside countries should not be forbidden if the security level in that country is adequate. The proposed transfer rules, which imply that the law is more closely related to the directive, suggest that processing of non-sensitive personal data is exempted from the demand for consent when transferred. It has been suggested, however, that this has been achieved at the expense of unclear regulation. The individual has more opportunity to process personal data on the Internet without consent after the amendment. In return, it is more difficult to know when consent is required (personal communication, government official in Ministry of Justice). The amendments were proposed for enactment in January 2000.

5.3 Personal Data Act

In October 1998 the Personal Data Act replaced the world's oldest data law. The act, which largely adheres to the EU directive's text and disposition (but not articles 25 and 26), governs all automated processing of personal data and manual processing of personal registers. This means that the Personal Data Act is independent of technology.

Particularly strict regulations apply to the processing of sensitive personal data. Such sensitive personal data are, for example, health, political opinions and religion (Justitiedepartementet 1998). In order to ensure the patient's right to integrity, the Medical Registers Act was enacted.

Section 18 of the Personal Data Act determines when handling of personal data is permitted within the health and medical services (Regeringens proposition 1997/98:44). Accordingly, sensitive personal data may be processed for medical purposes if the processing is necessary for

- preventive healthcare,
- medical diagnoses,
- care or treatment, or
- administration of medical services.

The Personal Data Act regulates an important area of processing within health and medical services – IT security. The Personal Data Act states that those responsible for personal data shall employ appropriate technical and organisational measures in order to protect the personal data that is to be processed. The Personal Data Act also regulates the patient's right to participate in retrieving health service register excerpts that contain personal data about that patient. Also the demand for consent when transferred is regulated in the Personal Data Act.

The restrictions that prohibited transferral of personal data to countries outside the EU and European Economic Area (EEA) have restricted county councils and counties from distributing public information via the Internet for example. According to the Swedish principle of public access, Swedish citizens are guaranteed integrity of personal data and legal security through proper management of records. Furthermore, publishing of non-sensitive personal data on the Internet was prohibited. In other words, the legislation entailed the most comprehensive regulation of information transferral ever in Swedish legislation.

The Personal Data Act was amended on January 1st 2000. The purpose of the amendment is to make it easier to use modern information technology. The restriction in § 33 in the Personal Data Act regarding transferral of personal data to countries outside the EU is softened, as is the possible prosecution for crime against this prohibition, which will not be prosecuted in minor cases (§ 49).

The amendment allows transferral of personal data to a third country, provided that the recipient country maintains an adequate level of security for personal data. This is partly in reference to transferrals from public registers in order to protect the county council's and municipality's interests concerning information distribution, and partly in reference to transferrals of personal data which do not imply any risks for the registered patient and where exceptions can be made in urgent matters because of a common interest (for example, personal data distributed via the Internet).

5.4 Medical Registers Act

In October 1998 simultaneously with the Personal Data Act, the Medical Registers Act came into force. This Act is a special law in relation to the Personal Data Act. The Medical Registers Act governs all processing of personal data in medical registers. If personal data is to be processed with help from IT for one or several of the following purposes, processing includes references to medical registers (Datainspektionen 2000):

- patient care documentation
- administration relating to care on an individual basis
- economic administration resulting in individual care

The data that is recorded in a medical register may even be processed for the following purposes:

- compiling of statistics
- follow-up, evaluation, quality assurance and administration of the area of activity
- provision of data stipulated by law or regulation

A health and medical services register is thus regarded as a medical register if it has been established for administration or documentation of healthcare in individual cases. Patient journals created with help from IT sources are considered medical registers.

Healthcare is, according to this law, care in accordance with the Health and Medical Services Act, the Dental Care Act, the Compulsory Psychiatric Care Act and the Forensic Psychiatry Act plus the prevention of infectious diseases according to the Infectious Diseases Act. The Act has no provisional regulations. This means that the Medical Registers Act governs the registers concerned from 24th October 1998. When the Medical Registers Act was instituted, it immediately replaced the Data Act regulations and those regulations and instructions present in the Medical Registers Act for those medical registers as stipulated by the Data Inspection Board. Personal data recorded before 24th October 1998 that is not protected by the Medical Registers Act can be governed by the Data Act and the Data Inspection Board (Datainspektionen 2000). Those parts of the Medical Registers Act that do not stipulate any restrictions are governed by the Personal Data Act.

Safety precautions taken to protect personal data in medical registers and that allow free flow of data between Member States are controlled by the Personal Data Act (Figure 1).

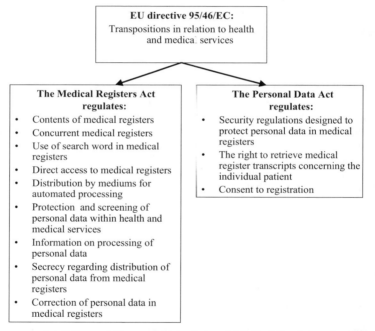

Fig. 1: Areas regulated through Personal Data Act and Medical Registers Act transposing EU Directive 95/46/EC in Sweden

Information about personal registration is regulated by the Medical Registers Act. The body responsible for personal data shall take precautions that the registered person receives information about the data processing. This information should include:

- who is responsible for the personal data
- the purpose of the register
- what kind of data the register contains
- the obligation to inform stated in the Medical Registers Act

- the secrecy and security regulations which apply to the register
- the right of access to information according to the Personal Data Act § 26
- the right to rectify incorrect or misleading data
- the right to claim damages for the processing of personal data in violation of this Act
- what applies with regard to search concepts, direct access and handing out data stored on a computer medium for automated processing
- what applies with regard to storing and sorting out, and
- whether the registration is voluntary or not.

Enactment of the Medical Registers Act means taking into consideration those relevant regulations stipulated in the Official Secrets Act, the Health and Medical Services Act, the Law of Patient Records and legislation governing gainful employment in the medical sector (Datainspektionen 2000).

5.5 The Data Inspection Board's role and implementation

The Data Inspection Board is the supervising authority when it comes to the processing of personal data. The responsibility for the supervision is applied to the Personal Data Act and the Medical Registers Act. Article 28 of Directive 95/46/EC also regulates the obligation to have a supervising authority. Only in recent years has the Data Inspection Board shown any interest in IT within healthcare (Ahlberg & Palmberg 1999).

The Data Inspection Board's main task is to find the correct balance between the individual's need for personal integrity and society's requirements for the effective processing of data. Protection of the sanctity of private life should be guaranteed without unnecessarily obstructing or complicating the use of new technology.

When the Personal Data Act came into force in 1998, a new way of working was introduced at the Data Inspection Board. The new legislation does not require permission for automated processing of personal data, as the Data Act did, but only a report to the Board. The main rule is that all computerised processing of personal data should be reported to the Board. Exceptions apply if a personal data proxy has been appointed, and for some processing within the health and medical services. Processing which is particularly integrity-sensitive should always be reported in advance to the Data Inspection Board for assessment. This applies to

- sensitive data processed for research projects without the consent of the registered person, unless the processing has been approved by a research ethics committee;
- processing of data concerning genetic predispositions which have been found by means of genetic examination.

Thus, the new legislation has changed the Data Inspection Board's role from controlling data processing by granting permission or licensing data processing to supervision and provision of information. Since the Personal Data Act came into force, the Board has therefore reorganised its activities.

In regard to its new role in supervision the Data Inspection Board carries out inspections and follows up inspection activities and complaints. With the Personal Data Act the number of licensing matters have decreased. This leaves more scope for supervision projects and field work and offers an opportunity to check whether the relevant bodies and institutions comply with the Personal Data Act and the Medical Registers Act.

The second new role of the Data Inspection Board is the provision of information about the existing rules. In connection with the implementation of the Personal Data Act there was a great deal of information activity. The Data Inspection Board organised two conferences for the bodies responsible for personal data before the Act came into force. Other conferences have been organised after 24th October 1998. They have dealt, for example, with the Personal Data Act and data security, the Personal Data Act and the Internet, what happens in Europe in view of the Data Security Directive and the role of the personal data proxies. It has been reported that the need for information in connection with the new Personal Data Act has been great.

A large part of the Board's activities now consist of providing authorities, companies, organisations, media and the general public with information. The Data Inspection Board's web site has become an important and extensive channel of communication.

5.6 The bodies responsible for personal data and personal data proxies

According to the Personal Data Act the bodies responsible for personal data have a greater responsibility than that which was stipulated in the Data Act. In the Personal Data Act there are a number of rules which the bodies responsible for personal data must abide by to achieve reliable protection of these data. The bodies responsible for personal data can appoint a personal data proxy. In § 3 of the Personal Data Act a personal data proxy is defined as "a physical person who, commissioned by the bodies responsible for personal data, shall independently see to it that personal data are processed in a correct and legal way".

It is a voluntary measure to appoint a personal data proxy, but the idea is that the proxy should be an asset to the bodies responsible for personal data with regard to the protection of personal integrity when processing these data. The proxy is to supervise the bodies responsible when processing personal data, list the processing sessions and help registered people to obtain rectification. The job can be compared to that of an internal auditor and the proxy must have such a position that he or she dares to call attention to errors and deficiencies. The Data Inspection Board has the ambition to offer the proxies advice and support and when required a proxy should consult the Board. The proxies should function as key persons in the workplaces and be a direct channel to the Data Inspection Board.

Compared to the previous Data Act, the Personal Data Act places greater demands on the county councils to interpret the wording of the Act themselves. In some cases the legislative history may be helpful. There, the personal data proxies have an important mission. If the body responsible for personal data appoints a personal data proxy, it will not have to report the processing of personal data to the Data Inspection Board. The proxy must, however, keep a record of the processing sessions.

The Personal Data Act states that the body responsible for personal data must report to the Data Inspection Board when a proxy has been appointed. The dismissal of a proxy must also be reported. The Board files the reports. In September 1999, 14 of Sweden's 20 county councils had registered 35 proxies distributed among 62 committees.

5.7 The role of the Swedish Healthcare Standards Institution for the IT development

The HSS is responsible for Swedish standardisation within the health and medical services, dental care, medical technology and aids for the disabled. The standardisation work has been of great importance for the implementation of the EU Directive 95/46/EC aimed at creating a common high level for the protection of the right to personal privacy and thereby facilitate a free flow of personal data between the member countries. A significant part of the standardisation efforts is thus to ensure that all exchange of and access to common information takes place in accordance with existing laws and regulations.

Representatives of HSS participate in the CEN and ISO technical committees and can thus influence the creation of standards. These people represent the manufacturers of information systems within the health and medical services, medical devices and materials and also the users: doctors, nurses, paramedical personnel, medical technicians and computer technicians (HSS 1998).

Standards for Health Informatics must be established to allow different systems to communicate and exchange information which has the same significance to the supplier as to the receiver. Therefore, in 1990, CEN decided to form the Technical Committee for Health Informatics – CEN/TC 251 (Petersson & Rydmark 1996). Each member country has in turn organised its work so that there is a mirror organisation organised in exactly the same way.

Sweden's mirror organisation within this field is TK Health Informatics, a technical committee within HSS offering expert knowledge in the field of computers within healthcare. TK includes representatives of the Federation of County Councils, the National Board of Health and Welfare, the Swedish Institute for Health Services Development (Spri; until its closure in 1999), the Data Inspection Board, the Swedish Association of Health Professionals, the Swedish Society of Medical Information Processing, the Association of Suppliers of Medical Devices, the county councils and suppliers of information systems (HSS 1998). TK's work is divided among four working groups, which have their counterparts within CEN.

The EU has allocated funds, which has made it possible to set up various project teams. These will have defined tasks and will work for a limited period of time. Collaboration between the EU and CEN when it comes to research and development in the field of medical informatics has been considered to be so important that a special coordination body, Accompanying Measure on Consensus Formation and Standards Coordination and Promotion (ACOSTA) has been formed (Petersson & Rydmark 1996).

The purpose of standardisation in the field of health informatics is to solve communication problems within health and medical services and in order to allow a joint utilisation of patient information. The standards of health informatics should allow the construction of new systems built according to standardised interfaces and thus able to make use of data as a shared resource. A significant part of standardisation is to develop standards to secure and protect information. That must be done in relation to the existing directives.

Standardisation work aims at achieving uniformity with regard to terminology and concept systems. The terms and concepts of the models become a significant part of the common language which is to be used between the information systems of the health and medical services.

CEN/TC 251 works out preliminary European standards and technical reports. Such a standard is valid for three years. A review must be initiated after two years in view of a possible promotion to a regular standard. Representatives of HSS finds it important that the Swedish medical sector participates and in consensus supports the established standards. Nothing can be done that doesn't work according to the existing directives. Sometimes, standardisation efforts take precedence over the directives.

The standardisation work will be of great significance as a basis for the expansion of the IT systems which will take place within the Swedish medical service in the future. The IT standardisation supports the application of the Data Security Directive.

Representatives for HSS are of the opinion that the Personal Data Act is very well in line with the Data Security Directive in regard to healthcare. Swedish healthcare complies with the Personal Data Act, but it is just as important that other laws regulating health and medical services are followed, such as the Medical Registers Act, the Official Secrets Act and the Patient Journal Act.

The European standard is important for the future. One of the interviewees described the current situation as follows:

"It is important that the area where this can be protected is extended [...] that's why this European standard is important...that medical records can be sent securely between Sweden and Spain; today this is not done to any greater extent [...] what is beginning to happen a bit is that they may start sending things in border areas between Germany and France or Belgium and Holland and to a certain extent Denmark and Sweden."

A project is used to describe the connection between directives and standards:

"I am working on the coordination of technology in a project [...] we are trying to introduce these cryptographic security techniques for protecting personal privacy, and to a great degree this should be seen in relation to the requirements of the Data Security Directive [...] adequate technical solutions which protect sensitive secret information [...] and we have based the standard within CEN 251 much on this and show how you can go about many of these development projects [...] then it will be very important to be able to lean on standards...so if there are standards that indicate methods and if you follow them, you could probably say that you have fulfilled the directives."

6. Outcome

Due to the only recent transposition of the European directive it is too early to assess conclusively intended and unintended outcomes. Nevertheless some outcomes are already evident. The County Council of Värmland was chosen to illustrate the current outcomes in very concrete setting. These outcomes refer to information security and experiences with personal data proxies. Additionally, more general considerations in regard to intended and unintended effects will be made.

6.1 Information security – County Council of Värmland

Within the County Council of Värmland (LIV) a number of questions relating to IT security and information security have been dealt with at a central level. During 1999 several documents concerning IT matters were published. A memorandum on IT strategies and security had been presented earlier. IT work is often conducted in the form of projects such as the information security project and the Visi project.

The largest investment is the information security project, which has been documented and presented in several reports. The project started in the autumn of 1999 and aims at producing a manual for information security according to the requirements of the legislation and the county council's needs, and to instil awareness, motivation and commitment into all employees with regard to security, and in the long term achieve a high level of security within LIV. The project is to be checked against various standards.

The information security work will continue for several years. The training input will be considerable and by June 2001 all employees were expected to have had basic training in information security. By the end of 2001 at least one unit is to be certified according to the information security standard SS 62 77 99.

The standard SS 62 77 99 describes how a management system for information security is established, implemented and maintained. The aim is that organisations and companies shall have satisfactory control of their handling of information and data, and protection against unwanted occurrences and threats; internal or external, intentional or unintentional.

A certification according to the standard will guarantee that the necessary measures have been taken to meet the authorities' and trade and industry's requirements with regard to information security.

The Visi project has been started to connect the various data systems now in operation within the county council. Within primary care there are 16 different systems at present. For institutional care the problem is uneven data maturity.

IT security is seen as a part of the information security work. The county council has many different activities with different needs. Certain information must have very strong protection against unauthorised access. Just as often staff may want to have information accessible via the Internet. In accordance with the principle of public access to official records there is an ambition to give as many people as possible access to certain information. The IT security work will be continuous. To achieve effective IT security, analyses of threats, vulnerability and risks must be carried out.

Based on, for example, the address register of the health and medical services, an authorisation control system will be developed. County council employees will have their individual roles and tasks, and a personal authorisation. This authorisation will grant access to certain information. To achieve this, technical solutions will be required, for example smart cards. The use of smart cards requires certification, allowing the county councils to become the certification authority.

As the Personal Data Act includes provisional regulations, the Data Act has applied in some cases until 30th September 2001. Interviewees did not believe that the Personal Data Act has had any effect on health services data processing as previous exemptions are regarded as valid even after the enactment of this law.

The Medical Registers Act is a concise legislation written to handle the specific problems faced by health and medical services. Information regarding this legislation has not yet been forthcoming from centralised authorities. No discussions regarding this legislation have been conducted, rendering the Medical Registers Act anonymous. The interviewees do not recognise any strong commitment to the law, which in turn may depend on the fact that the legislation does not stipulate meaningful demands nor does it give any indication on how it is to be interpreted.

IT matters are to a great extent governed by the legislation at a constitutional level but also by special acts such as the Health and Medical Services Act, the Patient Medical Records Act and the Medical Registers Act for the health and medical services. If you abide by this legislation, you will largely have fulfilled the requirements of the Personal Data Act. At the same time, standardisation has been of importance for IT efforts. The standard SS 62 77 99 is based to a large extent on Directive 95/46/EC.

According to the Personal Data Act the bodies responsible for personal data, i.e. the healthcare committees within the County Council of Värmland, have greater responsibilities than under the previous Data Act. To facilitate their work, they can appoint a personal data proxy. Within LIV a personal data proxy has been selected in 2000.

According to the provisional regulations in the Personal Data Act, certain registers within the health and medical services are governed by the Data Act. As a result, the County Council of Värmland's decision to select a personal data proxy, new registrations no longer need be reported to the Data Inspection Board.

The obligation to provide information for those registered is difficult yet realistic. It has been imposed by those responsible for personal data. The obligation is governed by the Medical Registers Act and was valid when the act went into effect. The patient's right to "register transcripts" was stated in the older Data Act. A similar regulation is found in the Personal Data Act – that those responsible for personal data must offer free information through the use of register transcripts provided in response to a written request. This regulation has caused uncertainty among patients. Less than honourable companies have tried to create a market by offering patients help by obtaining power of attorney in order to receive register transcripts containing uninteresting information.

The increased bureaucratic processes that are a result of the new legislation are seen as problematic by the County Council of Värmland. Nowadays, the County Council's Board of Directors are responsible for County Council archives. It is difficult to appreciate the consequences for the archive authority as long as the provisional regulations stated in the Personal Data Act are still valid. Only after the transitional period is over can any judgement be made. Requests to obtain register transcripts may increase which will lead to an increase in workload. The administrative process involved in identification and listing of all personal data processing and all health and medical services registers as stipulated by the Personal Data Act will increase the demand on resources.

Certain issues have been raised by the County Council archivist concerning medical research conducted. The Medical Registers Act covers evaluations and quality assurance conducted by health and medical services. The Personal Data Act covers research and stipulates that sensitive personal data may be processed in connection with research and for statistics purposes if the processing has been approved by a research ethics committee. Such difficulties are described in the following quote:

> "I'll use a personal example … a large eye study. In such a case, it is not possible to release data from identified journals to be used for large statistical purposes because every patient must give their consent … and how is it possible to get consent from everyone … in Sweden, much of the medical research that has been conducted assumes that journal information may be used without consent."

The purpose of the Personal Data Act is to prevent the violation of personal integrity in the processing of personal data. An important part of this protection is the notification of the person whose personal data has been processed and the specific processes that have taken place. Those interviewed believe that although information has improved, the new legislation has caused confusion regarding which law that is valid in particular situations.

Several interviewed persons would like to have more collaboration with national bodies. Increased cooperation between central and local authorities, first of all between the Data Inspection Board at a central level and the county councils at a regional level, is necessary in their opinion. Yet, the national IT work conducted by the Health Care Standards Institution and the Federation of County Councils enjoys little support in regional organisations.

6.2 Experiences of a personal data proxy

Certain county councils/regions selected personal data proxies directly after the Personal Data Act was enacted. To learn about their experiences, a personal data proxy in one region was interviewed.

Issues surrounding new data legislation are numerous and information provided by the Data Inspection Board is vague; any legal custom is not forthcoming. The Data Inspection Board has so far allowed the county councils/regions a great deal of freedom. Both the the Personal Data Act and the Medical Registers Act have been applied without direct controls.

The obligation to provide information according to the Medical Registers Act is regarded as unrealistic. The patient has difficulty getting information regarding registration, causing anxiety and insecurity in connection with a visit to the doctor. There are also many vulnerable persons in the health services as the mentally ill, infants, young children and so forth. This information obligation was earlier not stipulated by law but existed as a provision stated by the Data Inspection Board and outlined the release of registers.

The need for consent – that the registered patient, after having received information permits the processing of personal data – is seen as impractical and difficult to interpret. According to the Medical Registers Act, consent is not required while the Personal Data Act requires consent in certain cases. This has caused difficulty for healthcare service research in that the Personal Data Act is the legislation governing research. Register research is most problematic because the demand for consent is difficult to realise.

IT security provisions are regulated by the Personal Data Act. The Data Inspection Board has published general advice that is regarded as unclear and that does not lend any support to security efforts. The burden of debt – to act accordingly using the new legislation – has been removed from the Data Inspection Board and been placed in the hands of the personal data proxy. The regional responsibility has increased, causing in turn an increased work load.

Bureaucratic processes have been redefined in several different ways. Information obligations are time-consuming. The amount of register processing has increased because all registers must be signed by the personal data proxy. The purpose of the register is to show which groups of people that are registered and from which source the information has been procured. Subsequently, this information must be included in the register catalogue. The right to receive register transcripts may also bring with it an increased workload for authorities. The information must be turned over within a month after the request for a register transcript has been made.

6.3 Intended and unintended effects

The intended effect of the Data Security Directive was to facilitate secure and legitimate cross-border flow of data. Yet, due to technical, systematic and language problems this intended effect has not yet realised. But on the other hand, a variety of unintended effects can be observed. Some of these unintended effects are resulting directly from the interaction between European legislation and the institutional settings of the Swedish healthcare sector some of them are caused by the specific Swedish transposition.

The desired effect of the Data Security Directive was to allow secure cross-border flow of data within the SEM. But this has not been achieved yet and will not be achieved in the near future. Very bluntly, one interviewee revealed, the new legislation and the approximation of data protection laws is a necessary but not sufficient precondition to meet this objective:

> "Another thing which is required is that the information is intelligible [...] ordinary Swedish medical records written in Swedish are not that easy to read in Spain and vice versa; so it isn't very meaningful to send it over ... the work in progress to achieve a more general method of description if you use codes or this systematic analysis of concepts and terminology and standards [...] this is a gigantic task which you could say has just been initiated [...] so most of what we handle in computers as medical information in different member countries is not intelligible if sent somewhere else."

Today whole medical records cannot be transferred but only parts of them, for example laboratory results separated from X-ray images.

On the basis of the new legal framework patients are better informed then before. Information intended for patients regarding computer registration has improved insomuch that several more county councils inform patients compared to the earlier studies done by the Data Inspection Board (Renck & Sundh 2000).

Yet, various unintended effects, caused by the Data Security Directive are observable. Among the unintended effects are legal problems in regard to transferring data from public registers. The Data Security Directive, which was to be enacted in EU countries no later than 24th October 1998, was meant to create a uniform high level of protection in order to allow for the free flow of personal data between Member States. Member States have the freedom to state precisely those conditions which are to be obeyed when processing personal data within the framework provided in the directive (Regeringens proposition 1997/98:44). A common application of national measures is strived after in order to ease the free flow of personal data instead of a harmonisation of legislation. "The committee for the protection of individuals regarding the processing of personal data", established throughout the EU, will contribute to a common application of those national rules that have been accepted in order to carry the directive through.

When the Personal Data Act was enacted, the Swedish government chose to allow the legislation to follow the main outline of the directive's text and disposition. One exception was § 33 in the Personal Data Act on the prohibiting of personal data transferral to a third country. According to this paragraph, transferrals from public registers protecting the interests of the county councils and the municipality regarding the distribution of data were prohibited. The Personal Data Act was amended after an intense debate and is now annexed to the Data Security Directive.

The opinion of the county council is that the Personal Data Act is difficult to apply in conjunction with the Swedish principle of public access and that it will bring more long-term consequences than the EU directive. Information about the Personal Data Act provided by the Ministry of Justice (Justitiedepartementet 1998) points out that the provisions in the Personal Data Act may not be applied in such a way that the Personal Data Act restricts the Swedish principle of public access. Interpretation of the legislation is thus an important task both for the Data Inspection Board and the personal data proxy.

Sweden has been critical in its assessment of problems brought to attention by domestic debates and has taken the initiative, along with Austria and Great Britain, in starting a series of seminars. Spokespersons for Member States will have the opportunity to present their country's legislation and discuss the difficulty with application (Regeringens proposition. 1999/2000:11).

The Medical Registers Act is the regulatory legislation concerning IT use within health and medical services. The Personal Data Act regulates security of personal data in medical registers. Information from central authorities about the Medical Registers Act, which came into being on October 24th without transitional provisions has not been sufficient. Discussions about the legislation have not yet been conducted and it has become more anonymous than the Personal Data Act. Despite this, however, the Medical Registers Act is considered to be good legislation adapted for health and medical services built on the foundation of the EU directive.

The Data Security Directive states that a supervisory authority must be organised for the processing of personal data.

Another unintended effect, which was caused by the specific way Sweden has transposed the European directive can be seen in the above mentioned shift of responsibilities and burden form the Data Inspection Board to the personal data proxy within the data processing or keeping body.

As mentioned above, standardisation has gained a more important role, both in terms of representing Swedish interest and in swiftly adapting to new standards. Standardisation plays an an important role for the implementation of the EU Directive 95/46/EC. IT standardisation supports the application of the Data Security Directive. But this does not occur in cooperation with any other national authorities.

Another unintended effect is the change in data handling in medical research. The conducting of medical research as well as other research within the medical services field has become more complicated following the enactment of the Personal Data Act. According to the Medical Registers Act, personal data can be released via IT medium to other medical registers for the purposes of compiling statistics, quality assurance, evaluation and follow-up. The Personal Data Act governs research that has been scrutinised and approved by a research ethics committee. Patient consent is not required in these cases. In connection with other types of research conducted within the health and medical services field and regulated by the Personal Data Act, patient consent is required for the processing of personal data. This applies to that research which does not require approval of a research ethics committee yet exists in the borderland between evaluation/follow-up and that research which is more clearly defined. Examples of this named in interviews include register studies where the demand for consent is not realistic.

7. Conclusion

On 24th October 1995 the so-called Data Security Directive came into effect, which was to be fully implemented within three years, i.e. by 24th October, 1998. Sweden enacted the directive through legislation within a specific period of time. Before the enactment of the Data Security Directive, Sweden used an older data law from 1973. However, several specific laws were enacted during the 1980s and 1990s with regards to Health and Medical Services. Proposals for new data legislation were needed. With the entrance of Sweden into the EU and coupled with the knowledge that a new EU data directive was being composed, Sweden chose to wait until the new directive was enacted. When the Swedish legislation was written, the government used the directive as a model. Certain interviewees imply that by using the Data Security Directive as a model for the Swedish legislation, the resulting legislation became more detailed. The new legislation was also difficult to apply using the Personal Data Act in accordance with the Swedish principle of public access. On the other hand, the Data Security Directive states that the directive makes it possible, by applying regulations, to respect the principle regarding the right of public access to public documents. Regulations regarding the distribution of information were softened with the amendment made in the Personal Data Act in January 2000. The limiting of information distribution has only marginally affected health and medical services.

The Medical Registers Act was instituted to process the specific problems faced by healthcare services. If the Personal Data Act were the only legislation valid for health and medical services, the result would have caused circumstances deemed incongruous and unmanageable. Information regarding the Medical Registers Act, enacted 24th October 1998 without provisional regulations, is insufficient. The result has been unfamiliarity with this legislation. The enormous amount of publicity surrounding the Personal Data Act in relation to the Swedish principle of public access has also contributed to the Medical Records Act becoming more anonymous. The Personal Data Act's three-year transitional provisions have meant that the new legislation stipulated by EU Directive 95/46/EC have not yet reached a complete impact on an operational level. The Data Inspection Board has up to now given county councils/regions the freedom to apply the Personal Data Act and the Medical Registers Act without direct supervision or control.

Development in the areas of free transferral of patient data to other EU countries has been slow. Many technical solutions need to be applied. After the arrival of the EU directive, Sweden began to send journal data to Denmark. Laboratory results and x-rays are sent electronically using an international standard. Medical records cannot be sent in a uniform manner today. Here, the Swedish Health Care Standards Institution has an important role.

The results of this study indicate suggestions for actions that will lead to improved data security and that will provide the protection stipulated by EU Directive 95/46/EC regarding health and medical services.

– Collaboration between national authorities (HSS, the Federation of County Councils) and county councils/regions regarding IT issues must be developed and strengthened.
– Cooperation between the Data Inspection Board and the personal data proxy within the county councils/regions should be developed and intensified.
– County councils/regions should be active in standardisation efforts.
– Results from the standardisation must be made known and have an impact in the county councils/regions.

The above mentioned suggestions for action and cooperation will most likely hasten the development of the free flow of personal data/patient data from Sweden to other EU countries. This is also in regards to technical solutions for personal data transferral.

Currently the Swedish government and the Swedish parliament wish to amend the Data Security Directive and change it its character. The objective would be to focus on wrongful use instead of regulating the handling of personal data. The Ministry of Justice has already formulated such a proposal (DS 2001:27).

References

Ahlberg J, Palmberg L. Svensk sjukvård har tappat greppet om informationsteknologin [Swedish health care has lost the grasp on information technology]. Läkartidningen [Medical journal] 1999;96(38):3988-92.

Datainspektionen. Information om vårdregisterlagen [Information about the Medical Registers Act]. Rapport 2000: 5. Datainspektionen; 2000.

DS 2001:27. EG-direktivet om personuppgifter - En offentlig utvärdering [EC-directive about personal data - A public appraisal]. Stockholm: Justitiedepartementet.

Europaparlamentets och rådets direktiv 95/46 EG från den 24 Okt 1995: Skydd för enskilda personer med avseende på behandling av personuppgifter och om det fria flödet av sådana uppgifter [Protection of individuals with regard to the processing of personal data and on the free movement of such data].

HSS – Hälso- och sjukvårdsstandardiseringen . Utveckling av standarder inom hälso- och sjukvårdsinformatiken [Creation of standards in the health an medical informatics]. Rapport 20. Stockholm; 1996.

HSS – Hälso- och sjukvårdsstandardiseringen. Funktionskrav vid informationsspridning med IT-system i hälso- och sjukvården [Demand for functions when information in health and medical care is spread]. Rapport 22. Stockholm; 1998.

HSS – Hälso- och sjukvårdsstandardiseringen. Hälso- och sjukvårdsinformatik [Health and medical informatics]. Opublicerat material. HSS; 1999.

Justitiedepartementet. Information om personuppgiftslagen [Information about Personal Data Act]. Faktablad. Artikelnr. Ju 98.01. Sep 1998.

Petersson G, Rydmark M. Medicinsk informatik [Medical informatics]. Liber Utbildning; 1996.

Polit DF, Hungler BP. Nursing research – principles and methods. Third edition. Philadelphia: J.B. Lippincott Company; 1987.

Regeringens proposition 1997/98:44. Personuppgiftslag [Personal Data Act].

Regeringens proposition 1999/2000:11. Personuppgiftslagens överföringsregler [Transposition rules for the Personal Data Act].

Renck B, Sundh M. Datasäkerhet inom hälso- och sjukvården efter EU-inträdet [Data security within health-care after entry into EU]. Arbetsrapport nr 8. Karlstads universitet, Centrum för folkhälsoforskning; 2000.

Spri - Hälso- och sjukvårdens utvecklingsinstitut. Säkerhet i landstingens nätverk – Handbok [Security in the network for county councils– Handbook]. Spri-rapport 421. Stockholm; 1996.

Part IV

Free movement of goods and services

The European Union and Health Services
R. Busse et al. (Eds.)
IOS Press, 2002

A Swedish case study on the impact of the SEM on the pharmaceutical market

Clas REHNBERG

Abstract. This chapter analyses the consequences of EU membership for the Swedish pharmaceutical market. The EU legislative framework and directives regarding the pharmaceutical market have, to a large extend, been transposed to the Swedish health care sector. Experience shows that EU policy has mainly influenced various supply and input side aspects. Since health service organisation and financing are the responsibility of national governments, questions of pricing, subsidies and inclusion of drugs in benefit schemes are still regarded as national issues. However, the directives and verdicts of the European Court of Justice concerning general principles of free movement of goods have facilitated parallel trade and most likely reinforced the reduced price differences for pharmaceuticals among Member States.

1. Introduction

Pharmaceuticals are the most tradable of the major inputs used in the production of health care, since healthcare is a service which is normally both produced and consumed at regional or local levels. The pharmaceutical market has therefore been a focus of attention for the European Commission. The first directive concerning the harmonisation of regulations for the manufacturing and distribution of pharmaceutical products was introduced in 1965.

The purpose of this chapter is to present and discuss the transposition and impact of EU regulations for the Swedish pharmaceutical sector. The chapter focuses on the impact of regulations in general and the EU directives in particular on the financing, regulation and delivery of health services. In addition some of the verdicts from the European Court of Justice (ECJ) regarding pharmaceuticals are considered. The analysis aims to explore the overall impact on one geographical pharmaceutical sector rather than in-depth analysis of specific issues. The chapter begins with an overview of the role of the EU market within the context of the international pharmaceutical market. The characteristics, structure and major actors in the Swedish pharmaceutical market are then presented. The impact of relevant regulations, mainly EU directives, on institutional settings is then explored in relation to the system for market authorisation and safety, the distribution and public procurement and, finally, the trade of drugs between the Member States.

Sweden became member of EU in 1995, but had previously signed the Maastricht Treaty (as a member of the European Economic Area) in 1992. The EEA agreement required Sweden to follow certain rules concerning patent protection for drugs and to participate in a voluntary system for safety and for reciprocal approval of drugs sanctioned by EU. The agreements concerning patent protection of drugs were in line with general international obligations agreed by the World Trade Organisation (WTO). Apart from these commitments, there were a number of long-standing agreements between Nordic countries for free movement of labour and people across borders. These agreements did not change after EU membership, and the effects for the pharmaceutical market in Nordic countries are similar (see for example Norris 1999). When Sweden joined the EU, several of the pharmaceutical directives already corresponded to existing Swedish laws and regulations, although minor changes were made. Nevertheless, some EU directives had to be formally transposed into Swedish legislation.

The current Swedish health system is best described as a regionalised system with nineteen local governments – the county councils – each having the right to levy local taxes and to decide on the provision of health services. The major part of health service provision – including hospitals and primary health care centres – are operated by the county councils. However, during the last ten years, there has been a growing trend towards the use of market mechanisms within the public sector and to contracting out more services to private providers. Pharmaceuticals have traditionally been largely financed by central government through the Drug Benefit System (Läkemedelsförmånen). However, there is an on-going reform seeking to decentralise and co-ordinate pharmaceutical expenditures with other health services. The pharmaceutical industry has played a significant role in the Swedish economy with successful corporations as Astra and Pharmacia[1]. The workforce per population is one of the highest in EU and the pharmaceutical trade balance shows a positive and growing development. Swedish policy has traditionally been in favour of free trade and, as a small country with an economy consisting of a few large multinational corporations, it is highly dependent on international trade, not least the pharmaceutical industry.

2. The international pharmaceutical market

Pharmaceuticals are the most important goods in health services that are traded across the Member States. The production of pharmaceutical products has been specialised and concentrated in a few multinational corporations acting on the world-market for their specific products. The investment costs for developing new products and entities are increasing and the demand for returns on investment is becoming even more important. The importance of access to markets and the protection of patent rights are even more decisive for survival in the industry. The pharmaceutical industry has tried to influence EU regulations in order to facilitate entrance to the single market, but also to influence the protection of patent rights. The pharmaceutical market is probably also the most international of all the markets for input factors in health services.

The two major consumer markets of pharmaceuticals in the OECD area are North America and the EU. During the last twenty years the U.S. market has increased both in real terms as well as a percentage of the world market. The EU market and the Japanese market show some decline in relative size (Figure 1).

The pharmaceutical market can be analysed from either the consumer or the producer side (demand or supply side). Several of the problems that arise with harmonisation of the pharmaceutical markets can be explained by each country's interests in promoting (or not promoting) the pharmaceutical industry. As shown in Table 1, there are substantial differences between countries in balance of trade in pharmaceuticals. Generally, even if the relationship is not complete, patent protection and other measures to encourage investment in the industry are apparent in countries with a positive balance of trade for drugs. Spain and Portugal, on the other hand, were both faced with specific export restrictions due to an inadequate patent protection for drugs when they became new members of EU.

---

[1] Astra has now merged with Zeneca and Pharmacia merged with Upjohn in 1995.

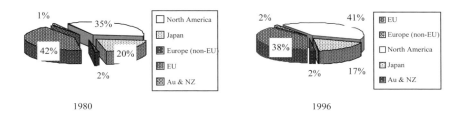

Fig. 1: Total expenditures on pharmaceutical goods, in million US$ (purchasing power parity), 1980 and 1996 (Source: OECD 2000)

Table 1: Export and import (manufacturing) for selected EU countries, in million US$ at exchange rate, 1996

Country	Export	Import	Balance of trade	Export/import ratio
Austria	980	1,047	-67	0.9
Belgium	3,313	2,202	+1,111	1.5
Finland	148	382	-234	0.4
France	5,581	3,293	+2,288	1.7
Germany	7,720	3,846	+3,874	2.0
Italy	2,714	3,266	-552	0.8
Portugal	78	663	-585	0.1
Spain	988	1,920	-932	0.5
Sweden	2,400	735	+1,665	3.3
United Kingdom	6,154	3,345	+2,809	1.8

Source: OECD 2000

France, Germany, Sweden and the UK show the largest net of exports and imports of pharmaceutical goods. Italy, Portugal and Spain all have a negative balance of trade. These three countries (together with Greece) also show the lowest drug prices among the Member States (Riksforsakringsverket 1999). Portugal and Spain also have a tradition with defective protection of drug patent (see section 4 below). The relationship between positive balance of trade in drugs is, however, not without exception. France, and to some extent Sweden, do not show a price-level above average. Still, countries with a relatively large pharmaceutical industry have in general encouraged investment in new research and development through patent protection and higher prices for new drugs.

3. Swedish health care and the pharmaceutical market

The pharmaceutical market as a concept could be misleading if specific characteristics are not demonstrated. Given the complexity of safety, price-regulation, and reimbursement from third-party payers[2], etc. it is far from a traditional market exchange between

---

[2] The concept of third party payer refers to the deviation of the standard market model with one group of consumers and one group of providers, and where there is a third party pooling the risk and handling the major part of the financial transactions with the providers. National and regional governments, sickness funds and private insurance companies could all play the role of a third party payer.

consumers and providers. The Swedish pharmaceutical market can be divided into five sections: production, distribution, retail sales, consumption and financing. The major regulatory agencies for approval and for pricing and reimbursement are also included in the figure. Figure 2 is a schematic representation of the major transactions and regulations of relevance for recent EU legislation.

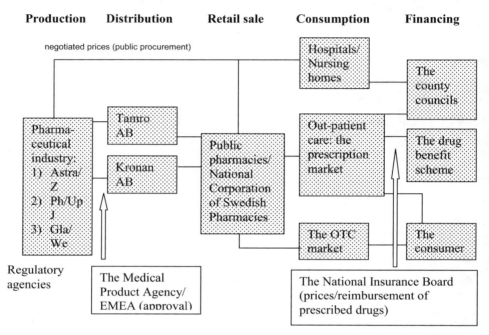

Fig. 2: The structure of the Swedish pharmaceutical market (based on documents from
        different regulatory agencies and financiers of pharmaceuticals)

Production covers both domestic and foreign pharmaceutical companies, including sales from generic products and parallel imports. Two corporations – Tamro and Kronan – handle almost all wholesale distribution. These corporations, previously owned by foreign producers and the state-owned Apoteksbolaget (the National Corporations of Swedish Pharmacies) respectively, have a legal monopoly of wholesale distribution. The monopoly situation in the distribution stage is partly explained by the monopoly in retail sales. Apoteksbolaget controlled the wholesale distribution through its part-ownership of the former ADA company (now part of Tambro AB). Retail sale is almost entirely carried out by the state-owned Apoteket AB (previous Apoteksbolaget) – a monopoly situation with respect to consumers and a monopsony with respect to producers.

The next sections in Figure 2 are consumption and financing. Total expenditure on pharmaceuticals includes all consumption of pharmaceuticals. However, it is possible to break this total figure down by exploring three sub-markets; the hospital market, the prescription market and the non-prescription market (often referred to as Over-The-Counter (OTC)). These sub-markets have different regulations, especially for prices and reimbursement. The market shares for the three markets have changed over time. As shown in Table 2, the prescription market is the largest market for pharmaceuticals. It has increased its relative share of total pharmaceutical spending from 73.2 % in 1985 to 81.6 % in 1996.

Pharmaceuticals consumed in hospitals decreased its market share during the same period, from 17.4 % in 1985 to 10.6 % in 1996. Non-prescribed pharmaceuticals on the other hand have kept a relatively constant share of the market, approximately 8-9 %, during this period.

Table 2: Expenditure in sub-markets as a share of total expenditure on pharmaceuticals, Sweden, 1985-1996

Year	Hospital (%)	OTC (%)	Prescription (%)
1985	17.4	9.4	73.2
1990	16.1	8.3	75.7
1995	12.1	8.6	79.4
1996	10.6	7.8	81.6

Source: Henriksson et al. 1999

The different sub-markets differ from each other with regard to financing. The hospital market refers to hospital purchase of drugs as an input factor to hospital production (mainly in-patient care). Hospitals are financed by their owners (the county councils) through contracts or budgets, which lead to budget restrictions regarding purchase of drugs and other inputs. Hospitals and county councils also have the right to purchase directly from the pharmaceutical industry and there is no price-regulation in this sector. Drugs for in-patient use can either be purchased by each hospital or by a centralised purchasing unit within the county council. In both cases, purchasing is regulated through the Public Procurement Act.

The OTC-market is the most "market-oriented" of the three pharmaceutical sectors. The presence of a third party payer is limited to a few drugs on the so-called positive list[3]. As OTC-drugs are mainly well-known, low-priced drugs they are financed by out-of-pocket money and there is price-competition among suppliers.

The prescription drug market is the most significant of the three markets and also shows the largest growth. This sub-market is financed by a complex reimbursement system paid jointly by the county councils and the central government through the drug benefit scheme. While patients have to pay a yearly deductible on pharmaceuticals and a decreasing co-insurance above that limit, pharmaceuticals beyond a certain limit per year are entirely free of patient cost-sharing. Price-control was abolished in 1993 and in principle free pricing is accepted. However, in order to qualify for reimbursement from the drug benefit scheme, pharmaceutical companies must apply to the National Social Insurance Board to have its products included in the reimbursement scheme.

Figure 3 demonstrates developments in the three sub-markets from 1985 to 1995 as part of total health care expenditure. The figure shows that all three markets increased gradually in the late 1980s, in particularly expenditure for pharmaceuticals sold on prescription, and more markedly in the 1990s.

---

[3] The positive list includes some OTC-drugs that are reimbursed by the drug benefit scheme.

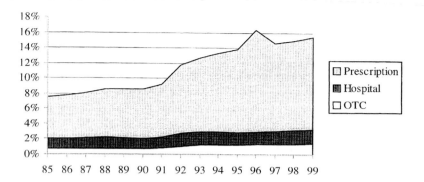

Fig. 3: The development for different sub-markets 1985-1995 in percent of total health care expenditures
(Source: Läkemedelsindustriföreningen 2001)

There are numerous reasons why pharmaceuticals sold on prescription have increased more than the other pharmaceutical markets. One significant explanation for the development is the differences between methods of financing between the three markets. Pharmaceuticals consumed in hospitals are financed by the hospitals and economic restraints within the hospital budgets have controlled these expenses. Issues of costs and benefits are, naturally, related. The hospital finance and planning department considers different health care inputs in order to derive maximum benefit from their budget. This procedure has probably had a restraining effect on pharmaceutical expenses in hospitals. No such incentives exist for prescription drugs. No upper level on the expenses exists, since the system has the characteristics of a National Insurance system. Expenditure for pharmaceuticals sold on prescription have mainly been controlled by price setting and through fees paid by patients. Pharmaceuticals sold over the counter (OTC) have been constrained by household budgets. This market has not increased significantly, probably because of economic recession, unemployment and an increased interest among households in savings, leading to a general lower purchasing power.

Technological advances can also partly explain the increase in pharmaceutical expenditures. Inpatient care has decreased during the last 10 years thanks to day-surgery, policlinic treatments and new and more advanced pharmaceuticals. Innovations in the pharmaceutical sector have replaced lengthy and costly hospital care with appreciably cheaper outpatient treatment. Given these facts, expenditure for pharmaceuticals is likely to continue to increase in the future.

4. Identification of EU directives concerning pharmaceuticals and their transposition in Sweden

The first European Community pharmaceutical directive was issued in 1965. The major concern underpinning Directive 65/65/EEC was the need to assure safety and authorisation of drugs in the wake of the thalidomide disaster[4] in Europe and Japan during the early 1960s which had shaken both the general public and public health authorities. Efforts, aimed at safeguarding public health, included drugs authorisation, with safety as the prime

---

[4] The thalidomide disaster among newborn children was a result of their mothers' unaware consumption of thalidomide during their pregnancy. Thousands of babies were born with limb deformities.

requisite. In terms of number of regulations and directives, most of the regulations concerning pharmaceuticals still focus on safety issues. In other words, efforts to harmonise regulations of drugs were originally aiming at protecting consumers by limiting side effects and assuring a proper use of drugs.

The efforts to develop a common system for authorisation and safety can be considered as a first phase in order to create a single market for pharmaceuticals. A general structure for approval of drugs was also along the lines of the Articles from the Rome Treaty concerning the free movement of goods.

Relevant Articles from the Treaty of Rome (Free Movement of Goods)

- Article 23 (Ex Article 9). 1) The community should be based upon a customs union which shall cover all trade in goods and which shall involve the prohibition between Member States of customs duties on imports and exports and on all charges having equivalent effect, and the adoption of a common customs tariff in their relationship with third countries. 2) The provisions of Article 25 and of Chapter 2 of this Title shall apply to products originating in Member States and to products coming from third countries, which are in free circulation in Member States.
- Article 24 (Ex Article 10). Products coming from a third country shall be considered to be in free circulation in a Member State if the import formalities have been complied with and any customs duties or charges having equivalent effect which are payable have been levied in that Member State, and if they have not benefited from a total or a partial drawback of such duties or charges.

Together with directives concerning authorisation and safety there are a number of general directives concerning patent protection and the incentives for research and development. This group of regulations is not specific for the pharmaceutical industry, but concerns all sectors where innovation and development of new products are an essential part of the business.

As the pharmaceutical market is one of the most regulated in the EU (and in most industrialised countries), the directives will overlap with each other and will also sometimes interfere with existing regulations for a new EU member such as Sweden. Most of the regulations deal with issues regarding approval, safety and standardisation of package and distribution. More recently the issues of efficient access to and organisation of a single market have been considered. Given specific attributes of the pharmaceutical market such as the existence of a third party payer, this development has raised concerns about price-control and reimbursement. In order to create a single market for products and services in health care, entry to the market is not enough to ensure sales. Issues concerning pricing and reimbursement mechanisms also have to be considered. The "transparency directive", 89/105/EEC, sought to ensure common principles for national decisions on pricing and reimbursement.

The directives and other relevant regulations can be grouped into three categories that will be analysed separately in this chapter:

- Market authorisation and safety
- Distribution and public procurement of drugs
- Price control, reimbursement and trade of drugs

The different directives that affect the trade and movement of drugs are illustrated in Table 3.

Table 3: Major directives and regulations affecting the movement of drugs

Type of regulation	Directives (excluding replaced directives)	Other EU regulations
Market authorisation and safety	93/39/EEC change the 65/65/EEC, 75/318/EEC and 75/319/EEC. 83/570/EEC, 87/22/EEC	Council regulation 2309/93/EEC
Distribution of drugs and public procurement	65/65/EEC, 87/21/EEC, 92/25/EEC, 91/356/EEC, 92/26/EEC, 92/27/EEC 93/36/EEC, 93/37/EEC	
Price control, regulation and trade of drugs	89/105/EEC for price control and reimbursement	The Treaty of Rome (Articles 23 and 24), verdicts from ECJ regarding trade and distribution

The directives and the subsequent decisions taken by the EU have been important for all types of regulations mentioned in Table 3, apart from trade of drugs and price control. The regulations concerning market authorisation and safety are, in particular, part of a conscious harmonisation strategy to implement common rules for all Member States. For trade of drugs there is no specific directive, but there have been a number of cases before the European Court of Justice that have had an impact on the movement of pharmaceutical goods between EU countries. In particular, the export of drugs from countries with lower drug prices has encouraged the development of parallel trade, i.e. a product that is launched in one country is re-exported to another country by another firm. Several parallel import cases have been considered by the ECJ, with reference to the principles stated in The Treaty of Rome, and where interpretations made by national and local courts have enforced the verdicts. In Sweden the Kammarrätten (the regional administrative courts) and Regeringsrätten (the national administrative court) have given a number of verdicts about the interpretation of decisions made by the ECJ. Overall, these administrative courts have accepted ECJ verdicts.

4.1 Market authorisation and safety

In Sweden, as well as in other EU countries, there has been a long tradition of reviewing the safety and scientific procedures of clinical trials during the development phase of a new drug or entity. The Medical Product Agency (Läkemedelsverket) has been responsible for this task in Sweden for many years. The agency is also responsible for the final decision to approve a drug for sale. For a number of years there has been co-operation between similar agencies in other EU Member States where the system of reciprocal approval has been used so that, if a drug is approved in a reference-country, it is automatically approved in the other countries.

The process to develop a general framework for drug authorisation and to facilitate a more simplified and improved access to the EU market started with the procedure for mutual recognition implemented through directive 75/319/EEC. The Committee for Proprietary Medicinal Products (CPMP) was set up to facilitate mutual recognition, i.e. the authorisation and approval in one of the Member States would give the producer access to all markets in the European Community. The main purpose of these amendments to Directive 65/65/EEC was to create a Community-wide single market for pharmaceuticals. However, the system was based on voluntary participation, which was handled differently across the Member States. The national approval agencies could arbitrarily decide whether to accept or reject an approval in another Member State and require new documentation for authorisation.

Several directives (83/570/EEC, 87/22/EEC) during the 1980s were intended both to develop a mutual recognition system and to initiate a process for shaping a single procedure for approval of new drugs for the entire EU market. The Member States were still not committed to accepting an approval made in one country, and there were many ways to circumvent approvals, through requirements about new information and references to differences in packaging of products. Overall, the harmonisation process was considered to be too slow and after several years of co-operation between national approval agencies at European Union level, the EU Council adopted directive 93/39/EEC, which replaced or changed the Directives 65/65/EEC, 75/318/EEC and 75/319/EEC. In June 1993 Council Regulation 2309/93/EEC provided the legal basis for the establishment of a new European system for the authorisation of medicinal products. The European Agency for the Evaluation of Medicinal Products (EMEA) was established in 1995 in London. This new organisation involves centralisation and stronger co-ordination of the approval and safety procedures. It also seeks to mobilise scientific resources throughout the European Union to provide high quality evaluation of medicinal products. It is intended to control the safety of medicines and develop speedy, transparent and efficient procedures for the authorisation and surveillance of products in the European Union.

The Swedish transposition of the directives concerning approval procedures has been entirely implemented. The first step was the decision to revise the Pharmaceutical Act (SFS 1992:859) and the Pharmaceutical Regulation (SFS 1992:1752). The major change resulting from this re-legislation is the joint procedure of drugs approval and the acceptance of the principle of mutual recognition. The Act also includes EU regulations regarding the fee for approval application, time limits for approval, etc. The Pharmaceutical Regulation (1992:1752) also gives the auditing and supervision function in Sweden to the Medical Product Agency (Läkemedelsverket). With the new legislation there were also some changes of specific instructions for application for approval and supervision of the pharmaceutical market. The major part of these legislation and changes of instructions came into force in 1995 through the Amendments in the Pharmaceutical Act.

4.2 Distribution and public procurement of drugs

The distribution of pharmaceuticals involves several stages between the production of drugs at the manufacturing companies, through different distributors and prescribers before it reaches the patients. EU regulations intended to influence distribution are aimed at securing a proper handling of pharmaceutical goods. The directives primarily concern principles for manufacturing, package and labelling of products as well as limiting advertising to educated or licensed health personnel only. In Table 4 the most relevant and recent directives are presented.

Table 4: Directives concerning the distribution of pharmaceutical goods

Directive	Subject
92/25/EEC	The wholesale distribution of medicinal products for human use.
92/26/EEC	Classification for the supply of medicinal products for human use
92/27/EEC	Labelling of medicine products for human use and package leaflets
92/28/EEC	Advertising of medicinal products for human use

All these directives were decided at the same time and were aimed at promoting an appropriate use of medicines. The directives primarily concern personnel (competent and appropriately qualified personnel), premises and equipment, documentation, production, quality control, contracting out, complaints and product recall and self-inspection. The consumer should be guaranteed appropriate information both through labelling and advertising, and from educated staff (pharmacists). Advertising to the general public for OTC products were accepted, but prescribed drugs may only be advertised to health professionals (doctors, prescribers and pharmacists). Directive 92/26/EEC also gives guidelines for when a medicinal product is subject to medical prescription.

There is no directive stipulating free access and competition in the distribution of pharmaceuticals. On the contrary, the importance of exercising control over the entire chain of distribution of medical products is mentioned in order to safeguard the appropriate distribution of drugs to consumers. This could be (and has been) interpreted as support for a monopoly in the distribution trade. Still, it is clearly stated in Directive 92/25/EEC that wholesalers should permanently guarantee an adequate range of medical products to meet demand. It is stipulated that wholesalers should, within a very short time period, supply new drugs that are approved and that have been launched.

All four directives mentioned above were transposed when Sweden became a member of EU. The transposition came into force through the 1992 Pharmaceutical Act. Furthermore, specific regulations regarding wholesale distribution are found in the Directions from the Medical Product Agency (Läkemedelsverket 1995:4). Most of the regulations regarding classification and advertising correspond to the Marketing Act of 1975:1418.

Direct purchase of drugs for use in the production of health care, such as in-patient hospital services, is regulated through public procurement legislation. Apoteksbolaget previously supplied most of the drugs used in in-patient care. With the Pharmaceutical Trade Act (SFS 1996:1152) the health authorities and individual hospitals were allowed to purchase drugs directly from the pharmaceutical industry. However, all public organisations have to follow the regulations in the Public Procurement Act (SFS 1992:1528) and Amendments in the Public Procurement Act (SFS 1996:433) which is the Swedish transposition of the Directives 93/36/EEC and 93/37EEC regarding co-ordination of procedures for the award of public supply contracts.

4.3 Price control, reimbursement and trade of drugs

As mentioned in the previous section, the movement of pharmaceutical goods is not only a function of access to markets through common authorisation and approval procedures, but is also influenced by different price regulatory measures. There are different approaches among the Member States both to limiting costs and to subsidising drugs. The continuous rise of pharmaceutical costs in OECD countries has caused concern about cost containment and has led to debates as to how pharmaceuticals should be financed in health care systems. There are various ways to monitor and control pharmaceutical costs. On the demand-side, there are a variety of models of cost sharing, as well as differing measures to control physician prescription patterns. Equally, on the supply-side, there are many different measures directed towards providers, such as profit control, price control, positive and negative lists, etc. All these measures could be regarded as efforts by third party payers to control overall health care spending in general and pharmaceutical expenditures in particular. Given the complexity and disparity of all these measures, it is an overwhelming task for the Commission to harmonise all these systems. This task will not be easier with the arrival of additional EU Member States. Hence, as patients rarely choose their medicine themselves and different third party payers pay wholly or partly for medicines consumed, the decisions made by national authorities to include a drug in the different national Drug Benefit Systems are crucial for access to the market and to sales.

Given this background it is understandable that the main directive addressing the issue of harmonisation of prices and reimbursement is rather vague. Directive 89/105/EEC relates to the transparency of measures regulating the prices of medicinal products for human use and their inclusion in the scope of national health insurance systems. The directive states that each Member State has the right to exercise control over national health expenditures and that the requirements in the directive should not affect national policies in this issue. There are a number of rules for price-setting in the directive stipulating that Member States should ensure that a decision on price should be given within 90 days of the receipt of the application. It also contains other regulations about information of the application procedure and management of profit and price control. Even if harmonisation of rules and decisions cannot be made, the intention of the directive is to give applicants – i.e. the pharmaceutical companies – better insight into the price-setting procedure. The purpose is to avoid restrictions on imports and exports due to control of prices and subsidises. The directive also requires that objective and verifiable criteria are used for the decisions to include a drug on a national Drug Benefit System.

The Swedish legislation has been judged to correspond to the directive concerning pricing of pharmaceuticals. The directive is judged to be entirely implemented through the Pharmaceutical Act and the Cost Containment of Pharmaceutical Act. The negotiation procedure between pharmaceutical companies and the National Social Insurance Board was not changed with the Swedish membership in 1995. The directive only concerns prescribed pharmaceuticals for which the patient is paying a fee. The use of drugs as inputs in hospital in-patient treatment is not affected.

The directives and other regulations of trade for pharmaceutical goods refers mainly to the original principles stated in the Treaty of Rome (Articles 23 and 24) regarding free movement of goods and services. There is no specific regulation that exempts pharmaceutical goods from these fundamental principles, apart from patent protection stipulated in various Articles and directives, which are valid for all goods (and services). However, the basic principle of transferring goods from one country to another of the Member States is more complex for the pharmaceutical market than in other markets. There are two features of the market that distinguish it from a traditional market. 1) the existence of a third party payer, and 2) the price-discrimination behaviour of the pharmaceutical industry combined with parallel import.

With a third party payer (such as the NHS, sickness funds, county councils etc.) the transfer of drugs across borders is not sufficient to provide real access to the market. The acceptance of the drugs from the third party payers is essential if it is to be included in any type of a drug benefit scheme. The decision to put a drug on the reimbursement list differs between Member States and Directive 89/105/EEC on harmonisation of prices and reimbursement does not stipulate a joint decision procedure, but recommends a step-by-step development where these regulations are co-ordinated. It is stipulated that once a drug is approved and an application for a drug in a drug benefit scheme is made, there is a maximum number of 90 days for a decision. If an application is rejected it must be accompanied by an explanation based on objective criteria, which should be published officially. However, it is clearly stated that these efforts must not interfere with each country's arrangement of their social security system (or equivalent). This means that the different third party payers can more or less independently design their own price and reimbursement principles for pharmaceuticals (and other input factors). The major impact of the transparency directive is a more open public control and insight into how national decisions regarding price control and reimbursement are made. In practice, once the approval process had been completed, the pharmaceutical industry has a number of clients to convince in order to sell their products in the market. First, the patient as a consumer (and his agent – the physician) and second, the third party payer which pays for the drug.

Given the disparity of the organisation and function of third party payers in the Member States and the established policy that price-regulation and the structure of social insurance systems is a national concern, harmonisation of price setting is found to be difficult. There are, therefore, no specific directives regarding the trade of drugs, but as mentioned previously, the Treaty of Rome provides the leading principles for free movement of drugs as well as other goods. The representatives of corporations engaged in parallel import refer to these articles in order to remove import restrictions that have been imposed by original manufacturers.

Due to imperfect patent protection in Portugal and Spain, restrictions on the export of pharmaceuticals until 1995 were imposed when these countries became members of the European Union (Spain joined the European patent system late in 1992). Cheap copies of new and more expensive drugs were sold on the market in Portugal and Spain and the pharmaceutical industry itself was involved in tough price-competition also for original products. Traditionally, prices on drugs in countries such as Spain and Portugal have been much lower than in other EU countries. The patent protection has now been somewhat harmonised among the Member States, but there are still differences. Belgium, France, Germany, Sweden, the Netherlands and the UK give a ten-year protection period and other countries six years or less. The weakest protection is found in Greece, Portugal and Spain where prices are still lower for the same product. The prohibition to export pharmaceutical products from Portugal and Spain has now also been abolished.

Swedish policy has traditionally been pro-competitive and has encouraged free trade, allowing imports from low-price countries. When in 1995 seven Member States, through the EU commission, tried to limit the import of pharmaceuticals from low-price countries, the Swedish government did not support the proposal, due to an internal conflict between the Ministry of Social Affairs and the Ministry of Industry[5], where the former at that time had the greatest influence. More recently, Swedish policy has emphasised patent protection in the pharmaceutical industry to ensure investment in research and development. Nevertheless, the Swedish government has explicitly followed the verdicts from the EU Court of Justice and allowed the parallel import given certain restrictions concerning distribution and packages of drugs.

5. Market authorisation and safety

The regulation of the pharmaceutical market in the European Union aims at creating a single market for the entire union. The complexity of the pharmaceutical market makes it necessary to cover the entire process from research trials to final approval, distribution, price setting and financing. The Commission is faced with differing national legislation in all stages of the process. It is clear, though, that national regulation of the pharmaceutical market differs depending on industrial policies, which frequently reflects the importance of the pharmaceutical industry in each country.

In all Member States the protection of public health and market authorisation of drugs are conducted through a set of regulations and agencies. Usually there is one central national agency that makes the final approval decision of new drugs. Since January 1995, common procedures for all Member States have been introduced, although parallel national

---

[5] This conflict of different objectives could be observed in other assemblages like the Bangemann commission.

applications for drug approvals were still possible. Since January 1998 it is only possible to market a new drug in more than one Member State through the common EU system for approval. The new European authorisation procedures includes the following areas:

– Applications and changes of authorisation to sell drugs
– Supervision of side-effects of drugs approved by EU
– Control of manufacturing procedures, laboratory and clinical standards

Almost all new drugs that are intended to be sold in EU are included in the new approval system. There are, however, two marketing authorisation procedures that have been in place since 1995: the centralised and the mutual recognition procedures. This work is co-ordinated by EMEA in London. Two committees assist EMEA, the Committee for Proprietary Medical Products (CPMP) focusing on pharmaceuticals for human use and the Committee for Veterinary Medical Products (CVMP) for veterinary products. These two committees work closely with the national medical approval agencies in the Member States.

The centralised procedure is compulsory for all medical products derived from biotechnology and optional for other innovative medicines. The application is made directly to the EMEA and evaluated by one of the committees mentioned above. The evaluation work is not made by the EMEA and the committees themselves, but by two national approval agencies of which one is appointed as rapporteur and the other as informant. The agencies report their evaluation to one of the committees and there is a maximum processing time of 210 days. During the evaluation process the pharmaceutical companies are given the option to respond to enquiries and to provide supplementary information if needed. The process is co-ordinated by EMEA, which forward the evaluation to the European Commission for final decision. The Community marketing authorisation is then valid throughout the EU.

The alternative is the Mutual Recognition Procedure where the applicant can choose one Member State for a marketing authorisation and then get extension to one or more other Member States. The rules for the evaluation procedure are the same as for the centralised procedure. If a Member State cannot recognise the original marketing authorisation, the dispute is handled by the EMEA. The option for the National procedure, i.e. an application for marketing a drug in only one Member State is still possible for changes of forms and doses of drugs and new indications for drugs that are already approved. This also includes drugs for parallel-import. In Figure 4 the number of drugs approved through the central procedure is presented since the start in 1995.

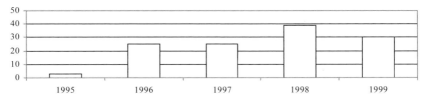

Fig. 4: The number of approved drugs executed by the European Commission 1995-1999
(Source: Lakemedelsverket 2000)

The evaluations that have been performed regarding the new system for market authorisation are by and large positive. the pharmaceutical industry also appears to value the new system. At the same time the pharmaceutical companies can be observed to act strategically in their choice of central or mutual recognition procedures. The central procedure will reduce the transaction costs for the entrance to the European market, but at the same time there is the risk of rejection and thus exclusion from the whole European market. There are also other reasons for choosing the mutual recognition procedure, such as country-specific traditions and regulations concerning doses and packages of drugs. From the perspective of national approval agencies the experience of collaboration between the agencies has also been positive and most decisions have been made in consensus. Overall the collaboration has strengthening the capacity building and competence of the agencies (personal communications).

The new European system for market authorisation is based on a partnership involving national approval agencies in all Member States. The Swedish Medical Product Agency (Läkemedelsverket) has as one of its objectives, to be one of the leading agencies in the European system for market authorisation. The co-operation is organised in a manner that causes some competition among national approval agencies. Apart from the prestige of being one of the most demanded agencies, there is a financial incentive, as regulatory fees from the industry become revenue for the agencies. The distribution of rapporteurs (or informants) across the agencies from the different Member States is shown in Figure 5. As each application sent for approval by the central procedure is judged by rapporteurs in two countries, one act as rapporteur and one as co-rapporteur.

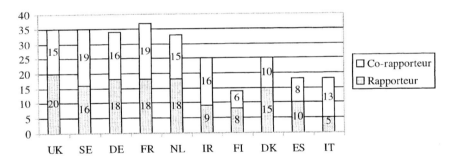

Fig. 5: Distribution of rapporteurs, central procedures 1995-1999 (Source: Lakemedelsverket 2000)

The figure shows that there is a large variation in the number of rapporteurs taking part in the central procedures, when consideration is given to the relative population size of the countries. The results also partly reflect the importance that is paid to becoming a rapporteur in various countries. In figure 6 the distribution across countries for handling the approval of new chemical entities among the agencies is shown. These results are mainly from the procedure of Mutual Recognition between the Member States.

The results from Figures 4 and 5 show that the UK, Sweden, Germany, France and Netherlands have won most of the missions. All these agencies represent countries with large pharmaceutical industries. In addition to approving new drugs, the new system also pay attention to control of safety and inspection of laboratory practice. This work is exercised by each national agency, with all information concerning abuse, complications, side-effects etc. stored at the EMEA. There are common guidelines for the reports about

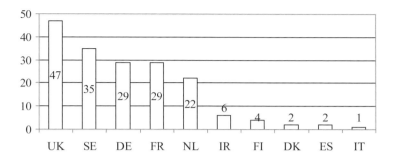

Fig. 6: Number of procedures for New Active Substances in Mutual Recognition
     Facilitation Group, until 1999 (Source: Lakemedelsverket 2000)

side effects and there are also requirements for the pharmaceutical industry to report such
effects.

5.1 Separation of approval and price decisions

Another institutional impact concerns the price-setting procedure. Even if some countries,
such as Sweden, do not have formal price-regulation, all prescribed drugs are subject to
third-payer coverage which affect the prices paid by consumers (and thereby the demand
for the drug). This procedure is to some extent regulated in Directive 89/105/EEC,
sometimes called the "price transparency directive". However, this directive has a greater
influence on the formal procedure but does not give guidelines about criteria for the
inclusion of a drug in national benefit catalogues. According to the directive the price
setting agency, in Sweden the National Social Insurance Office (Riksforsakringsverket),
should follow certain procedural steps before reaching a decision whether to include a drug
or not in the Drug Benefit Scheme. Of major importance is the regulation of the maximum
time for executing a decision for inclusion. According to the Swedish decision-making
authority this directive only implied minor changes of the procedure (personal communication). One peculiarity in Sweden is the separation of decisions about reimbursement/
subsidies (the National Social Insurance Office) and the financial responsibility for drug
expenditures by third party payers (the regional County Councils). The former agency
decides about the price/subsidy and the other takes the financial responsibilities. There is
currently a discussion about merging the decision to subsidise a drug and the decision to
finance the drug. An argument for keeping the subsidy decision at a national level is that
the decentralised structure of the county councils might interfere with the transparency
directive. On the other hand, the objectives of the directive could also be met if all county
councils meet the requirements for a price decision stipulated in the directive, i.e. a
centralised national decision-making is not a pre-condition.

5.2 New drugs on the market

The intention of this new drug licensing system is to improve access to the pharmaceutical
market, but also to ensure a rigorous safety and approval control. The new system is likely
to provide faster access to the EU market at a lower cost for the pharmaceutical industry.
For each new drug, a pharmaceutical company will only have to pay a single application
fee. Even more important is the reduction in time costs, since the joint access to all EU
countries will shorten the total administration period involved in the introduction of a new

drug. Hence, it is likely that (given no other changes) trade will increase as a result of the new drug licensing system. The volume of new registered drugs is an effect both of the mutual recognition system and more recently of the new central licensing system. From Table 5 it is obvious that there is an increase of new registered drugs in Sweden during the 1990s.

Table 5: Pharmaceutical specialities – registration in Sweden

Year (registration)	Number of newly registered drugs	- of which in force 1998
1980	123	79
1995	290	158
1996	252	115
1997	405	266
1998	507	--

Source: Läkemedelsindustriföreningen 2001

Even though there seems to be a sharp increase after 1996, which could be linked both to Swedish EU membership and to the new joint approval procedure, this rise could also be a global trend in the pharmaceutical market. The pharmaceutical industry worldwide shows an increasing investment in research and development of new products. The figures presented in Table 5 cannot be broken down to the pharmaceutical company's home country. It is more interesting to look at the export trade of pharmaceutical goods from Sweden after the membership in 1995 (Table 6).

Table 6: Swedish export and import to/from different markets, 1995-1997, in million Swedish Crowns (SEK)

Export	1995	1997	Percentage change from 1995 to 1997
EU	8,921	12,746	+43
USA	950	1,525	+61
Japan	1,964	1,635	-17
Eastern Europe (PL, CZ, H)	272	294	+8
Total export	16,777	21,710	+29
Import	1995	1997	
EU	4,979.0	5,631.0	+13
USA	143,0	182.0	+28
Japan	43.0	66.0	+52
Eastern Europe (PL, CZ, H)	1.6	1.8	+12
Total import	6,480.0	7,290.0	+13

Source: Swedish National Accounts, various years

The largest increase in export has taken place in the North American and in the EU market. Even if the number of countries in the other groups is low, there is a striking difference. The result could also be explained by the behaviour of the pharmaceutical industry and their focus on large markets. However, this behaviour is of course influenced by different regulations. It is obvious that the administrative cost for approval (and also income from sales) is much lower for applications at the FDA and the EMEA. The pattern for pharmaceutical imports is not that clear, which is natural since the Swedish pharmaceutical market as a share of the total international market is relatively small. Still, these import figures have relevance for the discussion of parallel imports (see section below).

6. Retail sales and wholesale distribution of drugs

The wholesale distribution of pharmaceutical goods has not been a controversial issue in Swedish health policy since EU membership in 1995. The principle and guidelines of good manufacturing practices for medical products for human use, and the objective for rational use of drugs were in line with the previous policy. The Medical Product Agency also has responsibilities for supervising the safety of the distribution of pharmaceuticals. This task is now part of the European authorisation system under the coordination of EMEA, referred to earlier. The main changes with respect to distribution are the centralised system for reporting problems, side-effects and inappropriate distribution, marketing and sales of drugs.

As was shown in the description of the Swedish pharmaceutical system previously, there are monopoly situations both in the wholesale distribution (a few private firms) and the retail sales (the state-owned National Corporation of Swedish Pharmacies). Since there are no specific regulations or directives about competition at the distribution stage, the issue of breaking up these monopolies is rarely discussed. However, there was a parliamentary committee that investigated the conditions and problems with a monopoly on retail sale, which suggested that the OTC-products and some prescribed drugs could be sold outside pharmacies. The Swedish Competition Authority (Konkurrensverket) has questioned the monopoly situation in the wholesale distribution, which is carried out by two companies. Traditionally the wholesale distribution in Sweden has been a "one-channel distribution system", which means that a specific drug could only be distributed by one wholesale distributor. One reason for preserving this system is the rather low cost for wholesale distribution (Figure 7).

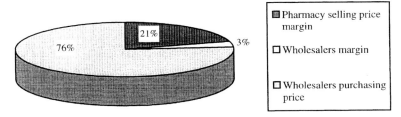

Fig. 7: The average price components of the pharmacy selling (Source: Läkemedelsindustriföreningen 2001)

The distribution costs in the Swedish pharmaceutical market is also rather low by international comparisons, which is explained by this one-channel distribution system. However, an inexpensive system is not the same as a cost-effective system since there might be consequences for the consumers in terms of time costs and poor levels of service.

Hence, it is not primarily the retail sale monopoly by the National Corporations of Pharmacies (Apoteket AB) that is the concern, but the wholesale distribution from the pharmaceutical industry to this corporation and to the hospital sector. The semi-private companies Tamro and Kronan have been given an exception from the rule of open entry to markets until the end of 2001, since there will probably be new regulations from either the Swedish government or the EU.

7. Public procurement

The public procurement legislation (the Public Procurement Act) is not aimed at pharmaceuticals specifically but has an institutional impact, which emanates from EU directives. Public health care providers are engaged in procurement processes where they try to find more efficient and new ways of purchasing drugs. Traditionally most providers have had drugs delivered from public pharmacies. With decentralisation and more autonomous providers together with the new legislation concerning public procurement, hospitals are finding alternative ways to purchase direct from the pharmaceutical industry. This development is at its initial stage, but might be a possible way for hospitals to negotiate rebates and establish contractual relations with manufacturers.

Since the county councils are given financial responsibility for prescribed drugs, several initiatives are also planned for a collective purchase of outpatient prescribed drugs. If this scenario becomes reality it will affect both wholesale distribution as well as the retail sales arrangements in the Swedish system.

8. The trade of drugs and parallel import

The trade of goods and services in the health care sector has been limited for a number or reasons: the specific characteristics of healthcare products, the financing system for health care, the ways in which services are provided to patients etc. As the major part of health care consists of services produced for a local or a regional market there are natural limitations when it comes to trade of inputs across borders (and also within a country). Given an extended freedom of choice for health care providers, the majority of patients choose to remain with their local doctors and hospitals. The main exceptions to these limitations are pharmaceutical products, which, due to their international characteristics and specialisations, are the most tradable products within health care.

Within the EU, the principle of free trade and movement and people and goods across the Member States has been a cornerstone for the creation of a single market. At the same time there is a great awareness of the need for incentive structures when it comes to investing and developing new products. The patent protection of pharmaceutical products and restrictions or conditions for sales of drugs has been considered to give a comprehensive protection. Regulations have been aimed principally at safety and security, which has made it difficult for new firms to market new generic drugs after patents have expired. One previous obstacle was the requirement to provide comprehensive documentation concerning a chemical substance, which was already approved for the market for an original product. After the patent expired the original manufacturer, who had access to the approval documentation, could easily launch their own generic product, which gave them a competitive advantage over other companies producing generic products without access to such documents. These types of EU regulations have been considered to impede both parallel imports and competition between original products and generic drugs. Until the 1980s this regulatory framework was not controversial and new firms did not challenge the system. The essential conditions for parallel import did not exist, as countries with low pharmaceutical prices such as Portugal and Spain, had not yet become EU members.

8.1 Parallel import

The issue of parallel trade refers to the import between Member States that is facilitated through the price differences for the same type of drug in different countries. This type of trade is not related to counterfeiters and other exploiters and it also does not violate the regulations regarding property rights and patent protection. It concerns trade in legitimate products, which are initially marketed by a company with patent rights for its product, but which are then bought by an independent operator who buys them in one country and sell them in another country. A prerequisite for this trade is the difference in prices due to varying Drug Benefit Systems and price regulations across the Member States. There are two circumstances that facilitate what is called price-discrimination in economic terms. First, different third party payers and agencies for price regulation have different principles and traditions for subsidising drugs, which have an impact on the negotiations with the pharmaceutical industry. Second, the industry itself is also engaged in strategic price-setting behaviour where prices are set according to the ability to pay in different countries. Such behaviour could very well be a profit maximisation strategy. It could also benefit countries with low ability to pay in terms of better access to new drugs. Still, the system is vulnerable for parallel import since the industry is not allowed to limit their sales in a defined market.

Hence, parallel importation arises when pharmaceutical goods are purchased by a separate company, usually with no production capacity, from a Member State where the price is low and imports it – without reference to the originator – into a higher price Member State, and then sells it in competition with the originator in that country. This trade goes from low-price countries (such as Greece, Italy, Portugal and Spain) and is exported to high-price countries (such as Germany, Switzerland, and United Kingdom). There are different types of parallel importation depending on how the drugs are re-packed and information to patients changed. The trade requires that a new label be put on the package with instructions in the language depending in which country it is sold.

Some governments in Europe, notably Italy, Portugal and Spain, set price controls having regard to the medical, economic and social impact of the product. In other European countries, primarily Germany, the UK, the Netherlands and, more recently, France, governments are exerting a strong downward pressure on prices through incentives and sanctions to encourage doctors to prescribe cost-effectively. Efforts by the EU Commission to harmonise the disparate national systems have been met with little immediate success, leaving the industry exposed to ad hoc national cost containment measures on prices and the consequent parallel trading of its products from markets with prices artificially depressed by governments into those where higher prices prevail.

As mentioned earlier, there is no pro-competitive directive or regulation aiming at trade of drugs across Member States. The primary target for the directives concerning trade is guarantees for safety, packaging, labelling, and overall a safe distribution. However, Articles 23 and 24 concerning free trade from the Treaty of Rome have been interpreted to be valid also for trade of pharmaceutical goods. Nevertheless, the major influence on the trade of pharmaceuticals does not come from directives but from various verdicts of the European Court of Justice.

Several cases concerning parallel importation have been judged by the ECJ. It is primarily the pharmaceutical companies, which have brought parallel distributors to the ECJ for violating patent protection. Some of these cases refer to infringement of regulations regarding safety and information to patients. The latter refers to re-packaging procedures and translation of instructions to the patients, which is necessary for parallel-import from one Member State to another. The parallel-distributors have made references to the Treaty of Rome about free trade movement of goods between the Member States. As there is no specific directive about this kind of trade, the verdicts from the ECJ have had a large impact on the trade of pharmaceutical goods.

The first major ECJ case *Centrafarm v. Sterling Drug* (1974) concerned a drug imported by Centrafarm to the Netherlands from the UK where the price was only fifty percent of the Dutch price. The original manufacturer referred to Article 30 in the Treaty of Rome where a number of reasons for introducing import restrictions were given - price differentials between the countries and claims that the sale of the imported drug, intended for another country, might lead to the diffusion of defective drugs among patients as information, pack sizes etc. were tailored to the conditions in the market of origin. The Court did not accept that any of these grounds were sufficient for the import restrictions according to the justifications mentioned in Article 30 (Cornish 2000).

Some of the most significant cases in recent years concern the Danish parallel importer *Paranova*. The case *Bristol-Myers Squibb and others v. Paranova* (1993) concerned the interpretation of Directive 89/104/EEC. This directive deals with the right of an original manufacturer to stop trade with its products (and brands) if the product concerned has been changed or distorted after being launched in the market. The crucial issue concerned the right of a parallel-importer to re-pack products already launched in the market and to attach new information material. The Court stated that, partly as a consequence of similar cases, re-packaging is not by itself a reason to implement import restrictions. This verdict has been interpreted by some domestic regulatory agencies in the Member States as an encouragement by the ECJ of parallel importing and intra-brand competition throughout the EU in order to achieve the objective of a single market. Thus a product, originally intended for a specific country or market, could be repacked by an alternative firm and then sent for importation to other countries and markets. In the later case *Paranova v. Pharmacia-Upjohn* (1999), the ECJ also accepted that the parallel-importer could also change the trademark to that of the original supplier in the imported country. The overall interpretation of the verdicts in a number of cases concerning parallel import shows that the ECJ has not accepted the conditions for different types of import restrictions that original manufacturers have tried to implement. All these measures have been interpreted as infringement with the principles of free trade. It is clear that the principle of free movement of goods and services has superiority over the protection of patent and the incentives for innovative research and development. It is, however, not specifically stated that parallel import is allowed or encouraged, but the verdicts have eliminated the potential and existing obstacles that have been or could been used against parallel import. It is also important to state that each Member State could interpret the verdicts in their own way and thereby influence the extension of parallel import. One such domestic regulation, which is in place in all Member States, is the decision to approve which companies should be allowed to act as parallel importers.

The Swedish regulatory agencies have, to a large extent, accepted the ECJ verdicts and have interpreted them in a way that makes parallel import increasingly feasible. Parallel imports in Sweden started in January 1997 with importation of the ulcer drug Losec from low-price countries within the EU, originally manufactured by Astra Hässle, by the parallel importer Cross Pharma, which is still the largest company among parallel importers in Sweden. Thereafter, the sales of parallel imported drugs have increased dramatically and the number of original drugs for which there are parallel imported drugs is estimated at approximately fifty drugs, but the number of parallel imported drugs is even higher. The number of parallel importers is at present around ten. The parallel importation in Sweden is estimated at approximately 8-9 % of the total pharmaceutical sales in Sweden (Table 7).

Table 7: The development of parallel imported drugs in Sweden 1997-2000

Year	Approved parallel imported drugs	Parallel-imported drugs (importation value in million SEK)	Share of total pharmaceutical market
1997	1	269	1.9%
1998	45	1,007	6.1%
1999	269	1,396	7.6%
2000	601	--	--

Source: Läkemedelsindustriföreningen 2001

The development shows a dramatic increase and the number of approved parallel imported drugs indicates that there is a potential for further increase. In order to make parallel importation profitable for the parallel importers it is necessary to achieve a minimum level of sales volume. Turnover varies substantially between specific drugs. The sales are highest for Losec (ulcer disease), Pulmicort (asthma), Plendil (hypertension/angina pectoris) and Sandimmun (immunisation drug) which together represent around 60 % of the total parallel importation within the Drug Benefit Scheme in Sweden. The share of parallel importation is largest for Sandimmun and Pulmicort, 84 and 78 percent respectively (Riksförsäkrings-verket 2000).

Within the EU there has been parallel importation since the 1970s, but on a very small scale. This trade was not regulated by specific directives and not subject for any court proceedings. It was mainly during the 1990s that a number of parallel-importers started to challenge the time-limited monopoly that patent protection gave to the original manufacturers. In Table 8 the share of parallel importation for a number of EU/EEA-countries is shown.

Table 8: The share of parallel importation as percentage of total pharmaceutical sales in some EU/EEA-countries (%)

Country	1995	1997/98	1999
Austria	--	<1	--
Denmark	9	11	--
Germany	2	2	--
Netherlands	12	14	--
Norway	--	5	--
Sweden[6]	--	2	9
UK	8	7	--

Source: Riksförsäkringsverket 2000.

The existence of parallel-importation is limited to a number of EU countries such as Denmark, Germany, Netherlands, Sweden and the UK. Even if the share of parallel-importation is limited and small, there is a clear trend of an increase of share of the total pharmaceutical sales within EU. The extent of parallel importation is determined by several factors. It requires a certain sales volume of the drug in question in order to make the import profitable. The regulations of the distribution system are also of major importance in order to facilitate effective parallel importation. The practices of wholesale distributors and pharmacies are regulated regarding the choice of products they have to offer and how the competition between drugs for same therapy should be handled. There are different

---

[6] The share in the Swedish market differs slightly between tables 7 and 8 due to different calculation methods.

practices between Member States due to traditions and norms when it comes to disposal and supply of drugs. Since both doctors and patients are accustomed to certain packages and doses for drugs, this heterogeneity makes replacement of products more difficult. The practices of wholesale distributors and pharmacies are sometimes also regulated in order to influence consumer choice and competition between drugs. Distributors might be regulated when it comes to informing patients about the differences between drugs included in a country's Drug Benefit Schemes. This monitoring of consumer choice will influence the choice of drugs. As an example, the public pharmacies in Sweden inform patients about the cheapest drug for a therapeutic group with similar products. Since parallel importation partly relies on comparability and homogeneity of products, all such differences in the distribution stage makes trade more difficult.

The favourable prices that can be observed for parallel-imported drugs do not necessarily imply corresponding savings for other part of the health care sector. There are also extra costs for parallel-importation. These concern costs for transportation and re-packaging drugs from low-price countries to high-price countries. The procedure of re-packaging and translation of information to patients is closely regulated and controlled by public authorities according to EU directives. In addition there are extra costs for storage of imported drugs. The distributors handle some of these costs, but an essential part is borne by retailers. These costs have not been calculated but there are concerns that these costs in some cases might offset the lower price of the imported drug. Hence, if one considers the total costs for parallel-importation the societal savings might be less than might initially appear. In order to be profitable it is estimated that parallel-importation of a drug requires at least a ten percent price-difference between the countries. For some drugs with a large sale smaller price-differences could be profitable.

8.2 Generic drugs

The parallel-importation of pharmaceuticals is not the same as the trade in generic drug, which refer to drugs with identical chemical substances as an original drug where the patent protection has expired. Parallel-importation could be accomplished for all kind of drugs, but given the necessity of a minimum price-difference it is concentrated on original drugs. The issue of generic drugs has not been as controversial as the parallel importation of original drugs. The pharmaceutical industry more-or-less accepts price competition after the patent protection has expired. The industry has also launched their own generic products after the patent expired for their original product. This has given manufacturers of original drugs a clear advantage over generic manufacturers, as generic products also have to be approved. By having access to documentation of test and clinical trials the original manufacturers could enter the generic market more rapidly. The EU Directive 87/21/EEC, which stated that the procedure for generic drugs could be shortened through a number of simplified routines, essentially reduced these differences in the entrance costs to the market. Generic products can nowadays be excepted from the documentation requirements regarding results of pharmacological and toxicological test in clinical trials, given that these results have been performed previously and the results published. If there are essential similarities between a generic product and a chemical entity already approved within EU, the generic application can be approved for the same indications. This directive has facilita-ted access and lowered the costs for entrance to the market for generic manufacturers.

8.3 Price differences and subsidises

The price-control system in Sweden was abandoned January 1, 1993 and price setting is in principle free. However, as stated before, it is not enough for a drug producer to trade a drug across the border and accept (or influence) a market price, without additional reimbursement from a third party payer. Hence, in practice there is price control through the reimbursement system[7]. The comprehensiveness of the drug reimbursement system has traditionally been rather generous. Once a drug is approved and accepted to be sold in the market, price-negotiations between the manufacturer and the National Social Insurance Board take place. Almost all approved drugs are automatically included in the reimbursement system. However, there is negotiation about the price in order to control total expenditures. The total sales effect in the pharmaceutical sector is a function of change in volumes, change in price and switch to new pharmaceutical products. The impact of these different explanatory variables is shown in Table 9.

Table 9: The cost increase components in pharmaceutical sales in Sweden, selected years
1989 – 1998, using pharmacy purchasing price incl. VAT

Year	Sales increase total	– of which due to price increase	– of which due to volume increase	– of which due to switch to new drugs
1989	10.3%	2.6 %	3.2 %	4.2 %
1995	12.7%	2.5 %	3.8 %	6.0 %
1998	16.2%	0.3 %	9.5 %	5.8 %

Source: Läkemedelsindustriföreningen 2001

According to Table 9, the price of drugs is diminishing as a cost-driving factor - one reason for abandoning direct price-control. The major contributory factors are the increased volume and the switch to new drugs. This development shows the importance of a third party payer aiming at controlling total expenditures through rationing the volume of drugs and controlling the price-setting of reimbursed new drugs. Since almost all financial responsibilities of pharmaceuticals covered by public reimbursement will be handled by the county councils system, it is likely that the control will be even harder in the future. Currently there is a division of the decision to set negotiated prices/reimbursement for new drugs and the financial responsibilities FOR pharmaceutical costs. In the future the same authority will probably make both decisions. One scenario is that the approval of a drug will not automatically mean that it will be covered by the benefit drug scheme.

As mentioned earlier, the price difference for pharmaceuticals between the Member States is the necessary condition for parallel importation. This condition has existed for several years and there are several explanations why prices for the same good differ across markets and consumer groups. In countries where the pharmaceutical industry has an important role in the overall economy and for employment, there is a tradition with higher prices and distinctive protection of intellectual property rights in order to encourage innovative corporations (e.g. Germany and the UK). In countries with small or insignificant pharmaceutical industries there are examples of weak or non-existent protection for patents. At the same time the price-regulating agencies have only strived for cost containment and low prices on drugs. Furthermore, the pharmaceutical companies set or negotiate different

---

[7] Still, it is possible for a pharmaceutical company to stay out of the reimbursement system and set its own price, since the reimbursement system is voluntary.

prices for the same drug in different countries depending on the ability to pay. This behaviour was possible as long as the market was marked off with little "spillover" of differences in price-strategy exercised by the pharmaceutical industry. One way to measure the effects of EU regulations and verdicts that have opened up parallel importation is to analyse the development of the price differences. Figure 8 presents the price differences for 150 most sold drugs in eleven European countries in a study conducted by the Swedish Pharmacies.

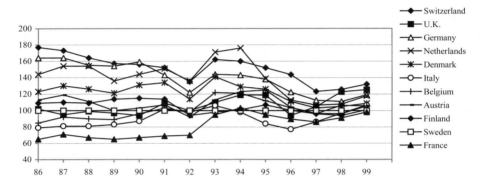

Fig. 8: Swedish prices of a set of drugs compared with ten European countries (Sweden =100, each year) (Source: Apoteket AB cited in Riksförsäkringsverket 1999)

The figure shows that there has been a "price-corridor" in Europe and the EU, which has been reduced during the late 1990s. This coincides both with the directives aiming at standardised packages and with verdicts from the ECJ concerning the interpretation of the conditions for introducing trade restrictions. The introduction of uniform rules for trade and expansion of parallel trade also coincides with this development. Price comparisons of drugs, however, suffer from several methodology problems and should be interpreted with some caution. There are problems concerning standardisation and size of packages, inclusion of different distribution costs, exchange rates etc. Nevertheless, the changes of a number of regulations have most likely forced the pharmaceutical industry to revise previous price-settings strategies and has reduced the scope for price-discrimination. It is uncertain what consequences a harmonisation of prices will have for access to drugs in countries with lower ability to pay for drugs. Within the EU it might be feasible to preserve a general price-level among the present Member States. The problem is much larger on a global level and also for an expansion of the EU to Eastern Europe where the ability to pay would differ from the EU average.

As was shown in the section on approval and trade of pharmaceutical goods, there was a contrast between Swedish export and import for different groups of countries. The export show high increases for EU countries and the North American markets, whereas the picture for import was more diversified. In Table 10 the development of the Swedish import of pharmaceutical goods is shown separately for those countries with high and low price levels respectively. The low-price countries are defined in two ways: one broader group (A) and a narrow group with only the countries with the lowest prices (B).

Table 10: The development of Swedish import of pharmaceutical goods from EU countries with high and low prices on pharmaceutical goods, in million Swedish Crowns (SEK)

EU countries	1995	1996	1997	1998	1999	2000	2000/ 1995	1999/ 1995
High price[1]	3,785	4,123	3,709	3,562	4,513	4,708	+24%	+19%
Low price A[2]	405	560	1,041	1,427	1,831	1,770	+337%	+352%
Low price B[3]	145	226	569	1,012	1,247	1,135	+685%	+762%
Total import	4,977	5,453	5,616	6,134	7,664	8,018	+61%	+54%

[1] Denmark, Finland, Germany, Netherlands and UK

[2] Austria, France, Greece, Italy, Portugal and Spain

[3] Subgroup of 2, namely Greece, Italy, Portugal and Spain

Table 10 indicates a sharper increase of imports of pharmaceutical goods from countries with a low prices and limited pharmaceutical industry since Swedish EU membership in 1995. The countries with low price levels, especially group B above, also show a negative balance of trade for pharmaceuticals goods. It is also obvious that the import of drugs has increased at more rapid speed from countries with limited pharmaceutical sector and an increasing import from low price countries. Naturally the level of import is higher from countries with a large pharmaceutical sector, but the trend after EU membership is clear. These figures might also have been influenced by more recent decisions in EU. For example the already mentioned verdicts from the ECJ about parallel trade might be of equal importance.

9. Unintended effects

Unintended effects are consequences and outcomes that were not expressed in the directives or could not be concluded by referring to its content. Furthermore, these effects could be positive or negative for different actors including consumers and for a country as a whole. To what extent there are unintended effects due to directives is a matter of judgement since all potential effects are not clearly specified in the directives.

An objective of the system with collaboration between approval agencies was to create identical information about products approved within the EU. The centralised procedure for approval was mainly aimed at facilitating entry and access to one large market. In order to achieve this the central approval procedure was established through co-operation and joint approval decisions. This procedure has not only led to a more rapid approval process, but also to extensive collaboration and exchange of information between national approval agencies. From the approval agencies' perspective this procedure has increased their joint capacity to handle the dramatic increase in complexity and mass of knowledge that have been developed in biotechnology during the last decade. One important effect of the collaboration between the approval authorities among the Member States is the advantage of a critical mass and exchange of information. Due to increased complexity in the research process of new chemical entities, the single national authorities have difficulties in keeping up to date with the latest developments. Hence, the collaboration and exchange of information have put them in a better position in relation to the pharmaceutical industry, where the merger trend has created similar concentration of knowledge.

As competition exists among the approval agencies, there is a fear that this competition will lead to a shortening of the examination time and that the quality of the approval will be deteriorated. Earlier studies also shown large variation of the examination time for new drugs. In Table 11 the recent figures on number of approvals and examination time is presented.

Table 11: Number of trials and examination time for approvals, 1997-1999

Year	Number of protocols	Share executed within 6 weeks (%)	Median number of days until execution
1997	578	86	42
1998	531	82	40
1999	522	91	39

Source: Lakemedlsverket 2000

It is too early to judge the effect of competition between the agencies. So far, the results do not show any drastic change of examination time that would indicate that the procedure has changed or quality deteriorated. The pharmaceutical industry believes that the EU approval process has resulted in reduced time for market authorisation.

The criteria for approving a new chemical entity differed across Member States before the principles of reciprocal and/or joint approval were introduced. The Swedish criteria for new approvals were rather strict and the effect of a new drug has to be significantly better that the ones presently in the market. With the criteria used by EMEA and the mutual approval principle, a new chemical entity can be approved with only minor improvements of the effect. An unintended effect for some countries like Sweden has been that the number of brands for almost the same type of chemical entity has increased dramatically. Drugs with minor improvements compared with present ones have been approved and, as a result, an increased supply of drugs with similar effects is noticed. The consequences of this increase of supply has been discussed in terms of confusion among patients but also unnecessary costs for information and marketing of products with almost identical effects.

The decision to approve a new chemical entity is closely linked to the decision to subsidise the new drug in different Drug Benefit Schemes. Previously most countries automatically included newly approved drugs in their Drug Benefit Scheme. Most countries have now separated these decisions. However, in Sweden this seems to have had an unintended effect since the older criteria for new drugs limited the number of products. From this follows an unintended effect in terms of more approved drugs that are not subsidised. This might have several implications for the choice of prescribed drugs as well as consequences for the patient-doctor relationship for such decisions.

10. Closing remarks and conclusions

Health services are, given their characteristics, largely locally produced and consumed goods. The major input factor – labour – is geographically located closed to the production unit. As a service good it is also consumed in the same area as it is produced. Hence, there are natural limits for trade of inputs as well as outputs. People in general are also reluctant to travel long distance for obtaining health services elsewhere. The major exception from these characteristics is the production and consumption of drugs. Pharmaceutical goods are probably the most transferable input factors in the production of health care.

The EU legislative framework and directives regarding the pharmaceutical market have, to a large extend, been transposed to the pharmaceutical sector in Sweden. The domestic legislation follows closely the directives from the European Commission and the verdicts from the European Court of Justice. As shown in the report these measures focus on the supply side of inputs for the health care sector at large. The purpose seems to be that the health care sector, as any other sector, should have the advantage of a free market when it comes to the use of inputs, pharmaceuticals in particular, but also for labour and perhaps capital. Since this type of trade does not differ from other sectors where providers demand inputs, the general principle from the Treaty of Rome should be in place. The present of a third party payer makes this freedom more complex on the consumer side since patients demanding drugs and other treatments are not faced with the total costs of their consumption.

The EU legislative framework has mainly been concerned with the approval procedures, patent protections, standards for distribution and marketing, and less with influence of price regulations and the design of reimbursement and drug benefit systems. The centralised approval procedure and co-operation between national regulatory authorities have improved the position for these agencies in terms of better capacity to deal with the continuing increasing complexity in the approval process of new chemical entities. By co-operating and sharing information and knowledge about the same new products, these regulatory authorities are a par with (or at least little inferior than) the multinational pharmaceutical industry. Another important consequence is that the centralised approval procedure would lead to a clear separation of the decision to approve a new drug and the decision to subsidise it.

The other principal objective of EU pharmaceutical directives has been the development and competitiveness of the European pharmaceutical industry in the global context. For multinational pharmaceutical corporations, access to the U.S. market has been hugely important for many years. Access to the US market is gained through the approval process controlled by the Food and Drug Administration (FDA). With one single positive decision by FDA potential sales for the largest world market are opened up. The procedure with one application for the entire EU-market has reduced both the transaction and time costs for the industry. This might in the future contribute to increasing the importance of the European market in comparison with the U.S. market.

A set of EU decisions (directives about standardised packages, verdicts about parallel import) has clearly facilitated the development of parallel import of drugs. Without these EU decisions this type of trade of drugs would probably have been much less significant. The effects for pharmaceuticals also differ across the different sub-markets. It is clear that the major impact is found for the prescription market and to some extent the OTC market. The market for use of drugs in hospital inpatient treatment is a more straightforward seller-buyer relationship, whereas the prescription market is a complex system with the patient-doctor relationship and different arrangements for payments and financial responsibilities.

Overall the impact of EU directives and verdicts is mainly at the regulatory and delivery side. The regulation of the approval procedure is the major consequence of EU regulations, whereas the verdicts from the ECJ have had an impact on the delivery and trade of drugs. The financial arrangements are to a large extent intact although the issues have been raised regarding the appropriateness of the responsibility distribution and sequences of decisions.

The impact of EU directives and regulations on the pharmaceutical market has focused on both the supplier-side (input) and the consumer-side (output). The results from the Swedish case study show that EU policy has mainly influenced different aspects on the supply side or input side. Since health service organisation and health care financing is primarily the concern of national governments, questions of pricing, subsidies, inclusion of drugs and services in benefit schemes etc. are regarded as national issues by most policymakers. Pharmaceuticals as goods or parts of a service share this problem with any health services, in the same way as outpatient visits and inpatient treatment. As long as the patient bears the full cost of these services and goods the principle for a single market is almost fulfilled. However, around 70-90 percent of health services is financed through some type of third party payment, private or public. A harmonisation of prices and subsidies would require a fundamental change of the way in which citizens' right for health service is defined. The question could be formulated as follows: "Is a single market for drug treatment (or any other service) possible without a harmonisation of third party payers' policies?"

References

Abraham J, Lewis G. Harmonising and competing for medicines regulation: how healthy are the European Union's systems of drug approval? Soc Sci Med 1999;48:1655-67.

Andersson F. The distribution of pharmaceuticals in Europe – current and future trends in wholesaling. Health Policy 1994;27:271-92.

Cornish WR. The free movement of goods I: pharmaceuticals, patents and parallel trade. In: Goldberg R, Lonbay J. Pharmaceutical Medicine, Biotechnology and European Law. Cambridge: Cambridge University Press; 2000.

Earl-Slater A. Recent legal and policy developments affecting the EU pharmaceutical business environment. European Business Review 1997;97:267-78.

Henriksson F, Hjortsberg C, Rehnberg C. Pharmaceutical expenditures in Sweden. Health Policy 1999; 47: 125-44.

Lakemedelsverket. Arsredovisning [Annual report]. Uppsala: Lakemedelsverket; 2000.

Leidl R. EC health care systems entering the Single Market. In: Normand C, Vaughan JP, editors. Europe without frontiers: the implication for health. Chichester: John Wiley & Sons; 1993. p. 111-8.

Leidl R, editor. Health Care and its Financing in the Single European Market. Amsterdam: IOS Press; 1998.

Landstingsförbundet. Upphandling av läkemedel [Public procurement of drugs]. Stockholm: Landstingsförbundet; 1998.

Läkemedelsindustriföreningen. Fakta 2000. Läkemedelsmarknaden och hälso- och sjukvården [Facts 2000. The pharmaceutical market and health services]. Stockholm: Läkemedelsindustriföreningen; 2001.

Norris P. The impact of European harmonisation on Norwegian drug policy. Health Policy 1998;43: 65-81.

OECD. OECD Health Data 2000. Paris: Organization for Economic Cooperation and Development; 2000.

Riksförsäkringsverket. Prissättning av läkemedel – svenska läkemedelspriser i ett internationellt perspektiv [Price-setting of Pharmaceuticals – Swedish drug prices in an international compairson]. Stockholm: RFV redovisar 1999: 10.

Riksförsäkringsverket. Parallellimporterade läkemedel – inte till vilket pris som helst [Parallel imported drugs – not just to any price]. Stockholm: RFV redovisar 2000: 6.

Statistiska Centralbyrån. Nationalräkenskaperna [National accounts]. Stockholm: Statistiska Centralbyrån; various years.

Taylor DG. Europe without frontiers? Balancing pharmaceutical interests. In: Normand C, Vaughan JP, editors. Europe without frontiers: the implication for health. Chichester: John Wiley & Sons; 1993. p. 283-94.

The European Union and Health Services
R. Busse et al. (Eds.)
IOS Press, 2002

The impact of the SEM on the medical devices market in Sweden

Mona SUNDH and Barbro RENCK

Abstract. Until 1993 the area of medical-technical products in Sweden was only partially regulated. The move towards EU membership was seen as a chance to overhaul existing legislation and to develop a fully fledged system for standardisation and surveillance of medical-technical products. The chapter demonstrates a considerable impact of SEM directives on Swedish legislation and institutional settings. It appears that larger companies, compared with smaller ones, have had a somewhat easier time to adapt to the requirements, take part in standardisation processes and in deriving greater benefits from the CE labelling. Smaller companies producing exlusively for the domestic market are facing disadvantages due to the additional workload. Healthcare personnel is affected from the EU legislation too. Medical technicians are now covering larger areas of responsibility. The chapter also indicates that the system of reporting accidents and narrow escapes within the EU may not work sufficiently well.

1. Introduction

Healthcare in Europe is of a high technological standard and is rapidly developing. The rapidly expanding technological developments facilitate continual improvement in diagnostic techniques and treatment (Svenska Läkaresällskapet and Spri 1997), and medical technology and products are regarded as necessary components of modern healthcare. Internationally, there are estimated to be 400,000-700,000 medical-technical products or about 6,000 product types in the market (Liedström 2000). Most of these are relatively simple while others are complex combining different technologies (Socialstyrelsen 1998). Within the EU, Germany is the country representing the largest market for medical devices and which invests the greatest resources. Germany is followed by France, the United Kingdom, Italy and Spain (Altenstetter 1998).

The annual turnover in medical-technical products in Sweden is estimated to amount to 12-15 billion Swedish crowns. Sweden exports 8.5 billion crowns worth of medical-technical products each year (Liedström 2000). In 1999 the turnover in the sale of medical-technical products in the EU was approximately 41 billion Euros (Swedish Healthcare Supplier Association, oral information).

To guarantee a sufficiently high degree of quality and safety with the use of medical-technical products within EU Member States, the EU has developed three main directives within the area of medical-technical products. The directives are also aimed at protecting the free movement of goods in such a way that they have the goal of harmonising the laws and institutions of Member States as they pertain to security, health protection and the performance of medical-technical products to inhibit the dissimilarities which can occur concerning trade within the Union. Altenstetter (1998, p. 142) draws four conclusions:

"First, European integration in the field of medical devices is the result of a combination of scientific push factors and industrial pull factors, as well as strong commercial and political pressures in a climate of globalizing influences and the growing interdependence of national economies.

Second, to the extent that regulatory policy on medical devices existed in the past, it was largely intertwined with industrial and R&D policies in which state actors had an interest in.

Third, the rise in healthcare expenditures has placed political pressures on all actor groups involved in the delivery and management of healthcare systems to prove to the financing authority (payer) that they are getting 'value for money'.

Finally, as my review of the international literature on technology assessment in healthcare and the many gaps in knowledge [...] shows, scholars seem to be unaware that medical devices constitute a research field worthy of study."

As opposed to, for example, the United Kingdom, which is generally regarded as the most developed with respect to market surveillance of medical-technical products in Europe (Bergman 1999), until 1993 Sweden only regulated the area of medical-technical products to a limited degree (Liedström 1995). The first time the area was referenced in a Swedish state investigation was in 1977 (Liedström 2000). The National Board of Health and Welfare, which in Sweden is the central administrative authority for healthcare and which has responsibility for monitoring medical-technical products, established in 1977 an advisory panel for medical-technical safety. During the 1980s, however, a number of serious accidents occurred in Sweden, which also perhaps served as a wakeup call. The tragic dialysis accident in Linköping, which claimed the lives of three patients, became a warning signal. According to Liedström, these perhaps were most dependent on weaknesses related to the division of responsibility. Then came the accidents with the mechanical heart valves, which pointed to technical problems (Liedström 2000). These cost the lives of more than 40 patients.

In the spring of 1985 the Swedish government established a commission on medical-technical safety. The work resulted in a report on medical-technical safety (Social-departementet 1987). The report contains a proposal for a law on the control of medical-technical products. However, the government did not propose such a law until six years later. The reason for the long delay was the movement towards the EU and the European Economic Area (EEA) agreements. Through the EEA agreement to which Sweden gradually acceded, Sweden agreed to adjust its rules for the manufacture, control and sale to meet the requirements of EU directives (Hallgren & Westberg 1995). Liedström (2000) maintains that many of the rules which were later included in the EU's medical-technical directives were already a part of the 1987 Swedish report. Interest within the EU at this time had increased concerning the regulation of the whole medical-technical product field – approximately 700,000 products existed in the world market at the time (Liedström 1994).

According to Liedström (2000) an important consideration of the EEA agreement for the producers and importers was to remove eventual technical barriers to trade (TBT). A TBT is considered to exist when a country has, for example, special national technical requirements for a product or special requirements for trade in a good or product, which in effect make it impossible for international exporters to penetrate the market. Because of the problems concerning technical barriers to trade, a special TBT group within European Free Trade Association (EFTA) was empanelled which focused on the medical-technical product area. This group cooperated with the European Commission and they also worked to establish cooperation with the Commission's civil servants. The effort to cooperate was reflected later within the work on standardisation, which occurs in the Comité Européen de

Normalisation (CEN) and the Comité Européen de Normalisation Electrotechnique (CENELEC) as well as their governing bodies.

2. EU directives on medical products and definition of medical products

After a range of directives regulating particular technologies, three main EU directives have been adopted in the 1990s concerning medical-technical products (Table 1).

Table 1: Relevant European directives (main ones in bold)

Council Directive 76/764/EEC of 27 July 1976 on the approximation of the laws of the Member States on clinical mercury-in-glass, maximum reading thermometers

Council Directive 83/189/EEC of 28 March 1983 laying down a procedure for the provision of information in the field of technical standards and regulations

Commission Directive 84/414/EEC of 18 July 1984 adapting to technical progress Directive 76/764/EEC on the approximation of the laws of the Member States relating to clinical mercury-in-glass maximum-reading thermometers

Council Directive 84/539/EEC of 17 September 1984 on the approximation of the laws of the Member States relating to electro-medical equipment used in human or veterinary medicine

Council Directive 88/182/EEC of 22 March 1988 amending Directive 83/189/EEC laying down a procedure for the provision of information in the field of technical standards and regulations

Council Directive 90/385/EEC of 20 June 1990 on the approximation of the laws of the Member States relating to active implantable medical devices

Council Directive 93/42/EEC of 14 June 1993 concerning medical devices

Council Directive 93/68/EEC of 22 July 1993 amending Directives 87/404 EEC (simple pressure vessels), 88/378/EEC (safety of toys), 89/106/EEC (construction products), 89/336/EEC (electromagnetic compatibility), 89/392/EEC (machinery), 89/686EEC (personal protective equipment), 90/384/EEC (non-automatic weighing instruments), 90/385/EEC (active implantable medicinal devices), 90/396/EEC (appliances burning gaseous fuels), 91/263/EEC (telecommunications terminal equipment), 92/42/EEC (new hot-water boilers fired with liquid or gaseous fuels) and 73/23/EEC (electrical equipment designed for use within certain voltage limits)

Directive 98/79/EC of the European Parliament and of the Council of 27 October 1998 on in vitro diagnostic medical devices

The first directive (90/385/EEC dated 20 June 1990) concerns active medical-technical products for implantation. By active it is meant that the products are powered by some form of electrical energy source or other source of energy other that that which is directly produced by the human body.

A considerably more encompassing directive for medical-technical product types such as expendable supplies, dental materials and handicap aids as well as medical-technical appliances and equipment is the Commission Directive 93/42/EEC dated 14 June 1993. This directive specifies the requirements and regulations for testing, certification and labelling of such products.

All medical-technical products (except for specially adapted products and products which shall undergo clinical testing) shall be CE labelled in order for them to be marketed within the community. The requirement for CE labelling is that they have undergone certain verification requirements. CE is an abbreviation of the French name for the EU, Communauté Européenne. CE labelling does not, as noted above, infer that a registration entity has approved the product or that the product has a certain quality or performance. CE labelling must instead be regarded as evidence that the product has the right to circulate within the community, that is to say a sort of passport for the product in the EU. A further prerequisite to receive the CE label, if it is not manufactured within the community, is that there is an authorised representative for the product within the community. If a registration entity participates in product verification, the numerical code of the entity is provided with the CE label.

This directive, as well as the others, shall be introduced into the Member States in such a way that the spirit and intent are not lost. National special requirements above those included in the directive are not acceptable with few exceptions (Liedström 1995). The primary purpose of the directive is to ensure product safety (Socialstyrelsen 1998). The introduction to the directive refers to varying procedures for the testing and certification of medical-products from Member State to Member State. This served to create obstacles to trade within the Community. The purpose of the directive is therefore also to make the four freedoms a reality, in other words the right for free movement over borders for goods, services, capital and people (Liedström 2000). This presupposes that a harmonisation will be achieved. In the product directive, the general definition of medical-technical products is complemented with a more precise determination of, among other things, complementary definitions of active medical-technical products, active medical-technical products for implantation, specially adapted products, products intended for clinical examinations, products intended for clinical testing as well as for in-vitro diagnostics.

A third directive – the directive for in-vitro diagnostic medical-technical products (98/79/EC) – was adopted by the European Parliament and Council of Ministers on 27 October 1998. It concerns an area which is undergoing profound development involving, according to Liedström (2000), almost a fifth of all medical-technical products. The directive encompasses medical-technical products for in vitro diagnostics which are manufactured from tissue, cells or substances of human origin. Several new aspects in the directive also concern the above mentioned directives. One of the aspects is that the directive provides for the establishment of a European database of registered manufacturers and products. Also included are the provisions for special measures concerning health monitoring and new responsibilities for the reporting entities.

The Swedish Law on medical-technical products (1993:584) provides in § 2 a general definition of medical-technical products, namely as every product which according to manufacturer's information shall be used, separately or in combination with another, on people exclusively or mainly to

–   show, prevent, monitor, treat or alleviate an illness
–   show, monitor, treat, alleviate or compensate for an injury or functional disablement
–   examine, change or replace an anatomic or physiological process or
–   check fertility.

The term product refers to 'loose items' (Liedström 2000). Examples of medical-technical products include sterile one-time use items and other disposable items, needles, knives, dialysis appliances and various forms of implantation.

It should be noted that certain products are on the borderline as to whether they fulfil the requirements for and are controlled by the directive, which applies to medicine or medical-technical products. Such products are referred to as combination products, by this is meant that medical-technical products most often combined with medication. For this type of product, it is very important that the manufacturer clearly reports the purpose of the product because it can be decisive which directive applies to the product.

Whether or not a product is counted as a medical-technical product is also dependent upon the information listed in the manufacturer's product declaration. One exception, in which the directive for medical-technical products does not apply, concerns individually manufactured or 'in-house production', that is to say those products which are manufactured or modified within healthcare and which are not intended for the market. Examples of this type of product can be those for research and/or development work or a product adapted to a particular physician's requirement for a special solution. Each individual member country has the prerogative to regulate these types of product for safety. In Sweden the National Board of Health and Welfare has composed the regulations and general advice (SOSFS 1994:21) for these types of products.

3. Purpose and methods

This chapter investigates the impact of the legislation and rulings introduced to implement the single commodity market for medical devices and to allow suppliers to cross borders and sell their products in other countries. Another goal is to describe how the central authorities and organisations have worked with implementation questions concerning medical-technical products in healthcare in light of Directives 90/385/EEC and 93/42/EEC. Further, it aims at describing how the directives for medical-technical products and its Swedish implementation really function in a healthcare district using the county council of Värmland, Sweden.

Directive 98/79/EC only went into effect on 7 June 2000. The instructions and general advice of the Swedish National Board of Health and Welfare (SOFS 1999:24) implemented the directive in Sweden. This directive was adopted at a time in which the major portion of the data in this study had already been collected. It was also not possible to conduct supplementary interviews to research this directive, as the timing of the adoption did not provide an adequate opportunity to generate effects in the operation during the period under study. Therefore, the study does not address the effects of this directive in healthcare and on the public authorities, manufacturers and so on.

Qualitative methods using the technique of network sampling or snowball sampling were used to get in touch with prospective subjects for this study. This involved the sampling of subjects based on referrals from other subjects already in the sample, an approach that may be used when the research population consists of individuals with specific knowledge in a field who are difficult to identify by ordinary means (Polit & Hungler 1987). The data have been collected at the national level through telephone interviews and personal interviews. Representatives for the Federation of County Councils, the National Board of Health and Welfare, Health Care Standardisation Institute (HSS), Healthcare Suppliers Association (SLF) and Siemens-Elema AB as well as Swede Rescue AB were interviewed. In addition an interview was conducted with a consultant who has many years of experience at the regional, national, international levels. Data has even been collected at the regional level in the County Council of Värmland in which interviews were conducted with medical technicians, purchasing officials and a head physician. The choice of Värmland was based on practical considerations in light of the limitations on time among others.

In order to study as carefully as possible how those at the regional and national levels work with medical-technical products and the laws and regulations in the area study information was collected through reports, brochures, diverse information materials, fact sheets among others. Current information available on the Internet has also been reviewed. In the following text, interviews and other sources of information will be presented together.

A semi-structured interview guide was used for the interviews, which were recorded on tape and transcribed. The interviews were analysed manually. All the transcriptions were coded according to the interview questions but also in relation to other sources of information. When appropriate, quotations from the interviews, which sometimes give a more detailed picture of an occurrence or opinion, have been included in the text.

4. Impact on national legislation and national authorities

To assess the effects of the Single European Market on the health services of Member States, an analytical distinction between impact and outcomes has been made. While outcome refers to the direct effects on financing, managing, delivering and regulating health services, impact analytically focusses on intermediate issues such as juridical and institutional settings. Therefore, in this section the impact of Single European Market interventions on national legislation, institutional settings and the economy will be analysed.

4.1 Impact on national legislation

The main law transposing Directives 90/385/EEC and 93/42/EEC into Swedish law is the law on medical-technical products which encompasses all products with a medical purpose

Table 2: Transposition of Directives 90/385/EEC, 93/42/EEC and 98/79/EC into Swedish legislation

Law by Number	Title
	Transposition of Directive 90/385/EEC
SFS 1993:584	Law on medical-technical products; changed through SFS 1994:860 and 1997:1236
SFS 1993:876	Ordinance on medical-technical products; changed through SFS 1994:1518, SFS 1995:1158
SOSFS 1994:2	The instructions and general recommendations of the National Board of Health and Welfare concerning active medical-technical products for implantation
SOSFS 1994:3	The instructions and general recommendations of the National Board of Health and Welfare concerning the obligation of the manufacturer to report accidents and narrow escapes involving medical products.
SOSFS 1994:21	The instructions and general recommendations of the National Board of Health and Welfare concerning the responsibility for medical products in healthcare among others
	Transposition of Directive 93/42/EEC
SFS 1993:584	Law on medical-technical products changed through SFS 1994:860 and 1997:1236
SFS 1993:876	Ordinance on medical-technical products; changed through SFS 1994:1518, SFS 1995:1158
SOSFS 1994:3	The instructions of the National Board of Health and Welfare and general requirements concerning the obligation of the manufacturer to report accidents and narrow escapes concerning medical-technical products
SOSFS 1994:20	The instructions of the National Board of Health and Welfare concerning medical-technical products, changed through SOFS 1998:12 and 1999:23
SOSFS 1994:21	The instructions of the National Board of Health and Welfare and general requirements concerning the responsibility for medical products in healthcare among others
	Transposition of Directive 98/79/EC
SOSFS 1999:24	The instructions of the National Board of Health and Welfare and general requirements concerning medical devices on in vitro diagnostic.
SOSFS 1999:23	The instructions of the National Board of Health and Welfare on changes in the regulations and general areas (SOSFS 1994:20) Medical-technical products.
Responsible department: Ministry of Health and Social Affairs	

(Liedström 1995). The law covers both CE and non-CE labelled products, specially adapted products as well as products for clinical testing. The law on medical-technical products has been in effect since 1 July 1993. It was complemented later in year with an ordinance. In addition, an ordinance (1994:1518) was issued concerning changes in the previous ordinance (1993:876) on medical-technical products. The laws and ordinances were adapted to the three medical-technical directives of the EU that were introduced successively. Further came the statute book of the National Board of Health and Welfare, SOSFS 1994:2 respectively SOSFS 1994:20 (complete transposition cf. Table 2).

Since 1 January 1995 active medical products for implantation are certified, that is to say, subject to a judgement of the register entity in order to be marketed. Verification commenced for other medical-technical products at the same time. The other products that are covered by the medical-technical directive have been divided into four different classes. Class I encompasses those least risky products that do not require any evaluation by a third party such as, for example, a registration entity (see the section on registration entities for an explanation) in order to be released in the marketplace (the participation of registration entities however is required concerning sterility and measurement accuracy). The overwhelming number of products falls into this class. Class IIa refers to those having an increased risk and requiring evaluation by the registration entity. Products in class IIb and III have a high risk potential and must function well in order for patients or others not to suffer injury and they must therefore be evaluated by the registration entity.

The directives which were issued for medical-technical products are written according to 'the New Approach' which among other aspects denotes that it is the responsibility of the Member State authorities to ensure that the various actors work according to the rules but that they do not have the task of granting permission to companies to market and sell their products.

4.2 Impact on the distribution of responsibilitites and accountabilities

The class to which a product belongs is determined by the manufacturer, but if the manufacturer and a registration entity are of different opinions the National Board of Health and Welfare will decide. It can also happen that a product, after it has been on the market for a while, is transferred to another class because injuries or narrow escapes have occurred or because technological progress and research has rendered the earlier class designation suspect.

The use of technology places high demands on those who work in healthcare and with technology. Accidents and narrow escapes can occur if the products on the market are not safe or if those who use them do not have sufficient knowledge concerning how the technology works and for what the product is intended. Appendix 1 to SOSFS 1994:20 (a Swedish adaptation of directive 93/42/EEC) contains a description of how risk is measured during the use of medical-technical products. It reads as follows:

> "the risks in using products shall be acceptable with regard to the advantages to the patients and consistent with a high health and safety level."

To ensure that there is as little risk as possible during the use of products the manufacturer shall ensure that the risks are eliminated or reduced as much as possible. If the risks cannot be completely alleviated sufficient protective measures shall be taken. The user shall be advised concerning remaining risks. One way, among others, to reduce risk is the recommendation that the manufacturer's declaration of medical-technical products should (Liedström 2000) contain information concerning the purpose of the product and who may use the product, that is to say physicians, nurses or other professionals. The declaration shall also indicate where the product may be used as well as which environmental requirements apply. Through the written declaration the manufacturer can limit its responsibility, among other ways, in the event the product is used in way that is not intended and an accident should occur, in which case the manufacturer has in essence no responsibility. Another requirement for the product instructions is that they shall be in writing or translated into the language which is used in the country of intended sale. An exception for the requirement of product instructions exists for class 1 and class 2 products under the condition that they are so simple to use that they can be used without more guidance. A European register of the products that are in compliance with the CE requirements and Vigilance reports, that is to say all products, is under construction. According to Liedström (2000) there are over 24,000 products in class 1 register maintained by the Swedish National Board of Health and Welfare.

The responsibility for showing that the product meets the product requirements for CE labelling rests with the manufacturer of the product. However, when the product has a higher class than class I this judgement must be done in cooperation with the registration entity (see below).

Two reasons exist (Liedström 2000) for a product not requiring CE labelling. One is that it is a specially adapted product that is manufactured according to the written instructions of an appropriate medical professional and according to the needs of a specific patient and such not for the market.

The second reason is that it is a product that shall undergo clinical testing. The requirement for clinical testing is relatively new and applies to those products whose attributes cannot be verified in any other way except through clinical testing. Those products that perhaps are most likely to be in need of clinical testing, according to the instructions of the National Board of Health and Welfare, are those active medical-technical products for implantation and products in classes IIb and III. To commence a clinical test of a product, an ethical committee must approved the design and an application must be filed with the authorities in the country in which the test shall be conducted. This authority the has 60 days in which to grant the required permission for the test or to reject the application. A fee of 10,000 Swedish crowns (approximately € 1,000) is required upon filing the application and is paid to The National Board of Health and Welfare. Then the National Pharmaceutical Authority reviews the design of the clinical test on a consultant basis.

Registration entity refers to the national administrative entity which reports the names of testing laboratories to the Commission, which have sufficient competency according to the applicable directives in the area to conduct third party certification. Table 3 provides an overview of the differences in responsibility between state-based authorities and notified bodies.

The Swedish government has appointed the Swedish Board of Accreditation and Conformity Assessment (SWEDAC) to test laboratories. SWEDAC reports the names of approved laboratories to the Commission and they receive a unique identification number which always must be provided in conjunction with the CE label. The authority which appoints the registration entity has a responsibility for ensuring that the registration entity has sufficient competency with which to carry out its responsibilities. Because of its responsibility, for example SWEDAC in Sweden, they must carefully follow the registration entity's work. They must also, if it is so required, to demand improvements and changes in the activity and they also have a responsibility to halt the work of registration entities if they are not performing their work satisfactorily.

Table 3: Breakdown of responsibilities by tasks and implementing agent

	Notified bodies	National authorities
Focus of EU intervention	Pre-market stage	Implementation
		Enforcement
		Post-market stage
Tasks	Conformity assessment	Surveillance of the market
	Quality assurance investigations	Vigilance
	EC Type examination	Clinical systems
	Statistical verification	
Decision is within	EU and EEA	Territory of the Member States

Source: N. Anselmann, European Commission, personal communication and Altenstetter 1998, p. 121

The requirements that are placed on registration entities are that they shall be competent and impartial. They many also not be directly involved in the construction, manufacture or marketing among other aspects of products. Nor may they represent the company or partner which is occupied with these activities. The requirement for integrity denotes also that the representative entity and those that work there "shall be free from all pressure from people and companies with an interest in the final result, especially of the economic kind, which can affect judgement" (Liedström 2000, p. 25). Furthermore the personnel of the registration entity have a confidentiality obligation. The requirements that they place on the registration entity shall also be place on eventual sub-suppliers. In Sweden there are three registration entities: Semkom AB, the National Pharmaceutical Authority and the State Testing Establishment. The applicable registration entity has the responsibility for cancelling or recalling a manufacturer's certificate if they are guilty of departing too radically from the requirements that are placed on medical-technical products.

A manufacturer has the right to choose a registration entity and can thus use an entity from another EU country. Germany has the highest number of CE-approved notification bodies and private certification bodies. Following Germany are the United Kingdom, Austria, the Netherlands and Belgium. These countries are in contrast with many other EU countries in which there are only a few notification bodies. In some of the new and potential EU countries there is a need to build up this activity from the ground up (Altenstetter 1998). Within the EU the problem has aroused awareness of the problem that even if all of the registration entities are accredited according to the same quality standards, there can occur differences between the entities depending upon, for example, the experience and abilities of the personnel. To counter these differences, emphasis is placed on common training of evaluators, common meetings and the possibility for exchange of work visits. Even the registration entities and the defined businesses which are on the threshold of applying have provided recommendations concerning how the medical-technical directives shall be applied.

On the level of healthcare institutions, the responsibility for ensuring that the laws and regulations concerning medical-technical products are followed rests with the head of healthcare. The operational responsibility for the use of products resides usually with the directors of the healthcare facilities (Liedström 2000). The personnel who work within healthcare and who use medical-technical products also have a certain responsibility. Their obligation is to perform functional checks as needed of the products before they are used, to use the products in the way intended by the manufacturer and to not use such products if they do not feel they are capable of using them.

4.3 The National Swedish Board of Health and Welfare

While the previous sections focused on the impact of EU-legislation on Swedish legislation an general institutional questions the following sections are more specific in regard to two Swedish key institutions.

The National Swedish Board of Health and Welfare is the authority performing the function of oversight concerning medical-technical products. This is provided for in ordinance 1994:1518. The Medical Products Agency's corresponding responsibilities during a transitional period concern factory sterilised one-time use articles and contraceptive produces which are not CE labelled. The National Board of Health and Welfare (through ordinance 1993:876 on medical-technical products as well as ordinance 1994:1518 on changes in ordinance 1993:876) is assigned the right to decide if the law on medical-technical products should also apply to other products that are used in the medical-technical system or in another way are closely similar to medical-technical products in use.

The National Board of Health and Welfare shall communicate instructions on the requirements for medical-technical products and the conditions that are needed for the protection of life, personal safety and health for the patients, users and others (Liedström 1995).

As the responsible authority with the area the National Board of Health and Welfare handles specific matter which can concern, for example, the assignment of product classes and the requirement of labelling as well as the decision concerning clinical tests among others. Another task is to raise the issue concerning the payment of fines. A further extensive task for the National Board of Health and Welfare is to coordinate with other authorities and organisations which are currently active both within and outside the country. Much of the resources of the National Board of Health and Welfare with the area are used for information to manufacturers, users and others. They also participate in the international work on standardisation. Under discussion at the time of writing was the proposal to transfer the review of the medical-technical products to the Medical Products Agency. If implemented, this should result in the National Board of Health and Welfare reviewing product use and the Medical Products Agency receiving the assignment to handle registration.

Since the 1930s Swedish healthcare has reported the number of deaths and serious injuries as well as the risk for such in accordance with the Lex-Maria system. However, the problem with the Lex-Maria system is that they only report narrow escapes or accidents which lie outside known problem areas or do not result from known complications. The cases which are reported are investigated and collected afterwards in the National database. Accidents and narrow escapes involving medical-technical products were reported during 1974-1994 to the National Board of Health and Welfare advisory council for medical-technical safety. After analysis they were published in yearbooks. The National database thereafter has included the reports. However, this situation changed with an EU directive and currently it is required that all serious events and/or narrow escapes with CE labelled medical-technical products be reported by the manufacturer to the responsible authority according to the so-called Vigilance system. In Sweden the professionals are even obliged to report serious incidents. The manufacturers are thus obliged to immediately commence an investigation of the reason for what had occurred. Further, the manufacturer is obliged to establish and maintain a "Post Market Surveillance System" which means that they continually monitor the practical use of the products they sold (Liedström 2000).

Another way to acquire knowledge and information concerning accidents and narrow escapes with medical-technical products in Sweden is the collaboration within the Foundation Kanalen (the channel) which exists between medical-technical departments in healthcare. Even the National Board of Health and Welfare has access to this information.

A difficulty with the manufacturer's obligation to report accidents or narrow escapes to the responsible authorities is that it presupposes a close contact between the user and the manufacturer. This contact is not always so close and can therefore result in the system of reporting accidents and narrow escapes to function ineffectively. Furthermore, the interviews in the study illustrate the difficulty in eliciting reports of accidents/narrow escapes from personnel. Perhaps this results from a fear on the part of the personnel that they will be held responsible. This occurred during an accident involving dialysis in the 1980s. Also the workload of healthcare personnel may serve to cause them to choose not to report near misses in the absence of a serious accident. The interviews in the study show that this can be some of the reasons, so few accidents/narrow escapes are reported within Swedish healthcare.

In 1998, 259 Vigilance reports were filed in Sweden (Liedström 2000). The corresponding number in the United Kingdom was 6,298, and in Germany 1,134 reports were made the same year. Swedish experts find it difficult to explain the difference in the number of reports, but of course a partial explanation may lie in the actual differences in the size of population among the countries. A further factor may be, according to Liedström, that the United Kingdom has the most developed system for reporting accidents/narrow escapes. With respect to Germany, the system functions differently among the various German states.

4.4 The Swedish Healthcare Standards Institution

A new method – "the New Approach" – has been developing for EU law making, and the directives which exist in the area of medical-technical products are fashioned according to this method. The methods means that the European Commission limit their influence to setting in certain basic, general requirements which are placed upon products, that is to say to avoid technical solutions in its rules system. The directive requirements are aimed at ensuring the health and life of people (Liedström 1994). When a directive is issued the Commission can, in accordance with "the New Approach", delegate the task of developing specific technical specifications to the European organisations on standardisation CEN, CENELEC or the European Telecommunications Standards Institute (ETSI). Liedström (2000) defines a standard as a voluntary agreement between interests who want to find a common solution to a problem which is often of a technical nature. The purely technical descriptions of the requirements of the directives may be found in the standards.

Within the European healthcare context 20 technical committees and 38 working groups consisting of scientists and specialists work to develop and produce standards in the area. In addition to the European standards that developed by CEN and CENELEC there are also global, national and industrial standards. A European standard is of great importance among other things because Member States have six months, after a standard has been adopted, to introduce the respective standard and then it is common for all of the Member States. Standards that are ordered by the European Commission are referred to as mandated standards. One of the interviewees from the Swedish Healthcare Standards Institution expressed the following views concerning standards:

> "The standards are a help, an implement, for the companies so that they can acquire CE labelling for their products. A sort of security instrument for knowing that close instructions are there and exactly what applies, for example, for wheelchairs. How the safety shall be adapted."

The same individual also pointed out that the standards also have great importance for purchasing because the law on public purchasing places requirements that existing standards shall be referred to, that is to say the required specifications shall be based on standards if such exist. He still points out that the knowledge concerning this can be insufficient.

The HSS is responsible for Swedish standardisation within the health and medical services. HSS is also Sweden's official spokesman in the European standardisation work within healthcare and represents Sweden in the CEN (1994).

Approximately 120 Swedish businesses, which in various ways work with medical-technical products, participate in the work on standardisation. Those at HSS identify three very clear reasons why companies should participate in the work on standardisation despite the fact that it costs them time and money:

1. The companies have an interest in influencing technical requirements in the standards, as they will want to assure themselves that the standards contain requirements which coincide with how they think in their company.
2. Through participating in the work one gains access to information which other firms only receive after the standards are complete. Those companies which participate in the work thus have a head start as they have had more time to adjust to the requirements which will be included in the standard.
3. Through participating in the work companies develop many contacts and a useful network.

Technical standardisation is a central part in European cooperation and many barriers to trade have been removed through the common standards which have been created. If the Commission approves the work the standards are published in the Official Journal and it is referred later as a harmonised standard.

According to (2000) as of the autumn of 1999 approximately 200 mandated CEN and CENLEC standards became harmonised standards within the medical-technical area. Liedström (2000) maintains in his book that the need for standards in European is great and there is an actual need for a further approximately 50 product type standards.

5. Intended and unintended outcomes

The impact of the Single European Market on Sweden in regard to medical devices is undeniable. As argued above, far reaching changes in terms of adapting Swedish legislation, introducing new tasks and redistributing institutional responsibilities and accountabilities, has taken place. Yet the question remains, to what degree the intended objectives hves been met and if uninteded effects can be observed.

In general, there is a clear trend towards the effective adaption of the standardisation and surveillance mechanisms proposed by European law in the day to day routines of the Swedish health service. Nevertheless, for various reasons the effective implementation takes some time. This is especially due to the fact that the dissemination of the new rules of standardisation and surveillance requires considerable time and, especially for techinicians in healthcare institutions, the new law attributes new roles and responsibilities and implements new processes.

Yet, not all of the elements of the new rules on standardisation and surveillance seem to work sufficiently. As a matter of fact, the new legislation creates an unwillingness among healthcare personnel to report all accidents and narrow escapes since the messenger is afraid of taking the blame. While this problem might be fixed in the future, it has been reported that small and medium sized companies are facing difficulties to adapt to the new circumstances and are facing competitive disadvantages. While the evidence provided is partly derived from interviews and therfore not as robust as statistical figures, the argument behind the complaint is highly plausible. It deserves attention, especially in the light of the fact that the Commission has always put an effort into the support of small and medium sized companies. Moreover, there is some concern that the SEM in the field of medical devices may turn out as a disadvantage for Swedish research in and production of medical devices. While it is difficult to tell wether this danger would have occured with or without European integration, the SEM does not seem to give Sweden in this field a stronger position.

5.1 Slow but steady process of dissemination

The interviews show that the authorities and organisations together with others have invested much work on information. Before and just after the law went into effect most of the information was aimed at companies because they regarded them as needing a longer time to be able to redirect production so that they were able to follow the new law. During the work to get out the information before the law on medical-technical products went into effect, a certain worry was noted, above all from the small companies. There were also those who, despite much information, still had not digested the contents of the new law. Through the information work of the National Board of Health and Welfare and the Healthcare Supplier Association, the situation is now much better. One of the interviewees, who works as a consultant in the area, put it this way:

> "Today I know that the members of the Healthcare Suppliers Association are well out front. They have handled this well and they supply approximately 80 percent of all the products to healthcare, so the situation is calm in this corner."

The next priority group for the information work were the caregivers and in this instance the interviewee suggested that there had been problems. This could depend upon those responsible within healthcare: hospital administrators, politicians, head physicians among others had a poor understanding of the law and its resultant regulations. The insufficient knowledge was described by the interviewee as serious but difficult to correct as this group of leading actors prioritised other questions. Written information worked poorly as it could often end up collecting dust on the shelf. A system is necessary to reach the right person directly. The problem is that they often have too many other tasks to manage or handle with greater priority. This problem remains to a great extent and much is necessary to solve it according to the interviewee consultant. Another problem area, which the interviewee raised, concerns the weakness in purchasing. During the interviews with the companies they expressed the desire for greater knowledge about, among other things, the requirements that products must meet to include them in the activity which is responsible for the purchase of products. They suggest that the lack of knowledge sometimes contributes to a buyer placing incorrect demands which can increase costs and so on.

5.2 New roles, tasks and uncertainties for medical technicians

Those directives which have been introduced into the Swedish law on medical-technical products have meant changes for medical technicians. Among others, the broader definition of medical-technical products has meant that the medical technicians are now responsible for a larger area of responsibility. A medical technician interviewed indicated that he himself had not had the possibility to work with everything but instead chose parts. A very current discussion within the profession is who shall implement repairs and handle the maintenance of the medical-technical products.

The work of medical technicians have become increasingly of a theoretical nature since the new law on medical-technical products was introduced. This is illustrated by the following quotation:

> "That which we do in the workshop on a daily basis concerns more and more theoretical job functions for which the clinic needs support. Ten years ago we turned on the soldering iron when we came in the morning ... today we turn on the computer when we come in the morning."

The interviewed medical technician notes that a time-consuming and important part of the activity is currently to check that the manufacturer specified the use the equipment has and to monitor that those at the hospital keep to these uses. Another important task is to be responsible for the personnel receiving adequate training for the apparatus that is being used. To participate in purchasing is also time-consuming for the medical-technicians.

One of the interviewees who represented HSS comments also that the directive has involved great changes for medical technicians. Before the requirement for CE labelling, professional medical technicians could personally decide on modifying apparatus or building a new one. Currently, this is impossible. The interviewee maintains that the medical technician could regard the change brought about by the new rules as taking away parts of their responsibility. The technical developments within healthcare are considered to have made it more difficult for medical technicians to master everything. The developments also change the work of the medical technician.

The medical technician commented also that it is now less usual that medical technicians manufacture their own products or make small changes in finished products because of the requirement of CE labelling. This can result in increased cost to healthcare because they are thus forced to buy new products when earlier it would have been enough to adjust existing equipment.

5.3 Unwillingness to report accidents and narrow escapes

An unintended outcome of Directive 93/42/EEC is that, according to legislation, the manufacturers have the obligation to report serious events. However, many countries within the Community lack a national law according to which the user has the same obligation to report. Businesses can find it difficult to maintain such tight contact with customers such that it is not possible to fulfil the reporting obligation effectively (Liedström 2000). Liedström holds that the system of reporting of accidents and narrow escapes within the EU may not work sufficiently well until the National Board of Health and Welfare (or corresponding authority in other Member States) demand that users of medical products are obliged to report accidents and narrow escapes to both the manufacturer and the oversight authority. According to Liedström it is likely that only about one percent of all the narrow escapes are reported or this situation is on its way to occurring. However, during an interview it was commented that there are problems even when users are obliged to report accidents and narrow escapes. The interviewee maintains that it depends upon the fact that during earlier accidents (for example, the accident involving dialysis in the 1980s) personnel were pointed out as the guilty parties. This has led to the unwillingness of personnel to report incidents or narrow escapes as long as they do not result in obvious injuries. The unwillingness to report also results in manufacturers not receiving information which could lead to improvements in their products. According to Lindström, one solution of the problem could be to introduce what exists now in the air force, that is to say "no-fault reporting". This denotes that the person who reports an incident shall not automatically be released from responsibility but it shall be regarded as a merit that the person reported the incident.

During an interview at HSS doubt was expressed concerning how the National Board of Health and Welfare can monitor that businesses classify their products in a correct way. The interviewee reported that there are companies which deliberately attempt to classify their products in a lower risk class to reduce the demands, for example, of involvement of the registration entity.

A further problem brought about by the directives on medical-technical products is that several of the interviewees pointed to a certain insecurity concerning what applies during the transition period between the time a directive is decided and until it begins to apply. Here there exist problems for the manufacture, user, seller among others. The following citation is from an interview with a medical technician which illustrates that people in the activity also have problems with learning everything about the legislation. The citation is an excerpt from a conversation concerning how local manufacture at the hospital is documented:

> "I have a personal manufacturing routine here and this routine requires that a risk analysis and evaluation protocol and other things which come about be kept and collected. We have it but, for example, this type of ad hoc construction which always worked for these years; we do not today have documentation and a review. We don't have time and space in healthcare to go so far with something as we always have done and which we know works."

The above citation points even to the directive causing increased need of trained medical technicians and the medical technician maintained that much of his work day was devoted to following directives and legislation. This can be viewed as a paradox as the directive is mainly aimed at the manufacturers. That it takes so much time, he maintains, depends upon the need to "interpret" the text in the directives and the legislation in light of the activity as well as the consequences they get. According to the interviewee is not self evident from the beginning but it takes time and effort in the activity so that everything is ready.

According to Liedström (2000) many acute care hospitals, healthcare centres, municipal home healthcare and so on is under supplied with technical competency. At the end of the 1990s there were medical departments at only half of Sweden's acute care hospitals. One way to work with the shortages is that the National Board of Health and Welfare has begun to formulate the requirement that the user shall be sufficiently competent to operate special equipment. One idea is to introduce a "driving license" for personnel who work with technical equipment. The shortage of medical technicians in the activity can also, according to the interviewee who now works as a consultant within the field, lead to people within healthcare not performing a so-called arrival check when a new technical apparatus arrives at the facility. A person cannot know if, for example, an electorcadiogram machine (ECG-machine) delivers a correct measurement. It is a problem, according to the interviewee, as studies show that more than every other product has faults or shortcomings upon arrival. The reason thus far can be that the company's quality control is deficient.

Another problem which arises is that the ethical committees in the respective countries who evaluate applications for the commencement of clinical testing command varying degrees of knowledge and competency and that they therefore can shift in their evaluations of applications for clinical testing. According to Liedström (2000) this weakness has not been recognised sufficiently.

The work of developing standards and the origin of standards is regarded as positive and there are among all the parties an orientation that recognises this as very important work and that everyone benefits when common standards are developed. Despite the positive orientation, worries and problems can nevertheless be discerned. According to Liedström, one problem is that there are too few competent people within the area who can work in the technical committees. Risks can also exist that competing companies and their interests will complicate the work with the origin and form of different standards. The work to develop standards often takes a long time depending upon if there are many who shall agree and for it to work for all the parties in all countries. Furthermore, some of the interviewees maintain that language can be a problem for some countries, especially for us Swedes and others who do not have any of the "major languages" as a mother tongue.

5.4 Larger companies adapt easier to new circumstances

According to the interviews for this study manufacturers and others prefer standards which describe performance and what a person will achieve with a certain product. The interviewees also thought that it would be better to transfer to the companies how to decide how the technical details can be best solved. The businesses interviewed maintain that if the standards were not formed according to this system, instead they risk slowing developments.

The investigation revealed that the larger companies have as a general policy to participate in the standardisation work. Perhaps they are over-represented in relation to smaller companies who do not have enough resources to participate to the same extent. One interview with a smaller company confirmed the problem with resources which can hinder participation in standardisation work. The smaller companies can also find it difficult to participate for such a long period which is often the case when a standard is being developed. This can mean that a certain skewed division in the standardisation work as well as the smaller companies finding it difficult to follow developments in the area. Another difficulty is that the users of medical standards seldom if ever have the possibility to affect the design by contributing their experiences and needs.

5.5 Smaller and medium sized companies struggle

The interviews with representatives for the authorities and companies revealed that for smaller companies that did not have any ambition or possibilities to sell their products outside their own country, the law has involved major problems and few profits. This is illustrated through the following citation:

> "If you are a small manufacturer in Gnosjö, for example, and stand and bend iron which is sold somewhere in the hospital and do not have any ambition to sell it anywhere else, perhaps only to the nearest hospital. Then all these European regulations and CE labelling is a curse, purely and simply."

Obstacles to the free movement of goods may exist when it come to selling one's products to other countries even if one has a good product and the ambition to sell to the whole of Europe. This can be because the buyers sometimes have unexpressed demands to buy products from their own country. Language is regarded as another obstacle. Small and medium size companies do not have sufficient resources to answer quotations, advertisements or to respond to questions which are written in language other than Swedish or possible English. In an interview with a representative for a small company it was expressed that they experienced the directives and standards sometimes leading to over regulation. Within the same company they experienced that the EU sometimes regulates events that they never believe will happen. That small businesses experience the situation in this way is, according to the interviewed consultant, hardly surprising because the form of the directives essentially has been a question between the large companies and the public sector in Europe.

A representative for a large medical-technical company maintains that for the enterprise he represents the new directives have not caused any problems. This is regarded as to a large degree being dependent on parts of their products being adapted to American requirements since a few years back. The knowledge therefore already exists within the company. Nor has the registration entity caused any major problems for this company.

> "Knowledge and experience of both the business leaders and the organisation and our way of writing quality system handbooks and corresponding materials, it is been a modest, shall we say, expansion of that. It has not involved any extremely large steps which I could imagine it might be for a number of other companies that do not have this experience. … But the adjustment takes time and involves training and it costs money and such. Against the background of the 'Green Papers' we've seen that it pays gradually but we haven't seen it yet."

Another problem for the companies, especially the small and medium-size businesses has been to follow up sold products, how they work, eventual accidents or narrow escapes and so on. According to the law on medical-technical products, this is the responsibility of the company. The medical technician expressed it this way:

> "The suppliers are supposed to check on sold items afterwards and shall really go out in some way and learn how good the equipment is and withdraw that which is faulty. But I don't know how ... I have not seen our suppliers out and learning about it – in principle we do it for them and tell them about it if it is not good."

The same individual also points out that it is ultimately the head of the clinic or other activity that is responsible for all of the medical-technical products in the facility and which are used there. However, the manufacturer has the supreme responsibility. One head of a clinic that was interviewed noted how difficult it is to live up to the requirement. A tough workload and lack of knowledge were offered as excuses.

5.6 Sweden as a research and manufacturing location for medical devices

The representative of a large medical-technical firm maintained that companies in Sweden did not lose anything through the directives or their implementation. On the other hand, he noted that Sweden as a nation has lost some of its previous possibilities for development of new products. This, he says, is connected to the idea that when there many new products were developed, healthcare in Sweden was under development. New hospitals and clinics were being built and investments in machines were made, among other things. There was also time for certain research and to test and develop new products for technicians and others who worked within healthcare. Often this occurred in cooperation with business. The interviewee noted that, on the other hand, today the company he represents only cooperates with a very small number of university clinics and often the test of new products "worldwide" also begins very early.

> "Germany is more important than Sweden and France is more important than Sweden and the USA is more important than Sweden. We are a small country. The unfortunate fact is that we are beginning to lose the initiative a little bit for developing new things in Sweden. I do not believe that companies suffer so

much, because business is big, multinational and so on, but we as a laboratory and manufacturer here in Sweden suffer from it and Swedish researchers and clinics suffer from it. But the company does not suffer so much from it; it is that which is the regrettable part of this equation. Businesses make it, the big companies and the multinational companies make it better than individual nations, unfortunately."

6. Conclusion

The report maintains that three important directives concerning medical-technical products have been adopted by the EU. It should be noted that manufacturers of medical-technical products have been very positive to the directives and that the manufacturers have even served as a driving force for their adoption. The great question and the one which this report has sought to illuminate is the effect the directives have had on healthcare and manufacturers among others. The studies identifies both intended and unintended effects.

Before Sweden adopted the law (1993:584) on medical-technical products and other legislation within the area, a massive information effort was made by the National Board of Health and Welfare as well as the industry organisation – the Healthcare Suppliers Association.

According to the interviews which were conducted for this study, the application of the legislation functioned satisfactorily among manufacturers and distributors among others. The study however shows that the smaller companies have the greatest difficulty in meeting the requirements. The companies which do not have the goal of selling outside the country in which they are located now must comply with a number of extra reporting requirements under the directive while the positive effects have been of marginal benefit to this type of company. The interviews with representatives for the larger companies indicate that they have not had any appreciable problem in fulfilling the requirements of the directives, but they also indicate that the expected great benefits have not been realised as, for example, access to the whole EU market for CE stamped products should have entailed. The representative interviewed however suggested that these benefits may be realised in the long run.

One difficulty is that the responsible parties within healthcare have problems in living up to the undertaking which resulted from the directives. The study shows that there is also a problem that the information concerning the directives and their effects does not reach the responsible parties in healthcare. Further, the study points to the need for a deeper understanding of the requirements concerning medical-technical products among those involved in the purchase. Sometimes incorrect requirements are placed on products which, for example, can result in the equipment costing more than is necessary.

The directives and the subsequent national legislation have meant great changes for the work situation for Swedish medical technicians and purchasers in that the scope of their work has expanded. Their work has also become more theoretical in nature. This development is something of a paradox in that the directive in the first instance is focused on manufacturers. The study however shows that the directive's text must be "interpreted" by healthcare personnel and this takes a good deal of time and effort from other aspects of the organisation's activities. This has also resulted in many emergency hospitals, primary healthcare centres, municipal home health services and so on are not sufficiently endowed with technical competency. The lack of medical technicians in the organisation can result in those within healthcare, for example, not performing so-called arrival checks upon the acquisition of a new piece of medical technology. If these checks are not performed, it is not possible to confirm if the apparatus was delivered with the correct measurement calibrations and so on.

The study also shows that the work with standards is important and that a number of standards are necessary. The work of developing standards and the origin of standards is regarded as positive and there are among all the parties an orientation that recognises this as very important work and that everyone benefits when common standards are developed. Despite the positive orientation, worries and problems can nevertheless be discerned. Smaller companies can have problem with resources that can hinder participation in standardisation work. This can mean that a certain skewed division in the standardisation work as well as the smaller companies finding it difficult to follow developments in the area. Another difficulty is that the users of medical standards seldom if ever have the possibility to affect the design by contributing their experiences and needs. Risks can also exist that competing companies and their interests will complicate the work with the origin and form of different standards. The work to develop standards often takes a long time depending upon if there are many who shall agree and for it to work for all the parties in all countries.

The study shows further that efforts need to be made to ensure that the system of reporting accidents/narrow escapes functions satisfactorily. Experts estimate today that only one percent of all accidents/narrow escapes which happen, or are in the process of happening, are reported.

A further area which displays shortcomings concerns the ethical committees in the respective countries who shall evaluate applications for the commencement of clinical testing command varying degrees of knowledge and competency and that they therefore can shift in their evaluations of applications for clinical testing. According to one of the experts interviewed, this weakness has not been sufficiently recognised.

Acknowledgements: *The authors are grateful to Göran Liedström for all of his help and excellent advice during the conduct of the study. We also wish to thank him for taking the time to review the contents of the report, a contribution which greatly facilitated its preparation. Furthermore we wish to thank the Federation of County Councils in Sweden for economic support during the project.*

References

Altenstetter C. Regulating and financing medical devices in the European Union. In: Leidl R, editor. Health Care and its Financing in the Single European Market. Amsterdam: IOS Press; 1998. p. 116-49.

Bergman SE. Myndighetsuppgifter för medicintekniska produkter [The authorities' task concerning medical-technical products], Socialstyrelsen [The National Board of Health and Welfare]: Stockholm; 1999.

Hallgren M, Westberg U. Teknik i vården [Technology in healthcare]. Natur och Kultur [Nature and culture]. Stockholm; 1995.

Liedström G. Medicinteknisk säkerhet och ansvarsfrågor [Medical-technical safety and questions of responsibility]. Vård [Healthcare] October 1994: 3.

Liedström G. Lagen om medicintekniska produkter. Kommentar och handbook [The law on medical-technical products. Commentary and handbook]. Stockholm: Fritze; 1995.

Liedström G. Lagen om medicintekniska produkter. Kommentar och handbok. Andra upplagan [The law on medical-technical products. Commentary and handbook. Second edition]. Stockholm: Nordstedts Juridik; 2000.

Polit DF, Hungler BP. Nursing research - principles and methods. 3rd ed. J.B. Philadelphia: Lippincott Company; 1987.

Renck B, Sundh M. Datasäkerhet inom hälso- och sjukvården efter EU-inträdet [Data security within healthcare after entry into the EU]. Working report no. 8. Centre for Public Health Research: Karlstad University; 2000.

Socialstyrelsen [The National Board of Health and Welfare]. Nya regler för medicintekniska produkter [New regulations for medical-technical products]. Stockholm; 1998.

Socialdepartementet. Medicinteknisk säkerhet. Betänkande av utredningen om den medicintekniska säkerheten [Medical-technical safety. Report of the investigation concerning medical-technical safety]. SOU 1987:23. Stockholm; 1987.

Svenska Läkaresällskapet och Spri. Kvalitetssäkring vid användandet av medicintekniska produkter [Swedish Medical Society and the Swedish Institute for Health Services Development. Quality assurance during the use of medical-technical products]. Stockholm: Spri; 1997.

The European Union and Health Services
R. Busse et al. (Eds.)
IOS Press, 2002

179

The SEM and the public procurement of goods and services in the Andalusian Health Service

Fernando SILIÓ VILLAMIL, Nuria ROMO AVILÉS,
Maria Angeles PRIETO RODRIGUEZ[1]

Abstract. This chapter presents the analysis of the impact of the legal norms in the area of public procurement of goods and services on Spanish healthcare services, using the case of the European legislation on the public procurement services of the Andalusian Health Service (AHS). Two sources of information were used: descriptive data provided by AHS's Public Procurement Service and interviews with the persons in charge of the economic and administrative services of the hospitals and primary healthcare centres. Of the total expenditure on goods and services by the AHS in 1998, approximately 68 % was done via public procurement. The new procedures have led to an improved organisation of the services, greater objectivity and improved advertising and transparency when purchasing. At the same time, there have been a number of negative consequences, e.g. it is more difficult to detect needs, it takes longer to make a purchase; in other words, there has been an increase in bureaucracy, or the lack of adaptation to the healthcare sector.

1. Introduction

This chapter consists of an analysis of the impact that the legal regulations on the public procurement of goods and services have on the health services of the European Economic Area. In the first part, public procurement in Spain from a legal point of view is analyzed. The main section of this report presents the case of one of the member states of the European Union, Spain, through a study of the impact of the European regulations on the public procurement mechanisms of the Andalusian Health Service (AHS). At the end, a number of conclusions and recommendations are presented, followed by comparative data for Germany, Sweden and the UK.

2. Public procurement of goods and services: a legal analysis of the Spanish case

2.1 Background

It is estimated that up to 15 per cent of the economic activity of the European Union's member states originates in the public sector to fulfil needs such as public works and supply and services demanded by the public administration. Public procurement, in addition to being one of the essential tools of each administration for its own functioning, has a great deal of influence in the evolution of the industrial and commercial structure of

---

[1] The authors acknowledge the input of Reinhard Busse, Bie Nio Ong and Matthias Wismar, especially regarding section 8.

society. For this very reason, the inclusion of Spain in the European Community has provoked a substantial change in the way public procurement is regulated. The legislative process began in 1986 and concluded with the enforcement of the Public Procurement Act 13/1995 of May 18th.

One of the backbone policies of the European Union in the construction of a single internal market aims to "effectively open the public markets" with the purpose of ensuring transparency of information and contract award procedures. This enables greater opportunities to both suppliers and businesses for developing and carrying out their activities in the Community. The market expansion allows for cost reduction through economy of scale returns and improved efficiency due to the positive effects of competition. Also, the diverse public administrations benefit from greater choice which enables important budgetary savings. Finally, consumers and users benefit from services at a better value for money[2].

The basic principles of public procurement which derive from the directives are: equality, transparency and competitiveness. These are basic principles which have to be complied with in any contract. In the health sector, the new legal framework has caused a revolution, as there is a high level of public procurement in the health sector administration.

2.2. Public procurement in Spain: legal notes

Public procurement in Spain has specific regulations. In fact, the awarding of public works and purchasing of goods and services contracts by public authorities and entities has resulted in a specific category of contracts with its own set of rules. These contracts, called administrative contracts, can be differentiated from private contracts regulated by the Spanish Civil Code.

The most recent legislative precedent is the Spanish Law of Contracts passed by Spanish Decree 923/1965 of April 8th, as well as the Spanish General Regulation of Contracts passed by Decree 3410/1975 of November 25th (Table 1). Both provisions were modified when Spain became part of the European Economic Community. With the Spanish Royal Legislative Decree 931/1986 of May 2nd, the aforementioned law was adapted to the communitarian legal framework while the regulation was modified by Spanish Royal Decree 2528/1986 of November 28th. Thus, the communitarian legal framework has had an impact on the public sector contracts since the accession of the Kingdom of Spain to the European Community.

The most important modifications changed in order to apply fair, transparent and non-discriminatory award procedures with more publicity and openness. This was the mandate included in Directives 77/62/EEC on supply contracts and 71/305/EEC on public works contracts in force at that time.

---

[2] During the time our research was being conducted, the European Commission adopted a package of amendments to simplify and modernise the public procurement directives. The Lisbon European Council acknowledged the importance of this legislative package for the competitiveness of European companies, effective allocation of public resources, economic growth and job creation, and recommended its adoption and implementation by 2002.

Table 1: Spanish legislation on "Public procurement"

– Decree-Act 2/1964 of 4 February concerning the revision of prices in public procurement contracts of the State and autonomous entitities; **currently in force as statutory norm.**
– Decree 923/1965 of 8 April 1965 passing the contents of Public Procurement Act; **abolished.**
– Decree 3637/1965 of 26 November 1965 concerning contracts performed and attached in a foreign country; **abolished.**
– Decree 461/1971 of 11 March 1971 developing Decree-Act 2/1964 of 4 February 1964 concerning the inclusion of revision clauses in public procurement contracts of the State and autonomous entities; **currently in force as statutory norm.**
– Act 5/1973 of 17 of March 1973 amending the statutory law of public procurement; **abolished.**
– Decree 2572/1973 of 5 October 1973 passing the the List of general administrative clauses for contracting equipment and systems for the processing of information; **currently in force as statutory norm.**
– Decree 1005/1974 of 4 April 1974 concerning the contracting of consultancy companies and services; **currently in force as statutory norm.**
– Decree 3410/1975 of 25 November 1975 passing General Regulations in public procurement; **abolished.**
– Royal Decree 1465/1985 of 17 July 1985 concerning the contracting of specific and particular non-customary works in the Administration; **currently in force as statutory norm.**
– Royal Decree 2357/1985 of 17 July regulating the contracting of specific and particular non-customary works in the Administration; **currently in force as statutory norm.**
– Royal Legislative Decree 931/1986 of 2 May 1986 amending the Public Procurement Act to adapt it to the European Economic Community Directives, **abolished.**
– Royal Decree 2528/1986 of 28 November 1986 amending the General Regulations in Public Procurement to adapt it to Royal Legislative Decree 931/1986 of 2 May 1986 and the European Economic Community Directives; **abolished.**
– Act 13/1995 of 18 May 1995 on Public Procurement Contracts; **currently in force.**
– Royal Decree 390/1996 of 1 March 1996 partly developing Act 13/1995 of 18 May on Public Procurement Contracts; **currently in force.**
– Act 53/1999 of 28 December amending Act 13/1995 of 18 May 1995 on Public Procurement Contracts; **in force from March 2000.**

The aforementioned directives were modified by Directives 88/295/EEC and 89/440/EEC respectively. Subsequently, the European Community adopted Directive 92/50/EEC on service contracts, as well as Directives 93/36/EEC and 93/37/EEC on supply and works contracts Such modifications and the signing of the European Economic Area Treaty which entered into force on 1st January 1994 and the Government Procurement Agreement of the World Trade Organization forced the modification of the Spanish legal framework on this subject (Table 2).

For various reasons, and to comply with those directives and agreements, the Spanish Public Procurement Act 13/1995 of May 18th was passed. However, very quickly the new regulation proved incomplete and insufficiently adapted according to the Community's perspective. Directives 93/38/EEC and 92/13/EEC, referring to the so called "excluded" or utilities sectors were not incorporated in time. This shortfall has been corrected by the Spanish Act 48/1998 of December 30th on award procedures in the water, energy, transport and telecommunications sectors, which confirmed their legal independence from the rest of the public sector contracts.

Table 2: Single European Market directives on "Public procurement"

Supplies

– Commision Directive of 17 December 1969 concerning the supply of products to the State, regional bodies and other legal persons in public law (70/32/EEC).
– Council Resolution of 21 December 1976 coordinating procedures for the award of public supply contracts (77/62/CEE).
– Council Directive of 22 July 1980 adapting and completing Directive 77/62/EEC on the coordination of procedures for the award of public supply contracts concerning certain awarding entities (80/767/EEC).
– Council Directive of 22 March 1988 amending Directive 77/62/EEC coordinating the procedures for the award of public supply contracts and derogating some provisions of Directive 80/767/EEC (88/295/EEC).
– Council Directive of 14 June 1993 on the coordination of procedures for the award of public supply contracts (93/36/EEC).

Public Works

– Council Directive of 26 July 1971 concerning the abolition of restrictions on freedom to provide services in respect of public works contracts and on the award of public works contracts to contractors acting through agencies or branches (71/304/EEC).
– Council Directive of 26 July 1971 on the coordination of procedures for the award of public works contracts (71/305/EEC).
– Council Directive of 22 August 1978 amending Directive 72/305/EEC concerning the coordination of procedures for the award of public works contracts (78/669/EEC)
– Council Directive of 18 July 1989 amending Directive 71/305/EEC concerning the coordination of procedures for the award of public works contracts (89/440EEC).
– Council Directive of 14 June 1993 on the coordination of procedures for the award of public works contracts (93/37/EEC).

Reviews

– Council Directive of 21 December 1989 on the coordination of the laws, regulations and administrative provisions relating to the application of review procedures to the award of public supply and public works contracts (89/665/EEC).
– Council Directive of 25 February 1992 coordinating the laws, regulations and administrative provisions relating to the application of Community rules on the procurement procedures of entities operating in the water, energy, transport and telecommunications sectors (92/13/EEC).

Excluded sectors

– Council Directive of 17 September 1990 concerning the procurement procedures in the water, energy, transport and telecommunications sectors (90/532/EEC).
– Council Directive of 14 June 1993 coordinating the procurement procedures of entities operating in the water, energy, transport and telecommunications sectors (93/38/EEC).

Services

– Council Derective of 18 June 1992 coordinating the procurement procedures of public service contracts (92/50/EEC).

Services, supplies, works

– European Parliament and Council Directive of 13 October 1997 amending Directives 92/50/EEC, 93/36/EEC and 93/37/EEC concerning the coordination of procedures for the award of public service contracts, public supply contracts and public works contracts respectively (97/52/EEC).

Also excluded from the public procurement regulations are the contents of the Directives 89/665/EEC and 92/13/EEC on resources. These are control mechanisms set up by the European Community in order to allow bidders to appeal when any discriminatory measures are put into practice in the awarding of public contracts. However, in the Spanish legal framework, such a possibility is facilitated through diverse lawsuits, regulated by legal procedures – mainly the Spanish Contentious/Administrative Statutory Act – which do not require any specific transposition as they are already included in the aforementioned legal procedures.

On the other hand, the European Parliament and Council's Directive 97/52/EEC of October 13th has been adopted. It modifies the current directives on supplies, public works and services. This has resulted in the need to adapt the Spanish legislation to the communitarian legal framework once again. This adaptation can be seen in the recent Spanish Act 53/1999 of December 28th which modifies Act 13/1995 of May 18th on public procurement. Due to the magnitude of its contents and even the necessity, with a few small exceptions, to adopt other provisions to make it viable, the new regulations did not come into force until March 2000. Strictly speaking from a formal point of view, the late incorporation of this sirective into our legal framework is an infringement of European law by the Spanish State, since the deadline for its effective incorporation was October 13th 1998.

Regarding content, the adaptations fulfil two essential aims. First, they reinforce the communitarian principles of publicity, non-discrimination, and competition in order to increase transparency and objectivity in the award procedures. Second, they fulfil the aim of simplifying such procedures as much as possible, as in practice the existence of excessive bureaucracy does not conform with those principles and hampers competition.

The first aim can be achieved by fostering competition. Therefore, even the area of influence of the law has been enlarged, by including even non-public contracts such as banking, financial, purchase of real estate, insurance and intellectual property contracts. All of these areas will come under the rule of the new law concerning their award, despite the fact that in their execution they are ruled by private law. Certain administrative practices are believed to hamper competition, such as the modification of contracts (e.g. extension of their scope), their deferral, the exaggerated length of some contracts, their fractioning to avoid advertisement, or pacts among corporations of the same group which could lead to price agreements or reductions. Thus, under the new law, a contract cannot be extended, low value contracts cannot be renewed or have their prices revised, and they cannot have long execution terms. The terms are limited for public services management contracts, and, as a general rule, unwritten deferrals are forbidden and the concept of price undercutting is defined in greater detail, as well as the ways in which a certain bidder can submit a tender. If such measures are satisfied, there will be an increase in the number of contracts.

As mentioned before, the reverse side of the coin is the excessive bureaucracy in the administration. This is the reason why the proceedings are to be simplified, e.g. with a reduction of the advertising periods, removal of certain requirements such as being up to date in tax and social security payments in order to bid, the non-requirement of award tables in negotiated proceedings, or the new rules for guarantees, both provisional and permanent.

Furthermore, the current reform tries to fulfil certain needs of the public administrations by establishing a clearer distinction between public works contracts and administrative awards of public works by eliminating some contractual forms such as the specific, concrete or unusual works contracts, as well as including, with some limitations, other forms such as financial leasing, leasing with purchase options, and contracts with agencies for temporary jobs. In addition, some strictly technical deficiencies are solved in this reform, although these are not relevant to our study.

The communitarian directives have meant a new concept of contracts in the public sector. As has been pointed out, they have not only enlarged the concept of public contract objectively, but also subjectively. While before, public procurement was essentially defined as being undertaken by a public administration or entity, currently it is also understood to mean those contracts undertaken by private entities but financed by the state budget. Such is the case that, entities under the rule of private trading forces that have purchases financed by public money are also included under the scope of the directives.

If the purpose sought by communitarian law was to foster competition and non-discrimination in order to achieve free movement of capital, goods and services in the public sector, in the internal legal frameworks, especially in those of the so called *Droit Administratif* (France, Netherlands, Italy, Portugal, Spain), the new regulations have also been taken advantage of as corrective mechanisms for certain administrative practices contrary to the law, and which have been named "anti-corruption rules". Despite this apparent coincidence, the truth is that the communitarian legal framework has established a tendency contrary to the public sector's at this time: to increasingly privatise the management and the organisational form of public administration deeds, a fact that has particular repercussions in the case of health services.

2.3 The purchasing system in Spain

The system of purchasing goods and services by the Spanish health centres has undergone a series of changes over the last few years as a result of the Community integration process. The impact of European legislation on the system of purchasing goods and services materialises in Spain through the Act 13/95 on contracts of the public administrations, currently in force, and which derives mostly from Directive 93/36/EEC.

The Spanish Public Procurement Act 13/1995 of May 18th regulates the process of purchasing goods and services by the Spanish public administrations. The main stages in the process are summarised in Figure 1 which is the result of field work in Spain and is also the summary of the process, as described by the persons interviewed. In Book II, Act 13/1995 establishes the publishing regulations in the European Community for the types of contracts according to the amounts involved. It lays down the following criteria:

- Works Contracts: To be published in the Official Journal of the European Community (OJEC) if the amount is equal to or higher than 4,090,831 Euro.
- Supplies Contracts: To be published in the OJEC if the amount is equal to or higher than 163,633 Euro.
- Management of Public Services Contracts: Publication in the OJEC is not compulsory.
- Consultancy and Assistance Contracts: To be published in the OJEC if the amount is equal to or higher than 163,633 Euro.

Fig. 1: Process of public procurement

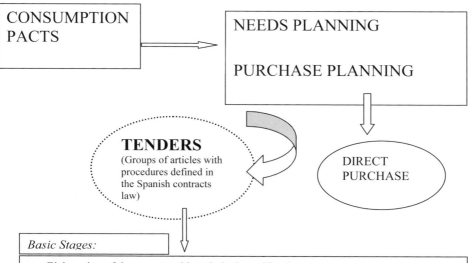

Basic Stages:

- ❏ Elaboration of documents with technical specifications.
- ❏ Elaboration of administrative documents.
- ❏ Agreements on the initiation of files.
- ❏ Report resulting from legal advice. (If it is not favourable, it must be corrected)
- ❏ Intervention through accounting proposal A.
- ❏ Approval.
- ❏ Dispatch to the central services for publication.
- ❏ Presentation of offers during the time limit for publication.
- ❏ Convocation of the opening table.
- ❏ Public reading of economic offers.
- ❏ Mechanization, classification and grouping of offers in the procurement department.
- ❏ Convocation of the technical committee for appraisal of offers.
- ❏ Grouping of the technical and economic report through the award report.
- ❏ Convocation of the award table.
- ❏ In case of approval, the award is proposed to the managing body and accounting document B.
- ❏ *Contract.*

3. Study objectives and methodology

3.1 Objectives

General Objective: To investigate the impact of legislation introduced to implement a more transparent market and fair competition, when the demand of the public sector meets the supply of the private sector, through the companies supplying goods and services in the Spanish health sector.

Specific objectives regarding demand:

1. To describe the main characteristics of the public procurement of goods and services in the AHS, differentiating centres and care levels.
2. To analyse the administrative procedures for the public procurement of goods and services, and to describe the modifications introduced with the implementation of the Spanish Act 13/95 (18th May), on the contracts of the Spanish public administrations.
3. To analyse the opinions of the directors of the AHS (central services, hospitals and health districts) about the impact of Community legislation on their purchasing system.

Specific objectives regarding supply:

1. To investigate the adaptation process of suppliers of goods and services to the new forms of public procurement.
2. To appraise the possible impact of the new legislation on companies supplying goods and services in the AHS.

3.2 Methodology

- Study setting: Andalusia.
- Design: Descriptive cross-sectional study.
- Study Population: Health centres of the AHS and companies supplying goods and services to those centres.
- Study Subjects: Intentional sampling of health centres of the AHS and companies supplying goods and services

In order to meet the objectives, the following quantitative and qualitative research methods have been used in two phases:

- Quantitative analysis of the database available at the central procurement services of the AHS. The analysis has been based on the following variables:
  - Volume of public procurement of goods and services.
  - Relation between the volume offered and the volume awarded.
  - Relation between the volume of public procurement published and total expenditure on the procurement of goods and services.
  - Percentage of tenders published in the Official Journal of the European Communities of the total number of those carried out.
  - Award by types of goods and services.
  - Percentage of centralised and decentralised expenditure.
  - Types of public procurement of goods and services.
  - Companies chosen.

– Qualitative analysis based on semi-structured interviews with economic-administrative directors taken from a sample of primary health care centres and hospitals in Andalusia. The analysis of these interviews has been carried out using the following variables:
    – *Purchasing process*
        – Reasons for the changes in this process
        – Expectations regarding these changes
    – *Volume of contracts performed through public tender*
        – Changes in the types of tender
        – Biennial tenders
    – *Publication in the Official Journal of the European Communities*
        – Volume sent for publication
        – Percentage of the total number of tenders
    – *Administrative process for public procurement*
    – *Call for tenders*
    – *Process of adaptation to European legislation*
    – *Consequences for the market*
    – *Subjective perception of the impact of European legislation and measures taken in order to adapt to the new provisions.*

Andalusia has a total number of 35 general public hospitals. Seven of these hospitals were intentionally chosen, and the decision was based on the size of the hospital and its location within the province. These hospitals are located in four Andalusian provinces and the number of beds available ranges between 530 and 1835.

Among the 34 primary health care districts existing in Andalusia, 8 were chosen. In this case, the selection criterion was hospitals with a higher expenditure than average. These hosptials are also representative of the different Andalusian provinces.

Thus, fifteen centres were selected in total which differ widely both regarding the number of doctors and nurses working in them and the budget available to purchase goods and services. This is an intentional sample, not really a representative one. It is believed, however, that it covers the different procurement services in Andalusia and shows the variations among centres regarding the acquisition of goods and services.

The semi-structured interview has been chosen as a research technique due to the need for information conceptualizing and appraising the impact caused by the European legislation on the purchasing of goods and services, as perceived by the personnel working in the administrative procurement centres. This type of interview was chosen as a qualitative technique to obtain information instead of in-depth interviews because of the need for structured information which could allow comparisons to be made among the different countries participating in the project.

The interviews were carried out in March 1999 in the different centres, in person and by a trained interviewer. Each interview was recorded and subsequently transcribed. The analysis of the information has been performed through a process of contents analysis, complemented by an automatic analysis performed by the computer programme NUDIST.

4. Quantitative results

The total value of tenders (€ 538.47 million) represented 68 % of the total expenditure on current goods and services (€ 786.66 million) in the AHS for 1998. Specialised care (i.e. hospitals) accounted for the biggest shares of both total real expenditure and tendered expenditure, followed by the Central Services of the AHS and their Province Delegations. All the purchase groups acquired their goods and current services mainly by public procurement and in all cases the untendered expenditure was less than 50 per cent: The blood transfusion centres put almost all purchased goods and services on tender (97 %), followed by specialised care (68 %), Central Services (60 %) and primary health care (51 %).

If the total amount tendered is analysed according to the purchaser, specialised care and health centres accounted for 77.0 % of the amount put on tender in the AHS in 1998. Going into further detail, the regional hospitals accounted for more than 50 % of the calls for tender in that purchasing group. The total amount of the calls for tender by the regional hospitals was not homogeneously distributed, varying between € 82.52 million from the Virgen del Rocio Hospital (= almost one fith of the whole amount within the AHS) and € 14.22 million Euro from the Virgen de las Nieves Hospital. Central services and province delegations followed in terms of tendered expenditure, while primary health care and blood transfusion centres were only responsible for relatively small amounts (Table 3).

Table 3: Distribution of calls for tender in the Andalusian Health Service 1998

Purchase group	Calls for tender (millions of Euro)	%
Specialised care (hospitals) & health districts (SC/HD)	414.76	77.0 % of total
- Regional hospitals (RH)	- 225.27	- 54.3 % of SC/HD
-- Virgen del Rocio Hospital	-- 82.52	-- 36.7 % of RH
-- Reina Sofia Hospital	-- 58.87	-- 26.2 % of RH
-- Carlos Haya Hospital	-- 45.52	-- 20.2 % of RH
-- Virgen Macarena H.	-- 23.92	-- 10.6 % of RH
-- Virgen de las Nieves H.	-- 14.22	-- 6.3 % of RH
- Specialised hospitals	- 139.61	- 33.7 % of SC/HD
- County hospital	- 49.88	- 12.0 % of SC/HD
Primary health care districts	12.04	2.2 % of total
Central Services	90.89	16.9 % of total
Province delegations	14.27	2.7 % of total
Blood transfusion centres	6.51	1.2 % of total
TOTAL	538.47	100 %

Source: Statistical and Information Services of the Andalusian Health Service

Distribution of calls for tender by type of procedure: In the AHS, calls for tender by the hospitals are classified by different types of procedure which are put on a numbered list. The contracts tendered for the purchase of goods and services are mainly for the following items: 10 "Perishable Medical Material", 71 "Cleaning Services", 50 "Medicines" and 30 "Analyses", with € 121.0, 75.7, 59.5 and 47.7 million, respectively, or 22.5 %, 14.15 %, 11.0 % and 8.9 % of the total respectively.

Calls for tender by purchase group can also be analysed. In specialised care, tenders are centred on 10 "Perishable Medical Supplies", 71 "Cleaning Services", 50 "Medicines" and 30 "Analysis", with 27.5 %, 18.1 %, 11.7 % and 10.7 % respectively, of the total tendered.

In primary health care districts, the largest volume of calls for tender are 10 "Perishable Medical Supplies", 61 "Transport" and 71 "Cleaning Services" which account for 33.4 %, 26.6 % and 10.7 % respectively. In health districts, procedures 10 "Perishable Medical Supplies" and 40 "Foodstuffs/Dietetics/Nutrition" stand out, accounting for 33.2 % and 27.3% of the total tendered. Blood transfusion centres use more than 50 % – exactly 52.1 % – of their calls for tender for 30 "Analyses".

Province delegations mainly tender calls for procedures of type 61 "Transport" with 65.4 % of the total and for those of type 01 "Works". Finally, in the central services of the

AHS, the calls for tender are centred in procedures of type 01 "Works", 06 "Rental of Equipment" and 75 "Logistic Services", with 28.6 %, 22.1 % and 20.0 % respectively, of the total tendered.

Publication in the OJEC: In 1998, 89.6 % of calls for tender were required to be published in the OJEC, compared with 10.4 % that did not require compulsory publication in the OJEC but were published regionally and/ or nationally. Table 4 lists the calls for tender in relation to their publication in the OJEC according to purchase group in 1998. In every case, the percentage of calls for tender published in the OJEC is higher than the percentage not published. Specialised care and central services stand out in particular with 90.5 % and 94.6 %, respectively. It can be observed that 96.6 % of the calls for tender by the regional hospitals were published, surpassing 95 % of the contracts in every hospital with the sole exception of the Virgen de las Nieves Hospital. The percentage of calls for tender published in the OJEC is markedly lower for the province delegations and especially the primary health care districts.

Table 4: Calls for tender by purchase group in relation to their publication in the OJEC, Andalusian Health Service 1998 (in million Euro)

Purchase group	Calls for tender published in the OJEC	Calls for tender not published in the OJEC	Total calls for tender
Specialised care (hospitals) & health districts	374.06 (90.2%)	40.70 (9.8%)	414.76
- Regional hospitals	217.34 (96.6%)	7.70 (3.4%)	225.05
-- Virgen del Rocio Hospital	81.47 (98.7%)	1.05 (1.3%)	82.52
-- Reina Sofia Hospital	57.84 (98.3%)	1.03 (1.7%)	58.87
-- Carlos Haya Hospital	43.37 (95.3%)	2.15 (4.7%)	45.52
-- Virgen Macarena Hospital	23.05 (96.4%)	0.87 (3.6%)	23.92
-- Virgen de las Nieves Hospital	11.61 (81.6%)	2.61 (18.4%)	14.22
- Specialised hospitals	123.53 (88.3%)	16.30 (11.7%)	139.83
- County hospital	33.18 (66.5%)	16.70 (33.5%)	49.88
Primary health care districts	6.67 (55.4%)	5.37 (44.6%)	12.04
Central Services	86.02 (94.6%)	4.87 (5.5%)	90.89
Province delegations	10.30 (72.2%)	3.97 (27.8%)	14.27
Blood transfusion centres	5.25 (80.7%)	1.26 (19.3%)	6.51
TOTAL	482.30 (89.6%)	56.18 (10.4%)	538.47

Source: Statistical and Information Services of the Andalusian Health Service

Regarding the distribution of the calls for tender, those published in the OJEC focussed around the same types of procedures as those put on tender in general, namely 10 "Perishable Medical Supplies", 71 "Cleaning Services", 50 "Medicines" and 30 "Analyses", with € 104.0, 75.4, 57.8 and 41.6 million respectively.

5. Qualitative results

5.1 Changes in the purchasing process

The transposition into Spanish law of the 92/50/EEC Directive of the Council – dated 18 June 1998 – was performed through the 13/1995 Law (18th May) on the Contracts of Public Administrations.

The main change perceived by the procurement departments and that has been attributed to the law by the managers of procurement services, is the increase of the purchase volume through the public procurement process. Before, the form most widely used to perform public contracts was direct purchase:

> "Everything has changed much, but especially the purchases made through the public procurement process, which have increased. The usual way to make these purchases was the direct method, that is, the "direct award" in the old legislative framework. Before, we used to have a maximum public procurement volume of 15-20 %, but now that figure is 75 % (last year's figure)."

In general, the proceedings are very similar to the ones existing before this law. The main changes are as follows:

- European publication is required.
- There are new criteria for the award of contracts.
- There are different costs to establish the type of procedure.

The changes in the process are seen as having both positive and negative aspects (Table 5).

Table 5: Positive and negative aspects of the new procurement process

Positive aspects	Negative aspects
Improvement of the organisation in a short period of time.	Increase in red tape, which affects speed. It is compulsory to go through a long, hard and difficult process.
An increase in objectivity of the awarding criteria.	The law fails to adapt to the sector and to the specific needs of health bodies.
Better publicity and more transparency.	There is little clarity in some aspects, such as the framework agreement or the proceedings required for the negotiation process.
Quicker procedures to negotiate exclusivity contracts.	It becomes more difficult to detect needs. There are more information needs, and this implies an increase in services and personnel.
Increase in quality, rigor and procedure according to protocol.	Discomfort among professionals as big tenders by hospitals might not take their specific needs into account.
	Extension of time limits to make the purchases.

5.2 Reasons for the changes in the purchasing system

Reasons for current changes in the purchasing system are frequently attributed to the European Union's influence in the integration process of its Member States:

"Changes in the legal framework are partly made to discipline Member States of the EU taking into account a common legislation for everybody, and also because we are talking about countries where a considerable percentage of the GDP is represented by an influential public sector. The eleven countries in the euro zone are countries with a public sector that has a considerable presence in the economy. Therefore I think everything is done to establish discipline and change the previous ways of doing things. Also to try and avoid corruption and deviation of funds, seeing what was coming with Maastricht: the control of budgetary deficit."

Changes and improvements can also be seen as a result of the enforcement of the Spanish Public Procurement Act which establishes the adaptation of services to the new situation. Another argument given by the people interviewed is to ascribe the changes as the result of an evolutionary process towards the improvement of public administration, meaning more budgetary control and a reduction of arbitrary decisions:

"We form part of the Public Administration. We deal with public money and we have to justify every expense. We have to establish valuation criteria for publication."

"The changes were implemented at that particular time in order to regulate what transparency was and guarantee the awarding of contracts, as well as improving advertising and competition."

In summary, the following reasons for change could be detected:

— Adaptation to the new legislation derived from the 93/1995 Law.
— Implementation of reforms from Community legislation.
— Evolutionary process that had to take place due to the improvement of the purchasing departments in the health services and to the evolution of the public administration in general.

5.3 Change in tenders towards biennial tenders

The increase in paperwork is one of the main consequences of the new contracting procedure, in particular when calling for a tender in order to purchase for the health sector. Multiple year tenders are a way of avoiding and delaying the increase of "bureaucratic tasks":

"Now we have pluriannual (multiple year) tenders, in this way we avoid the enormous bureaucratic task ahead of us, and the volume of contracting lowers the prices."

According to the people interviewed, tenders for multiple years have increased as a result of the new Spanish Public Procurement Act. This type of tenders have more complex procedures but also more advantages. One is an increase in the contracting authorities' loyalty towards the supplier who will supply the merchandise for longer periods of time. In return, there is an improvement in quality and better prices:

"What I mean is: if you call for a tender for prothesis and instead of a year you offer a three year deal, in a way you are also offering loyalty to the supplier.

> You are telling him 'you are going to work for three years with me' and that makes his offer to us more attractive both in quality and price, than for a year."

However, the interviewees also pointed to some restrictions and problems arising from these types of procedures, e.g. the impossibility of applying them to goods undergoing fast technological development and which require changes in their definition when purchasing them:

> "You can't call for pluriannual tenders for an item that you know has a technological level permanently changing in the market. For instance: haemodynamics, with all that it involves, catheterism and all that. Well, now there is an American company that releases a new product every six months, technologically tested, efficient and with proven results. With an administrative or management purchasing decision I am compromising the potential development of a clinical service. In those cases, we contract for a year period. For other clinical products, those we know don't change, like services and others in the same category, yes, we contract them for more than a year."

Among the procurement services contacted, there are some that do not apply this type of procedure to all the purchased goods and services. They are only applied for large contracts:

> "Currently, pluriannual tenders are applied only to services that are what we call large contracts: catering, maintenance, insurance and foodstuffs. Before they were not for so long and this solves so many problems. They are such a complex type of procedure that once you have dealt with them and have a one-year's contract, you might as well do it for four years, at least, if you are satisfied with them."

Sometimes the people interviewed said that these types of procedures already existed and cannot be attributed to the new legislation, although these cases were rare:

> "The only modification concerning pluriannual contracts is the fact that article 70 allows to award a tender before the start of a financial year and even before the term of the tender is awarded. Therefore, this is a change ascribed the new legislation, an improvement but only a slight improvement. It is going a bit to far to say that we can award a tender before or after the budgetary year. I think there is no difference in passing an award on January 2nd or on December 20th when you consider it but cannot decide until January 2nd. Anyway now you can decide and award it on December 20th."

In summary:

– There is an increase in the number of biennial tenders in order to avoid the higher complexity of the bureaucratic proceedings. "Imagine saying to the service manager, 'we are going to award contracts for catheters and six months later, we going to award contracts for catheters' and six months later the same! In this sense, there has been a complete change of strategy …"
– These tenders improve the quality of products and reduce their price.
– There are health centres in which these tenders are not applicable equally to all goods and services, only to big contracts: "It is very difficult to initiate a public tender. You

cannot do everything in a year. A great effort is being made to know the market, to establish assessment."

5.4 Changes in the types of procedure

The first sign of the impact that the legislative changes had in services was the increase in public tenders in the process for purchasing goods and services. The gradual increase in this type of procedure can be seen in the procurement services which are considered to achieve an institutional objective:

> "The Andalusian Health Service's institutional objective is to have 80 % of contracting through procurement by the 31st December 1999. We know from the start that this is a difficult objective to fulfil. It will be almost impossible to achieve it but that's not enough reason not to try. We estimate that we will achieve around 60 %. That would be approximately 8,000 million pesetas, which is quite a sum!"

In some procurement services, an increase in negotiated procedures for exclusive contracts has also been noticed:

> "Yes, practically all we do here is calls for tender. But we are also dealing with some negotiated procedures on medicines because there are many pharmaceutical specialities that are exclusive and there is no room for competition. We are also negotiating the contracts for the maintenance of technological items. Why? Because for instance, the maintenance of a gamma ray chamber can only be done by the company that builds that particular type of chamber. We have also applied the negotiated procedure in some competitions that had been declared void, and to tell you the truth, our experience with the negotiated procedure is quite positive as it gives you room for making offers, making counter-offers, or even sitting down together with two or more suppliers. In general there is more manoeuvring capacity."

Another change is the direct awarding of tenders that do not surpass 2 million pesetas. According to the people interviewed, the allocation of a larger budget has been the previous step for the increase in this type of procedure:

> "When a larger budget is allocated you can submit more tenders. The change in the regulations has not been a determinant factor for this, not at all. It could have had an influence in the area of pharmaceutical products. Now it has been established that it has to be done through tenders or procurement procedures. Quite a different situation from the general agreements existing until 1991 with the pharmaceutical industry, between the Spanish ministry of health and the pharmaceutical industry. In order to comply with the communitarian directive the Kingdom of Spain is obliged to call for tender all pharmaceutical products. This is the only area in which there is an increase of tenders. Something that before was not considered for tendering, now has to pass through that procedure. As far as the rest is concerned everything remains the same."

The increase in this type of procedure has negative and positive consequences on the services. Among the negative ones, the limitations that tenders have when trying to negotiate with the suppliers can be highlighted:

"Tenders are a very closed, time-specific procedure. In them, at a given moment when you have to publish, you have to draft a technical report and what comes out of that is all you get. While, with the negotiated procedure you are given more freedom."

There are some circumstances in the contracting process in which tenders have advantages for the contracting services. For instance, when the quantity of the item to be purchased is not fixed:

"It is an advantage when the quantity of an item is not an exact one. Then you can say an approximate figure. The modification procedure is long and now we can avoid it."

Regarding this fact, it should be mentioned that both the negotiated procedure and dividing an offer into various parts of less than 2 million pesetas could have increased as a defence mechanism within a more rigid context. In both cases, this could lead to unwanted cases of corruption. In summary, perceived changes were as follows:

– Increase in the number of tenders, which is considered as an institutional objective: "In 1997 in this hospital, the total volume of expenditure for administrative procurement was 2,910 million pesetas (either through public procurement or through the negotiated procedure). In 1999, we have reached 5,528 million pesetas, that is an increase of 64 % compared with 1998 and almost 100 % compared with 1997."
– Increase in the contracts negotiated in exclusivity.

The following consequences can be noted:

– Negative: It is a closed procedure that allows for little manipulation by the persons in charge of the contracts.
– Negative: Generation of new forms of corruption.
– Positive: It allows an approximation of the quantity to be given when it is not possible to establish an exact quantity.

5.5 Contracts published in the Official Journal of the European Communities

Publication of tenders in the Official Journal of the European Communities ranges between 11 % and 80 % among Andalusian health centres. Hospitals tend to publish more that Primary Health Centres. This difference is due to the volume of contracts. Among hospitals, the Virgen del Rocio Hospital in Seville published in the OJEC more than any other hospital in 1998. However, it has to be taken into account that this hospital has the biggest assigned population, number of beds and budget:

"Here we send almost everything to the OJEC as almost everything surpasses the limit and if not, it does by the end of the year...We control every tender that we have prepared and we know what stage they are at. Almost all of them are published ... some in BOJA [Official Journal of the Andalusian Regional Government] but the majority of them in the OJEC or BOE [Official Journal of the Spanish State]."

Publication in the Official Journal of the European Communities implies an extension of the period of time devoted to the award of contracts. Some of the interviewees admitted having divided tenders in order to avoid publication and thereby reduce time limits:

> "This is the year for cleaning services. We are careful to avoid tenders over a certain figure so as not to have to publish them. If we didn't do this it would take us a year just to buy cotton, wool or lint."

5.6 Changes in the criteria used for the award of tenders

The criteria for the awarding of tenders are different depending on the Andalusian health centre studied. It depends on the type of goods and services to be purchased whether more points are given to either price or to technical quality. There is wide scope for case analysis. Generally, the first distinction is made between supplies and services. When considering supplies, price is more important. When considering services, the main considerations are mostly technical.

> "Well it's all relative. When establishing the award criteria each procedure has different considerations. They are usually different, in an average situation we would give 40% to price, 40% to functional and technical considerations and 20% to criteria such as: time limit for deliverance, free telephone and fax services, where their warehouses are, etc. ... which are quite specific considerations. Or even any extra offers they could make us."

These criteria are established according to the type of goods and services, based on the decisions made by the departments in charge of the procurement services, and the usual practices in the awarding of contracts. There seems to be a general criteria in each centre for the different groups of items or services contracted.

In high-tech supplies and services, priority is generally given to the technical report, but for those goods which have an established quality and technology, money is the main consideration:

> "There are differences by group. A very important group for us are protheses, they have a very special consideration. They are within the same circuit but due to their economic value they are very important. Therefore, we try to put them first so that we can give more time and dedication."
>
> "The more specific the item is, specific in terms of technology i.e. pacemakers, hip replacement prothesis etc. the more important technical considerations are in relation to price. When dealing with items that are of standard use with a simple technology, generically more defined, what we consider is price."

Occasionally, considerations are being made to specific aspects that were not related to the technical report or price:

> "We have given value to the fact that they have an Andalusian branch as well as their warehouses, but not for all the procedures, only for some."

In other cases, the department making the purchase can fix the price before calling the tender. In that way, priority is given to the technical report because the start is by fixing a "reference" price according to market considerations.

In most of the cases studied, the technical information is provided by the centre's specialised staff. However, that is not always the case and it depends mainly on the type of centre. In the following quote a case is illustrated corresponding to a situation in which there was no separation between price and technical report when calling for a tender:

> "We try not to separate the information given to our technicians from the price that a product has. We provide both price and technical requirements to them. You ask: What's the best catheter? Well that depends on the price. It could be an excellent one, yes...but if it costs half a million pesetas... Is it worth buying it at that price? It will depend on the quality, the fact that other companies offer it too and also at what price they offer it. Independent of the technical report, we organise meetings with those responsible for services, or their number two people, to work out what the outcome of the tender will be. Taking into account the price and quality of the product. All because to blindly believe in the report makes no sense."

The fact that undercutting prices in tenders in order to obtain the award of a hospital service doesn't work, means that prices have to be as fixed as possible. This is done well before the preparation of a tender, then technical standards are taken into account:

> "So, if you have a price decided upon you probably give priority to other things like the work schedule, as happened here. Here we have cleaning services to which we could have given 40 % of the priority to price and 60 % to actual work, training plans, experience, in a few words, all the technical skills and know-how a company has in order to clean a hospital. Just the opposite was the case of medical gases, now with two year contracts. In this case, 80 % goes to the price. Why? Because the medical gas market has almost an oligopoly between two companies that share the market between them, both are technically proficient, both can guarantee quality. One is already with us and the other serves the hospital next door and is present in 40 % of hospitals."

In some hospitals, the impact of the European Union will have price repercussions and therefore criteria will be established when purchasing goods and services for health centres:

> "What I think is happening is that prices are already reaching a balance, prices are being established and it will be difficult to lower them. What's more, I think that prices will increase in a matter of years. In the rest of Europe, they are 20 or 30% more expensive than in Spain. So, with the harmonization of the currency in the next three years, the harmonization of interest rates, the tax harmonization which is already here... I believe prices will tend to balance out and it is easier to increase them in Spain than to lower them in the other countries. Here for instance someone was telling me about the case of the Kodak X-ray plates. Right now Virgen del Rocio Hospital is paying the lowest price in the whole of Europe. It was a negotiation that worked well for us. Kodak has its headquarters in London and in Europe – almost all the American multinationals also have their headquarters in London – and they are making it more difficult for us because they want to know why some prices are being maintained in Spain. That's the reason I think the trend will be to increase prices."

In summary, criteria for the award of tenders vary according to the price and the technical report: "For instance, if there is a tender for diet, the price is relative as they may be offering you only dirty water with vegetables. But with gauze, the price is an issue because the quality has been determined."

In general, for supplies, the price is more important than in services. The latter usually depend more on the technical characteristics:

> "It is complicated, because this Hospital (Virgen del Rocío) has 15,000 million pesetas and 900 suppliers; one of them sells heads of lettuce and another one sells you medical gases, therefore it is a completely different market. What is important is to know the market, or at least to know how it works."

In the supply of high technology, however, technical considerations (the technical report) are more important than the price.

5.7 Adaptation to the new legislation

Procurement services tend to adapt themselves to the time limits established by law in order to award tenders. That has been the most frequent opinion among the interviewees:

> "The time limit established by law is three months for the awarding of tenders. Yes, at least for these ones. There could be a procedure that gets blocked but in general we award them before the three month limit."

In hospitals or primary care centres where managers were interviewed, the first problem they mentioned was the formality of the tender itself and the technical report which has to be drafted by the centre. The main inconveniences related to the processing of tenders are: the length of time, usually long, the establishing of objective award criteria, the comparative analysis and the definition of the technical characteristics. Also, it is necessary to obtain consensus among professionals, which is also sometimes difficult:

> "Depending on the tender, technical reports also take a great deal of time. In the case of a complex tender, too many people have to come to an agreement or have to be willing to help or decide and that takes time."

Once the formalities are fulfilled in their own centre, the external time limits – mainly legal advice and publishing by the central services – are also mentioned as an obstacle to ensure compliance with legislation.

> "The biggest delay for us is the legal report as well as the publishing for the reasons I mentioned, but that's a very specific point."

Occasionally, specific problems arise with some companies when is time to sign a contract or deliver the goods. These problems also delay the fulfilment of the time limits. This is a result of the exclusivity that some companies have, resulting from the negotiated procedure:

> "I've got problems with some firms, it is difficult to sign a contract with them, more so if they have exclusivity. There are some pharmaceutical companies which have the exclusivity of a product ... there is no way out, you have to buy from them through a negotiated procedure. This procedure has legal formalities. You have to call them, negotiate, sign a contract and afterwards provide a series of documents. The negotiated procedure obliges the companies to be up to date with social security and tax payments, there are no exceptions, but that's not

always the case. When that happens they know that your only option is to buy from them. So until they solve their payments you have to wait, sometimes past the deadline, if so, you have to put forward a complaint and eventually you sign the contract."

It has to be taken into account that the publication of a tender is a process for the planning and scheduling of the services. This aspect is regarded as an advantage for the procurement department:

"In the long run, I think it's positive. It makes you think about what your needs are, both in goods and services."

As regards improvements derived from "better purchases", publishing increases the offer from different brands and products. The increase in competition lowers prices and sometimes there is even an improvement in the technological quality of some items. Also, service managers need to be better informed about the market:

"It obliges you to plan your work. You have to know what and when to buy. Concerning the publication it's an advantage. You have offers of different brands and products on the table."
"The increase in competition is lowering prices. The offered products are starting to come with technological innovations."

However, there are also cases in which the procurement departments studied consider the new directives as a path full of obstacles. Especially when they involve the publication process and compliance with time limits, which do not grant any advantages. These cases appeared to be very rare:

"Compared with the previous situation, no advantages at all. Time limits have been changed but the situation is practically the same. I think we still have to shorten the time limits because adding it all up we have a total of four months in a procedure that we want to complete as soon as possible. We can easily spend a month just waiting for the legal consultant's report and for the audit, the same ..."
"No advantages at all. It delays the arrival of the material when we need it."

In summary, regarding the adaption to the new legislation, the following problems can be observed:

— The conduct of the tender proceedings and the elaboration of the technical report by the Hospital or Primary Health Care Centre is sometimes considered as a problem to comply with time limits.
— The problems coming up during the conduct of the proceedings include: the time required, which is normally long; putting the criteria for the award in objective terms; the comparative analysis, and the definition of technical characteristics. It is also necessary that professionals reach a consensus, which is sometimes difficult.
— Time limits which are external to the conduct of the proceedings by the hospital, especially legal advice and publication by the central services.
— Specific problems with some companies, such as the difficulties signing contracts or with the stock supply. These problems are considered to be caused by the forced dependence of the health centre upon the company.

On the other hand, there are also advantages:

– Increase in the planning and organisation of services.
– Increase in the supply of different trademarks and products.
– Increase in competition.
– Possible decrease in prices.
– Increase in technological quality.

5.8 Consequences for the market:changes in the type of providers

In general, the people interviewed didn't remark on any substantial change in the type of providers that submit to tenders called by the AHS:

> "No, I think they are generally the same. I have been working for nine years in both the hospital division and the purchase division and have also been involved in their management, so I have met many suppliers over the years. They are still the same...there are very few who are new. The changes are mostly related to the fact that we don't know what to do with the money. We can perceive a movement in some entrepreneurial groups, all coming from construction companies, that are trying to penetrate the health market. They try to do this through the services."

A larger presence of big companies and multinationals compared to small and medium-sized enterprises was noted. This is due to the market's own dynamics and because of the latter's impossibility to tender:

> "It's all the same. There are four or five large companies and they keep growing."
> "I think that at an average supplier level they remain the same. What we can perceive is the merging of companies, but that is not because of the law but due to the market ..."
> "They are usually big. The great disadvantage is for the small companies, they can't compete. So they are mostly multinationals. Small and medium-sized ones are out, mainly because they neither know about nor can prepare the required documentation."

The arguments put forward in order to explain small and medium enterprises' (SMEs) difficulties for tendering are mainly due to debt but also because of not being able to prepare the required documentation for any tender.

Among professionals, there is a feeling of dismay because they had been used to working with the same suppliers from smaller companies for a long time:

> "The suppliers remain the same but what is noticeable is that there are less small suppliers. The reasons are not in the new contract legislation but in the lack of a budget in order to pay them. When they aren't paid for 300 days, 600 days or two years, some suppliers can't cope with it. Therefore, some small suppliers disappear.
>   Anyway, they have a shortcoming from my point of view. They are not pre-pared to deal with the required documentation for any tender. A multinational or a big national company usually has a department which only deals with

tenders. There they have, and can produce, all the required information and certificates. This gives them the capacity to respond efficiently and on time.

A small company makes use of various means. For example, an independent business manager or agency to prepare the documentation. Sometimes you have a supplier, you buy from him directly and on advantageous terms, quality and price wise. Then you call a tender and the independent agency can't be considered for it because it didn't fulfil the required documentation for financial reasons. You feel a bit powerless...a big distributor obtains the award, you know it's adding 20 % or more to the final price and on top of that, the product isn't as good, the quality is not the same."

The change in the type of supplier can also occur because of the improvements made by the departments in their purchasing. They take advantage of competition among suppliers and try to avoid dependency as clients:

"There is a simple explanation: when you become dependant on a certain supplier, they take advantage of you. The moment a company knows that the market offers better options, it actually starts competing, its prices drop and its offers improve. If a company knows that you use them exclusively or sales are guaranteed for any reason, their offers tend to be worse."

A case was found in which the changes occurred only in a specific type of contract and not in general:

"Large contracts for cleaning services have changed. Contracts for maintenance continue with local companies and so do the stationary suppliers. 'El Corte Inglés' is still contracted for clothing."

One of the main achievements of integration in the European Union could be a greater participation of foreign companies in tenders for health services. However, such a situation is not reflected by this data. In most cases, the main tenderers are multinational companies with branches in Spain or they are simply the same companies as before the process of European integration:

"What we have are foreign companies with branches in Spain and they distribute their products. The items we buy are the same that company is selling in Germany. The German company doesn't come here to sell. We work as usual and the majority of purchases from multinationals are through their Spanish branches, they sell to us."

"Some Dutch companies, for instance, have come to seek subscriptions for specialised magazines for the library, and that's all. In that field we deal with specialised companies not coming from Spain. In fact not a single Spanish company tendered, they have all been awarded to foreign companies. We didn't even need to pay in foreign currency or convert pesetas because they are multinationals with a branch in Spain. Many of them come from Belgium and the Netherlands but we buy them from a Spanish company."

In summary,

– no substantial changes are usually perceived;
– no increase in foreign companies competing for the tender has been detected;

- the number of small and medium-sized enterprises competing for tenders has decreased;
- those changes that have taken place are due to improving purchase departments;
- changes are perceived in a specific type of contract on some occasions.

5.9 Subjective view of the impact of European legislation on public procurement departments

For most of the people interviewed, their purchase systems have not registered any impact as a result of the new European legislation. Some exceptions can be found in the following; the obligation to publish in the Official Journal of the European Communities; changes in the awarding criteria; and changes in the procedures:

> "Now we have to put the amounts in Euro and it is compulsory to publish in the OJEC: No European companies have come."
>
> "The European legislation has altered the 'C endorsement'. Concerning public procurement, in the former law the procedure was similar, slightly different, but similar. The changes mostly concern the publication, the awarding criteria and the procedures, but they are minor ones."

In some of the procurement departments where staff were interviewed, they said that they had received phone calls from European companies interested in the tenders. No tenders by those companies were submitted after the calls:

> "I haven't noticed any change in attitude. I have only noticed an interest in knowing what we did. Sometimes, companies from Brussels or London call us, but not to make any concrete offer. My opinion is that information is spreading, but it hasn't gotten into the market yet. Perhaps only in some goods, in electro-medical equipment."

However, the impact can be perceived in the Spanish Public Procurement Act 13/95 which reflects European legislation. It can also be seen in the new formalities for calling a tender as established by law but not from the communitarian law. Some of the professionals interviewed, who work in public procurement in Andalusia, said that they felt they were under surveillance because the new law was brought into force to avoid corruption. Thus, it has caused some lack of confidence:

> "With regard to the law (13/95) nowadays in purchasing our job is to prove that you are not doing it wrong. You have so much that needs to be justified that in the end you only have to show you are not bending the law. It's like starting from the fact that there is a wrong side in public management and you have to prove just the opposite."

For some of these professionals, in order to apply the law in health services, its implementation should be more flexible and adapted to the situation and objectives of public services:

> "The great variety of items, their particular characteristics, the urgent need to have them and the regular changes in them are limitations which shouldn't exist in a hospital. Sometimes we are talking of real urgent needs, to give you an example: you decide to buy a pacemaker and tomorrow you have a new one in the market which is professionally more attractive. What happens? you can't buy it and that goes against you. I think it is great to comply with the law but

there should be room for some exceptions. If we only stayed within a framework in the end we wouldn't do a good job in many senses.

The law has improved a lot of things but there are still some restrictions that certain services don't permit. The ideal situation would be to find more flexible interpretations of the law. We should have more options when facing an emergency."

In some cases, there have been complaints about the lack of information that service managers have on the impact of the new European legislation on their departments. The following is an extract of an interview that illustrates this situation:

"First, I have noticed a lack of information within the health authorities. I do not think that there have been enough information campaigns. We haven't been well prepared, not concerning the hospitals at least."

In summary, the impact is not normally seen, except for:

- The obligation to publish in the Official Journal of the European Communities.
- Changes in the award criteria.
- Changes in the procedures.
- In some cases there have been requests for information by European companies.
- The impact is perceived through the 13/95 Spanish Law on Public Procurement derived from the European legislation.

Other aspects include:

- Professionals have a feeling of control which they attribute to the law.
- The implementation of the law should be quicker in health services, because of the characteristics and objectives of this type of services.

5.10 Measures implemented to adapt to Community policies

Compliance with the new legal framework implies implementing a series of measures. Among the most important of these measures are reorganising the procurement departments and increasing personnel:

"There are a lot more public procedures. We were obliged to put someone from our staff on full-time just to deal with them."

"Since I started, we have had eight people in the department. Perhaps now is the time to increase staff. Now, as well as having more quantity of work we require more quality of work. We might need a plan now to add reinforcements to this department."

In summary, measures implemented to adapt to the requirements of Community policy in the are of public procurement include re-structuring of procurement departments and increase in the personnel.

6. Effects derived from the transposition of the European regulations to the Spanish legal framework

6.1 Intended effects

The health sector's considerable amount of procurement emphasizes the effects that the communitarian rules will have in this area. Without including all possibilities, in the health sector there are important categories of contracts and it is worth mentioning the most important ones in a descriptive analysis.

Works contracts have a great deal of importance not only for building new health centres but because it is always necessary to reform and extend existing premises. However there is a great drawback in this type of contracts: insufficient formal budgets, as the investments budget is scarce if not non-existent. Apart from those works financed by the European Union's ERDF funds, this difficulty has been overcome with subsidies either from local corporations, companies or instrumental entities that are in charge of the negotiation of contracts. These types of contracts do not have any repercussions in the management within the centres themselves. This is because the negotiation of contracts is normally centralised due to the amounts involved. Over time, a gradual externalisation of the execution controls has also been observed. Before, the administrative services had their own team of engineers and architects as well as project supervision departments. Currently, these services are provided by professionals who do not belong to the organisation itself. So far, concerning the impact of the communitarian principles, there has been no effective opening of the market. The reasons can be found in the need to have branches in the area where the work is to be carried out or the need to purchase or transport machinery and staff belonging to a firm, which hampers the participation of foreign companies with very few exceptions. However, those exceptions are important as they have bided as temporary joint ventures usually with the participation of a Spanish construction company.

The administrative awarding of public works has not yet developed greatly in the sector, but now the need to improve access and equipment in health centres is starting to make this type of contract more commonly used, particularly in order to build and manage parking garages and power generation stations in large hospitals. Concerning tenders, they are also applicable to works contracts.

Another important category of contracts regards management of public services, strictly speaking "concerted health care." This type of contract implies indirect management of public services. This is the case when the administration, holder of the competency to provide the service, does not have enough resources to do it. In such cases, it is necessary to hire services from private firms working on the same activity. Thus, in concerted health care the aim of contracts is always to provide health services, though a distinction needs to be made between complete concerted health are, when a private hospital or clinic is contracted to provide the totality of the services involved, and specific concerted services, such as imaging diagnosis or particular services in order to treat certain pathologies. This could be the case when contracting services to operate on cataracts in a specific population group. Health transport is also included in this category. Concerted health care is categorised as an administrative contract regulated by the Spanish Public Procurement Act and also, as established according to its specific set of rules, by the Spanish Health Care Act 14/1986 of April 25th, article 90. Despite their economic and social importance, concerted health care contracts are irrelevant from the perspective of this study, as this type of contract already existed in the Spanish legal framework and is not subject to communitarian regulations.

However, there is a fact worth mentioning related to private health centres or institutions. It would be interesting to study the running of such centres as they are business activities linked to free entrepreneurial activities or movement of capital, as far as the investment of communitarian funds is concerned. From that perspective alone, concerted health care would be conditioned by the communitarian regulations.

In health services, the supplies contract can be categorised as the most important one due to the volume of activity that it produces. Among the purchase of goods, electro-medical devices can be highlighted. Such supply contracts have traditionally had the same financial problems as the works contracts, budget wise, as such purchases become an investment. New types of contracts have solved this problem. Now it is the hiring without a purchase option which prevails, which allows not only the use of equipment but its fast renewal. This is important due to scientific and technological improvements and at the same time, it enables depreciation of equipment that soon becomes obsolete to be avoided. The introduction of new contract types such as leasings and hiring with purchase options offer new possibilities for these purchases. These sorts of goods are mainly supplied by European companies as well as American and Japanese companies with branches in Spain, therefore the application of the communitarian rules is not modified by the nationality of the supplier. These companies (communitarian and those included in the European Economic Area and the World Trade Organization) benefit from the fact that they are able to bid directly from their countries without needing to establish themselves in Spain, which saves costs. But from the perspective of health care services, no change will be perceived in the short term.

Medicines are another important purchase for health care centres. Traditionally, health care institutions purchased medicines for hospital dispensaries through an agreement between the administration and the pharmaceutical industry. Also, the Spanish Medicines Act categorised these products as excluded from contract legislation. This practice and legislation caused a non-favourable judgement by the European Court of Justice concerning case C-328/1992 Commission versus Kingdom of Spain, Sentence of May 3rd 1994.

Regarding suppliers, this argument can also be applied to the case of electro-medical equipment. Large laboratories hold firm control over market forces which frequently makes free competition difficult in the supply of these products. In any case, in order to comply with the communitarian principles concerning the supply of medicines, harmonisation techniques are also necessary as the nature of the product demands that the corresponding authorisations and administrative checking procedures are in tune with fabrication and commercialisation.

This is also valid for the supply of all other health products: reagents, medical gases, surgical equipment, and so on, due to the fact that their technical features have already predetermined the market and therefore there is no variety in the type of supplier, though logically, purchase by tender could lower the product's prices. In the case of ordinary supplies, generally due to their low cost, they are considered as minor items with no communitarian participation. It is the local companies that are in charge of their supply.

In the section concerning services, as well as consultancy and assistance contracts, in which the range of communitarian influence is modest, some important services required by health centres are: cleaning, catering, maintenance and security services. Such services are contracted through tendering and competition is fostered due to their high value. However, because of their inherent characteristics requiring the availability of many workers, mainly Spanish companies and groups bid for the tenders. Compliance with the communitarian regulations has not attracted foreign companies. At another level is computing services, where participation of foreign companies is greater due to the sector's configuration.

Other contracted services, of lower economic impact, are publicity for health promotion campaigns, training services or legal services, for which there is no communitarian participation.

Insurance services are a recent addition to the Spanish health system. Communitarian regulations have an influence on the contracting of civil liability insurance policies due to their high costs which require advertising at communitarian level. This sector, though supervised, requires a mandatory administration authorisation in order to operate the various insurance categories and has been influenced by the regulations established by the communitarian institutions. This influence has forced the member states to adapt their internal regulations. In Spain, such adaptation has been carried out according to the Private Insurance Code and Supervision Act 30/1995. The contract type envisaged by the Spanish State Contracts Act of 1995 revealed itself as inadequate. This is why, after the reform, this service is considered a private contract, though its awarding should comply with the contracting communitarian principles.

To conclude this brief description, a series of contracts will be mentioned with patrimonial content and therefore excluded from the procurement legislation, but which have to be awarded in compliance with the communitarian principles. They are the awarding of contracts for the opening of cafes, press and lottery stands, cash lines and other business premises appropriate to health service buildings. In this contract category, rather unclear regarding its legal status, the communitarian regulations have not been applied and consequently, there is no communitarian competition.

6.2 Unintended effects

The analysis of the influence that public procurement has in the health sector demands that some determinant regulations are considered. First, basic legislation on public procurement, according to the Spanish Constitution – article 149.1.18 –, establishes it as an exclusive state competency. Being considered of a widespread nature, affecting the administration proceedings in various sectors and closely related to the market regulations, the Spanish regional governments will only be competent with regard to its legislative development. Nevertheless, in its sentence of April 22nd 1993, the Spanish constitutional rights court, in case 513/1987 regarding a conflict of competencies, established that regional governments have broad competency in the sectors which affect the organisation of their administrative proceedings and in those areas of competency which are granted by statutory dispositions. For instance, some Spanish regional governments can regulate the extent of competency of the contracting authorities, for example, the guarantee that bidders are financially and economically able, the securing and or exemption of guarantees in certain contracts, the reasons for ruling on a public service management contract, the leasing of real estate, payments in cash or other goods in a supplies contract etc.

On the other hand, concerning the health sector, the regional governments have major competencies in health service management. Together, the various regional health services form the Spanish National Health System.

It is probably in the health sector where the debate on new management forms and the need to overcome the traditional model under the administrative law has had greatest importance. The National Health System Analysis and Evaluation Commission appointed by the Spanish Parliament in 1990 advocated, in its summing up of the sector's problems, radical reforms which included, among others, the granting of greater autonomy to the health centres in order to transform them into public companies.

To put in Spanish jurisprudence, Muñoz Machado's, own words "... the trend for abandoning Public Law guarantees and the infiltration of Private Law in every aspect of the public services goes against the reality our times. Whilst we abandon some of those sorts of guarantees the European Union, to which we belong as full members, is imposing the necessary maintenance of a series of guarantees, that of course belong to Public Law, for the functioning of certain establishments or in order to configure certain activities" (Muñoz Machado 1995).

Definitively, this is what is happening in spite of concepts or differentiated organisational models in topics such as public procurement in which the working tools have to suit the forecasts of communitarian law independent from the role of such rules as determining factors in a management model. As has been said, regardless of the management model adopted, public procurement is fully submitted to communitarian law, and health managers, who have to combine effectiveness, efficiency and legality in their task, sometimes find themselves in difficult positions.

The impact of European regulations in the purchase of goods and services is important, as illustrated by the previous legal analysis, because it has changed some patterns in administrative management, bringing about some legislative modifications in the Spanish legal framework. These changes will be greater in the future. Planning for the purchase of goods and services has become an essential tool, permitting a greater rationalisation of procurement. On the other hand, such change, which has not been welcomed by an important portion of the management staff, has contributed somehow to the debate on new forms of organisation of the health services.

7. Conclusions and recommendations

The transposition of the European regulations to the Spanish legal framework on public procurement started in 1986 after the accession of the Kingdom of Spain to the European Economic Community. Since then, the extent of the influence of these transpositions has been gradual, although from a substantial perspective it can be asserted that communitarian law has been properly incorporated within Spain's internal rules. However, such incorporation has suffered delays in certain cases and formally has meant the non-compliance of obligations by the Spanish state as stated by the communitarian treaties. Such was the case of the directives on supplies contracts in the utilities sector, as well as those that modify and adapt the directives on services, supplies and works, both adapted after the deadline.

The communitarian directives have put forward a new concept in public procurement. Due to the diversity of legal frameworks in member states, the administrative organisation or the denomination of contracts is not an issue for the European regulations. On the contrary, what is actually important is an effective opening of the public sector's market. Thus, any contract, fully or partly financed with public funds, is considered as a public contract and contracting entities either from the public administration or not will be appointed as the awarding body.

From this perspective, the impact of communitarian law on the purchasing of goods and services in health care services has been as important as in the rest of the public sector. This is because procurement is a widespread subject that affects any activity involving public expenditure and investment.

The impact of the communitarian regulations has been immediately perceived in its intended effects. The incorporation of regulations within the Spanish legal framework has meant, procurement wise, a reinforcement in the application of the communitarian principles of transparency and competition, as well as the application of the equality and non-discrimination principles. This is evident if the new regulations concerning the contracting proceedings, award proceedings, the fixing of time limits and deadlines for publishing in the official journals are looked at, as well as the new rules for establishing the essential capacity and reliability qualifications of the contracted companies.

From the contracted parties' perspective, partly because of the market's configuration, there are no significant changes and because of this, the supplier's features remain the same.

Generally speaking, the contracting possibilities have substantially changed. Now new types of contracts and new possibilities for purchasing goods and services are available.

The unintended effects resulting from the application of the communitarian regulations have stressed the existing differences between the trend set up by the European Union and the need to provide health care management with alternative mechanisms.

Concerning the purchase of goods and services in the health care sector, the debate on the wrongly called "privatising trend" has been heightened. This is referred to as "wrongly called" because in fact, the trend does not imply the transfer or sale of resources and services to the private sector. What is actually being questioned is a management model subject to public law.

With regard to public service management and public order in general, the inherent nature of things establishes a series of limiting factors. Public administrations, as opposed to a private entity, cannot without further questioning do anything that is not formally prohibited. In fact, in the public sector, any activity always requires a qualifying rule. Every proceeding carried out by the administration is predetermined in rules according to the classical principle of legality; therefore there is no possible management model aside from the established rules and norms.

If the communitarian legal framework establishes a particular administrative concept in the public sector, implying the existence of public law guarantees which are mandatory for the functioning of certain establishments or for the configuration of some proceedings, it is worth taking advantage of. And it should be done with the right flexibility required for managing public services with more effectiveness and efficiency.

The formal limitations that a regulation establishes can be compensated with more decision power. In the case of health care, when public administrations have to contract services, they have to comply with certain requirements and they are under constant supervision, not only political, but also legal, financial and economic. However, when the administration contracts a service according to public law, it has a special regime not without advantages; it does not contract as a private entity among equals.

In summary, the assessment given to this situation is positive, although the limitations alluded to should be taken into consideration. The following recommendations can be made:

In general,

- encouragement from the entities involved in the management of health care services should be sought in order to foster legislative and initiatives.
- the regulation proposals should be formulated by the competent authorities of the regional governments as established in the Spanish Constitution and the Regional Governments Statutes which grant them with competencies in the development of rules in contract law.

Specifically:

- It is necessary to give managing entities mechanisms in the planning, co-ordination, and homologation of proceedings for greater effectiveness in procurement.
- It is absolutely necessary to define what is to be purchased and which services are needed before the procurement process starts. A very important mechanism is the preparation of a product and services catalogue. Catalogues define the technical features

of the goods and services included in it. These would be subject to constant modifications as the health care activities are linked to scientific and technological progress.

− Regarding the contracting systems, the simplification of administrative proceedings can be achieved by creating centralised entities that would catalogue suppliers according to contracting capacity. Contract forms would need to be approved, not for types of works contracts, services or supplies, but for specific contracts i.e. cleaning, supply of reagents, security, hiring of equipment, etc. As well as the approving, within the entities, of provisional and definitive security exemptions, the fostering of prototype contracts and tenders to decide on them, the creation of contracting boards, the preparation of contracting guidelines and the necessary moves to design management training courses need to be developed.

− Although budgets are issued on an annual basis which sets the pace of public expenditure, it is important to fix a planning mechanism in order to establish the appropriate purchase time.

− Finally, a redistribution of competencies would be recommended in order to establish who purchases. Despite the fact that autonomy in making decisions has proved to be an efficient mechanism, in certain purchases, more centralisation could save administrative costs and some services could benefit from the effects of economies of scale.

8. Public procurement of medical goods and services in other EU countries

8.1 Comparative data for Germany, Spain, Sweden and the UK

As public procurement rules are applicable to public institutions, it may be assumed that the degree of having public providers within a healthcare system will co-determine the impact of the SEM public procurement legislation upon the healthcare systems. To assess such a relationship, all tenders published in the OJEC between May 1st 1999 and Apriil 30th 2000 were analysed in regard to the Member State of origin and whether it came from the healthcare sector.

As can be seen in Table 6, the total number of all tenders found and analysed was 23,660. Using the population size to weigh the number of tenders, Sweden had 25 % more tenders than the EU average while the ratio was lowest in Spain. Looking only on healthcare tenders, differences were more pronounced. While in the EU on average 8 % of all tenders originated from the healthcare sector, this percentage varied between 5.5 % in Germany and more than 18 % in Spain. The number of healthcare tenders weighted for population size was about 60 % higher than the EU average in both Spain and Sweden while it was about 40 % lower than EU average in Germany.

These data clearly provide an empirical underpinning for the importance of organisational features of the healthcare systems. In decentralised public systems as in Spain and Sweden the public procurement rules lead to a high number of tenders in the healthcare sector while this number is substantially lower in the equally public, but centralised NHS in the UK (see below). The decentralised public-private mix of providers in "Bismarckian" countries such as Germany results in even lower numbers of healthcare tenders.

Table 6: Healthcare tenders in Germany, Spain, Sweden and the UK, May 1999 to April 2000

	Member State					
	Germany	Spain	Sweden	UK	Rest EU	EU 15
Population in million (1998)	82	39	9	59	186	375
Share of EU population	1/4.6	1/9.6	1/41.7	1/6.4	1/2	1/1
All tenders						
Absolute number	4,439	1,724	707	3,054	13,736	23,660
Adjusted for population (absolute number)	20,300	16,577	29,458	19,411	27,694	23,660
Ratio vs. EU (EU = 1.0)	0.86	0.70	1.25	0.82	1.17	1.00
Healthcare tenders						
Absolute number	242	318	72	293	969	1,894
Percentage of all tenders	5.5%	18.4%	10.2%	9.6%	7.1%	8.0%
Adjusted for population (absolute number)	1,107	3,058	3,000	1,862	1,954	1,894
Ratio vs. EU (EU = 1.0)	0.58	1.61	1.58	0.98	1.03	1.00

8.2 The public procurement process in the UK

In the UK, a body called NHS Supplies (NHSS) provides a service to most NHS Trusts (hospitals, community and mental health) for the procurement of goods and services. NHSS has the following capability:

- Customer services to trusts: outposted teams which offer generic and specialist advice for procurement (this includes everything from foodstuffs, stationary to medical supplies and highly specialist equipment);
- Contracts: the specification, negotiation and management of contracts;
- Warehousing and logistics.

There are a number of private companies in the same business which can compete for national contracts, especially in the generic businesses, such as foods, stationary etc. Arguably, NHSS has built up considerable expertise in the medical supplies business, but not all outposted teams have this specialist knowledge available. Currently, there is debate about the future of the customer services part of NHSS, and strengthening the specialist, clinical knowledge is one option.

In terms of procurement of goods and services, trusts are free to choose which of the following routes they choose:

- Go through NHSS for the specification, negotiation and management of a contract;
- Use NHSS customer services to utilize their specialist knowledge to secure the best contract, and then manage it themselves;
- Directly access, negotiate and manage the contract themselves.

Decisions on the above options depend on what is considered best for the local organisation in terms of price, quality, accessibility etc. Thus, in practice there is considerable variation between organisations.

An important advantage of using NHSS is the already mentioned expertise they have in the field, but also because they attempt to stay abreast of new developments and appraise the costs and benefits for trusts. Because NHSS works across many organisations, they also build up incremental knowledge of what works in practice. They maintain a database of the range of contracts held by NHS organisations.

NHSS offers "non-partisan" advice, and it is important that they develop the evidence-based aspects of their services in order to counterbalance the commercial sales talk of representatives, especially because consultants tend to believe the representatives of companies, especially when they have a medical/nursing background. The financial benefit of NHSS is the potentially lower overhead in comparison to operating with a dedicated trust-based supplies function.

The procurement process: There is no fundamental difference between the procurement of goods or the procurement of services. When a need has been identified within an organisation, it is the size of the contracts that determines the process:

– Below £25,000, the trust can decide itself what and where to buy. This is mainly decided by the Executive Team (esp. Director of Operations and Finance Director) and put to the Audit and Performance Committee, which is a sub-committee of the Trust Board. Mostly, decisions are made on the basis of comparing competitive quotations. At times, smaller purchases are done as single tender actions.
– Between £25,000 and £104,435, the trust puts contracts out for tender. The length of the contract can vary, but the total sum needs to be within these limits.
– Above £104,435, the contract has to be put out to tender and advertised in the European journal. This process takes a minimum of 77 days. If these are rolling contracts over a 4 year limit, they also have to be advertised in the European Journal.

For the contracts that have not been put in the European journal, the rules in the trust's own Standing Financial Instructions apply. These lay down rules for the tendering process and management of contracts and the framework is developed by the Department of Health (there is local variation about the size of the £25,000 limit depending on the total size of the organisation's budget). A number of routes are possible:

– NHSS may have a series of "packages" which can be bought. NHSS maintains a database of suppliers for a range of common services and can draw attention to these "packages", e.g. the management of maintenance for information systems or ward supplies. NHSS manages the process of supplies throughout.
– NHSS might offer advice for developing a service specification, manage the tendering process and be involved in contract negotiations e.g. competitive tendering for cleaning and portering services. Once the tender has been awarded to a specific company, the trust manages the contract directly or NHSS does it on behalf of the trust.
– The trust organises a contract directly with a supplier.

The main difference between goods and supplies lies in the fact that in general, it is easier to specify the quality of goods than of services. However, there are notable exceptions, such as highly specialized equipment such as MRIs or ultrasounds that are influenced by medical "preference". In terms of services, the issue of liability (health and safety) has to be considered.

In general, procurement depends on foresight and sound planning, good negotiating skills, credibility (expertise) and building up relationships within the organisation (visibility).

Impact of EU directives and regulations: Setting the financial limits has been one of the main influences of EU directives and regulations, and the process for Europe-wide tendering has to be followed to the letter. Thus, it is difficult to procure things quickly (77 days minimum) and long-term planning is essential. Safety issues concerning sterilisation have been influenced, especially regarding autoclaves. Another example is the storage of liquid gases to comply with a 14 day supply requirement. This means the expansion of tank capacity.

In the UK, the Medical Devices Agency issues up-to-date bulletins to NHSS and the NHS as a whole on EU regulations. In general, everyone appears to be well informed of the latest requirements.

At present, the procurement issue is becoming politically important as the government appears to want to move away from the "privatisation" of services. The idea of developing central coordination across all public services for integrated procurement is gathering momentum.

Reference

Muñoz Machado S. La formación y la crisis de los Servicios sanitarios públicos. Madrid: Alianza editorial; 1995.

Consumer choice of medical goods across borders

Matthias WISMAR, Jens GOBRECHT and Reinhard BUSSE

Abstract. Consumer choice in medical goods is examined in relation to the potentially relevant areas of pharmaceuticals, therapeutic appliances and dentures. Potentially, the impact of European legislation and jurisdiction on the Member States is very high, but in reality the outcome has been minimal. Four major factors account for this gap between impact and outcome: i) the restrictive handling of the pre-authorisation procedure, ii) differences in the health care baskets across Europe, iii) the "unusual" distribution systems of medical goods, and iv) the lack of the cost-reimbursement provisions.

1. Introduction

In this chapter, an attempt is made to analyse intention, impact and outcomes of both the TEC and secondary European legislation in regard to consumer choice for medical goods.

To analyse the impact of Community policy and ECJ rulings on consumer choice in medical goods, using the German situation as an illustration, a) the relevant European and domestic legal sources were analysed (see Table 1), b) medical goods were divided into three important sub-categories, c) structured telephone interviews were conducted, and d) secondary literature was used when appropriate.

Table 1: Major juridical sources in regard to consumer choice of medical goods

Legal source	Articles, paragraphs or rulings of relevance
European level	
TEC	Art. 23 (ex-Art. 9), Free movement of goods
	Art. 28-30 (ex-Art. 30, 34, 36), Prohibition of quantitative restrictions between Member States
Secondary legislation	EEC 1408/71 (Art. 13, 19, 22), modified/ extended especially by EEC 1390/81 [self-employed], 2791/81 [modification following the Pierik cases], 3095/95 [other insured], 1606/98 [special schemes for civil servants] and 307/99 [special schemes for students]
	EEC 574/72
ECJ	C-120/95 "Nicolas Decker"
	other ECJ cases (see next chapter)
German level	
Social Code Book V (SGB V)	§ 16 (1) 1, suspension of eligibility while abroad
	§ 17, provision for employed abroad
	§ 18, cost-coverage for treatment abroad

Germany was chosen as the analytical lead country for the topic of cross-border consumer choice in prescribed medical goods. The rationale for this choice is grounded not only in the fact that Germany has long and relatively densely populated borders to six other Member States (Denmark, the Netherlands, Belgium, Luxembourg, France and Austria) but also, more importantly, because for a brief period in 1998 cross-border consumer choice in prescribed medical goods was in principle possible – and took place.

2. Background

The subject of this section combines the topic of cross-border consumer choice for both medical goods and healthcare services (the latter are analysed in the next chapter).

2.1 Consumerism and patient sovereignty in healthcare

To conceptualise users of health services not only as patients, beneficiaries or insurees but also as consumers is a relatively new approach for most health services in the Member States. In market terms, the patient confronts suppliers of health care (physicians, hospitals etc.) with individual demands and preferences – which have to be distinguished from needs. It is assumed that the consumer is endowed with the power to make or influence decisions which would otherwise have been made exclusively either by the physician or the competent institution. Yet most health services only provide limited opportunities for patients to make choices in relation to prevention, diagnostics, therapy, or medical goods (Schwartz & Wismar 1998). Moreover, even if there is the chance to choose between different options, patients and consumers are faced with a severe lack of useful and valid information to make informed choices.

In terms of healthcare financing, consumer choice in goods seems at first sight a minor issue for health services, but this is not the case for the patient or consumer. Most health services have introduced user charges, reference prices or fixed lump sums for various goods such as glasses, pharmaceuticals, aids and dentures, leaving the patient to top up a considerable portion of the price. Differences in pricing between Member States can therefore serve as an incentive to acquire goods in another country. In addition, tourism and the tendency of pensioners to spend long periods in southern European countries make cross-border consumer choice in goods even more relevant even if not entirely necessary. Last but not least, frontier workers or people residing along densely populated European borders may choose to acquire prescribed medical goods across the border just for reasons of convenience.

2.2 International dimension in social protection

Cross-border provision of social services or international welfare-state arrangements are - in principle - not new, having developed before, parallel and independently from European integration. There are a variety of bi-lateral agreements on cross-border welfare state provision and some of them can even be traced back to the time before the First World War. For example, in 1912, Germany and Italy agreed on the co-ordination of pension schemes for frontier workers (Leder 1995). Similar activities took place between Belgium and France. Currently, Ireland and Northern Ireland are implementing measures for cross-border provision of services (McKee 1999). Germany has concluded Social Security Agreements with a wide range of countries which guarantee necessary treatments in case of emergency or illness abroad[1]. The attempt to co-ordinate health services by introducing minimal standards in regard to the equal treatment of nationals and foreigners is in line with

---

[1] Social protection arrangements are in force (January 2000) with Bosnia-Herzegovina, Bulgaria (pensions only), Yougoslavia, Macedonia, Croatia, Poland, Switzerland, Slovenia, Turkey, and outside Europe Chile (pensions only), Israel, Canada (pensions only), Marocco, and the USA (pensions only).

these developments. The International Labour Organisation (ILO), founded in 1919, and the Council of Europe have been active in this area (Leder 1995).

2.3 Co-ordination of social protection systems in the European Economic Community and the European Community

In this context, the co-ordination of social protection systems in the European Union has to be analysed. The necessity to co-ordinate social protection across the Member States of the EEA[2] can be best explained in terms of an example. In Denmark, all inhabitants – whether nationals or foreigners – are automatically covered by social provision. The welfare state is largely financed from taxation. In contrast to the welfare-state in Denmark, the German pension, health care, long-term care, unemployment and occupational accident schemes are statutory insurance systems financed jointly out of employers' and employees' contributions[3]. As a result the membership of the social insurance scheme is primarily workplace-related. A Danish citizen living in Denmark and working abroad in Germany would have to pay taxes both in Denmark for social protection and contributions in Germany for statutory insurance schemes. Vice versa, a German worker resident in Germany but employed in Denmark would neither pay contributions nor taxes for social provision. In terms of eligibility, the German worker would neither have access to the German or to the Danish health service while the Dane could enjoy the benefits of both.

To avoid such overlapping and excluding competencies, a common co-ordination of the social services was required, which is established in the TEC[4]. It was introduced immediately after the Treaty of Rome was signed – the third regulation ever to come in force in the EEC. In its latest version it is known as Regulation EEC 1408/7.

2.4 The Decker ruling

Meanwhile, the development of European legislation in respect to the issue of cross-border purchase of prescribed medical goods goes beyond Regulation EEC 1408/71 through the impetus of the preliminary ruling of the ECJ in regard to the "Decker case" (C-120/95). Nicolas Decker, a Luxembourg citizen went abroad to purchase a pair of glasses, prescribed by a Luxembourg ophthalmologist. He bought a pair of glasses in Arlon, Belgium. When he returned to Luxembourg he claimed the cost incurred abroad for the glasses from his sickness fund. This was denied on the ground that he had not gone through the normal pre-authorisation procedure. According to Regulation EEC 1408/71, patients who travel to another Member State with the express intention of purchasing medical goods at the expense of the competent institution have to meet this requirement. Otherwise, their costs are not covered. Decker took his case to a Luxembourg court, referring to the free movement of goods established by the TEC. In turn, the competent Luxembourg court asked the ECJ to clarify the interpretation of the TEC through a preliminary ruling. The

---

[2] Iceland, Liechtenstein and Norway as parts of the European Economic Area are part of the co-ordination of social protection in the European Union.

[3] Among the five statutory insurance pillars of the German welfare state, only the occupational accident insurance is payed exclusively by employer contributions.

[4] TEC Art. 42 (ex-Art. 51): "The Council shall, acting in accordance with the procedure referred to in Article 251, adopt such measures in the field of social security as are necessary to provide freedom of movement for workers; to this end, it shall make arrangements to secure for migrant workers and their dependants: (a) aggregation, for the purpose of acquiring and retaining the right to benefit and of calculating the amount of benefit, of all periods taken into account under the laws of the several countries; (b) payment of benefits to persons resident in the territories of Member States. The Council shall act unanimously throughout the procedure referred to in Article 251."

base line of the interpretation was that the free movement of goods is in principle applicable to health services, as long as neither the financial stability of the service nor the public's health is in danger (Wismar & Busse 1998). Yet, the Decker case is not the end of the story. Many questions arising from this and subsequent rulings remain unresolved or disputed.

3. Medical goods relevant for consumer choice

Medical goods for the purpose of this chapter are:

- pharmaceuticals,
- therapeutic appliances and
- dentures.

The potential impact could be very high since, as the German social health insurance (SHI) expenditure data show (Table 2), 19% of all SHI expenditure are for medical goods – a sum of almost € 24.5 billion (not including patient co-payments and direct purchases).

Table 2: Expenditure on medical goods in German SHI (1998) = theoretical impact

Goods	Expenditure in billions of Euro	Percentage of SHI total
Pharmaceuticals	17.06	13.4%
Appliances	4.38	3.5%
Dentures	3.02	2.4%
Sum of goods	24.47	19.3%
SHI total	126.89	100.0%

3.1 Pharmaceuticals

According to the German Pharmaceutical Act (*Arzneimittelgesetz*), pharmaceuticals are substances or manufactured substances which cure, soften, prevent or diagnose illness, sufferings or impairments in humans and animals.

According to § 31 of the SGB V, patients in Germany have a right to obtain pharmacy-only drugs at the expense of the SHI. The German pharmaceutical market contains several, partially overlapping segments:

- Pharmacy-only drugs: Pharmaceuticals which are only allowed to be sold in pharmacies (market data are only available for these drugs).
- Prescription-only drugs: Within the pharmacy-only drugs, prescription-only drugs form the largest segment. These are only allowed to be sold with a prescription and in a pharmacy.
- Prescription possible: Pharmaceuticals which may be prescribed at the expense of the SHI funds. These drugs may also be bought over-the-counter in a pharmacy but a prescription is needed if a SHI fund is to cover the costs.
- Non-prescription drugs: These drugs can be purchased without a prescription in a pharmacy and they cannot be obtained to the expense of SHI funds. The patient has to pay for these drugs in all cases.

Figure 1 visualises the various market segments by expenditure volume.

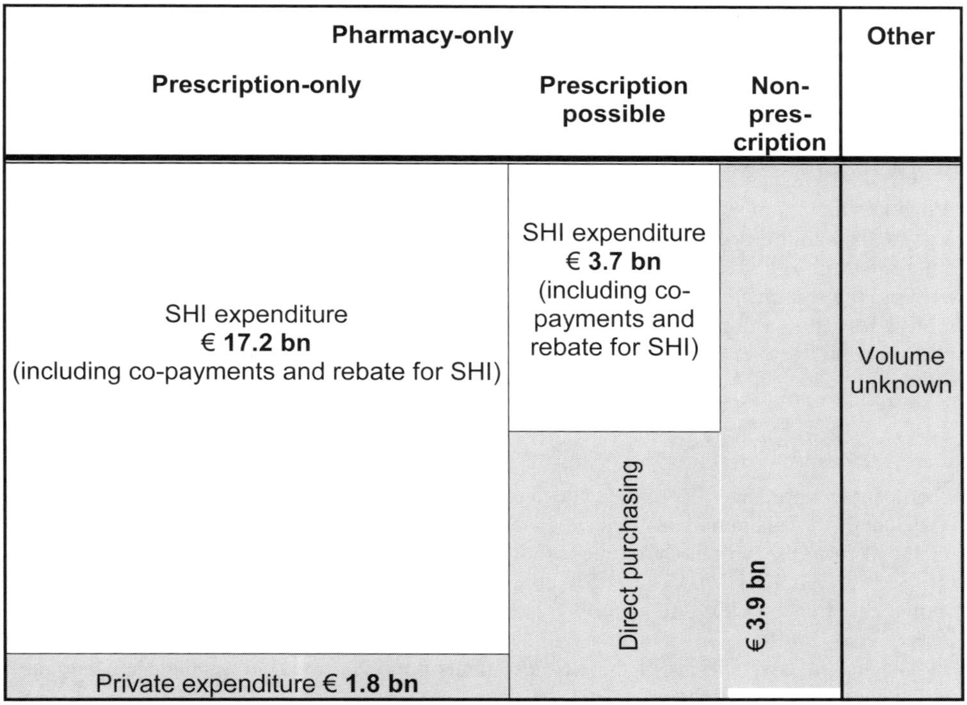

Pharmacy-only			Other
Prescription-only	Prescription possible	Non-pres-cription	
SHI expenditure € 17.2 bn (including co-payments and rebate for SHI)	SHI expenditure € 3.7 bn (including co-payments and rebate for SHI)		Volume unknown
	Direct purchasing	€ 3.9 bn	
Private expenditure € 1.8 bn			

Fig. 1: The German pharmaceutical market according to segments and market volume in Euro (1998); areas in white indicate the SHI-covered market, areas in grey unrestricted consumer choice

Most pharmacy-only drugs may be prescribed to the expense of the sickness funds. However, there are a few but important exceptions – which even include prescription-only drugs – and these are gaining increasing attention (Busse 2000):

– Since 1983 drugs for certain conditions (common colds, drugs for the oral cavity with the exception of antifungal drugs, laxatives and drugs for motion sickness) are legally excluded from the benefits' package for insured people over 18 years old (§ 34(1) SGB V).
– The Social Code Book allows the Minister of Health to exclude "inefficient" drugs (i.e. they are not effective (for the desired purpose) or combine more than three drugs the effect of which cannot be evaluated with certainty (§§ 2, 12, 34(3) and 70 SGB V). The evaluation of these drugs takes into account the peculiarities of homeopathic, phytotherapeutic or anthroposophic drugs. A negative list according to these principles came into effect on 1 October 1991. It was revised in 1993 and contains about 2 200 drugs.
– Additionally, drugs for "trivial" diseases (such as common colds) which can usually be treated by treatments other than drugs may be excluded (§ 34(2) SGB V). A list of this type has not yet been worked out.

The coverage of drugs is also regulated in the pharmaceutical guidelines of the Federal Committee of Physicians and Sickness Funds and forms part of the contract between the two sides at the federal level. These guidelines, which are legally binding, attempt to steer the appropriate use of different groups of pharmaceuticals. They limit the prescription of certain drugs to certain indications (e.g. anabolics to cancer patients), specify that they may only be used after non-pharmaceutical treatments were unsuccessful (e.g. so-called chondroprotective drugs) or in a few cases, disallow any prescription by the sickness funds (e.g. drugs to quit smoking).

In mid-1998, the Federal Committee amended its pharmaceutical guidelines to exclude drugs for the treatment of erectile dysfunction and drugs to improve sexual potency such as Viagra. The committee argues that individually very different behaviour does not allow the determination of a standard of disease upon which to base economic considerations. In its opinion, the responsibility of the sickness funds ends where personal lifestyle is the primary motive for using a drug. The Federal Social Court disapproved of the general exclusion of drugs for the treatment of erectile dysfunction and instead demanded measures against their misuse.

3.2 Therapeutic appliances

Therapeutic appliances comprise devices such as prostheses, glasses, hearing aids, wheelchairs or inhalators. Insured persons are entitled to them, unless they are explicitly excluded from the benefit catalogue through a negative list issued by the relevant ministry (§§ 33 and 34 SGB V).[5] The regulations for the coverage of non-excluded therapeutic appliances are complex and therefore are only briefly described (for further details see Perleth et al. 1999).

The federal associations of the sickness funds publish a medical appliances catalogue, which contains among others:

– a legal account of who may be entitled to medical aids debited to the SHI,
– an alphabetical catalogue of all medical appliances,
– the medical appliances listing which can be provided for the account of the SHI.

The medical aids listing represents a positive list of services which can be provided at the expense of the statutory health insurance (Table 3). The decision to include medical aids lies exclusively with the federal sickness funds' associations. The definition of the medical aids listing is established by law (§§ 126-128 and 139 SGB V).

In the German SHI, the insured person has a right to contact lenses in exceptional cases only. And in these cases the SHI only grants a subsidy up to the costs of spectacles otherwise needed.

3.3 Dentures

Paragraph 30 SGB V subsumes dental prostheses, caps (crowns) and bridges as "dentures". Currently 55 different goods/procedures in the area of prosthesis and denture are listed in the Unified Value Scale-Dentist ("Bema – Bewertungsmaßstab Zahnärzte"). The Federal Committee of Dentists and Sickness Funds agrees on the services provided under SHI coverage and their value relation in so-called value points. Table 4 provides an overview on the prosthetic procedures that matter most in terms of reimbursement value.

---

[5] The Federal Ministry of Labour and Social Affairs (the predecessor of the Ministry of Health) has explicitly excluded aids with small or disputed therapeutic benefit or low selling price (e.g., wrist belts, ear flaps etc.).

Table 3: Listing of therapeutic appliances according to § 128 SGB V by number of category

01	Vacuum devices	13	Hearing aids	25	visual aids
02	Adaptation aids	14	Inhalation devices and devices for breathing therapy	26	Sitting aids
03	Instruments and devices for the application of medicines	15	Aids for incontinence	27	Speaking aids
04	Bathing aids	16	Aids for communication	28	Standing aids
05	Bandages	17	Aids for compression therapy	29	Stoma-items
06	Radiation devices	18	Vehicles for sick persons	30	Splints
07	Aids for the blind	19	Nursing care items	31	Shoes
08	Orthopaedic insoles	20	Storage aids	32	Therapeutic movement devices
09	Devices for electrostimulation	21	Measuring instruments for status and function of the body	33	Toilet aids
10	Walking aids	22	Mobility aids	99	various items
11	Therapeutic appliances against decubitus (bedsore)	23	Orthotics		
12	Aids for patients with removed larynx	24	Prothetics		

Source Hilfsmittelkatalog einschließlich Hilfsmittelverzeichnis, 1.11.1996

Table 4: The ten prosthetic procedures/goods with the highest cumulative reimbursement value and the their frequency 1995 (western part of Germany only)

Bema-No.	Rank	Prosthetic procedure/good	No. of procedures in thousands
91b	1	full porcelain bonded bridge	4,039
20b	2	porcelain bonded crown on tooth	3,996
19b	3	provisional crown	12,609
91d	4	telescopic crown	881
20c	5	jacket or partial crown	670
97a	6	total upper jaw	481
96c	7	partial prosthesis (more than 8 teeth missing)	649
92a	8	bridge element	1,559
100b	9	restoring prosthesis	1,668
24c	10	removal and fixing of provisional crown/bridge	9,536

Source: Kassenzahnärztliche Vereinigung 1996

4. Consumer choice across borders in European legislation and jurisdiction

The surprising finding of this section is that even Regulation EEC 1408/71 contains in principle a far-reaching provision to facilitate cross-border consumer choice for prescribed medical goods.

4.1 Elements of consumer choice in EEC 1408/71: Population covered and rules and principles

Originally, Regulation EEC 1408/71[6] only covered workers. But from the early 1980s onwards, Regulation EEC 1408/71 gradually extended its scope in terms of groups covered. Regulation EEC 1390/81, which came into force on 1st July 1982, included the self-employed. The Regulation also covers members of workers' and self-employed persons' families and their dependants, as well as stateless persons and refugees. In 1991, the Commission submitted a proposal to extend the scope of the Regulation to include all insured persons, particularly students and others not in gainful employment. This proposal has been incorporated into Regulation 1408/71 through Council Regulations EC 3095/95 and EC 307/99.

Council Regulation EC 1606/98 extended the scope of Regulation 1408/71 in order to put civil servants on an equal basis with general statutory pension rights prevailing in the Member States. As a rule, the provisions of the Regulation cannot be invoked by nationals of third countries working in the Union. After pressure from the European Parliament, the Commission in 1997 presented a proposal for a Regulation amending Regulation 1408/71 as regards its extension to nationals of third countries (COM(97)0561).

Although complicated in detail (and terminology) Regulation EEC 1408/71 and the accompanying provisions of Regulation EEC 574/72 rest on two simple sets of rules and four main principles. The two sets of rules are:

1. It defines the competent state as the state in which the beneficiary is employed and has to contribute to social protection schemes either by contribution or by taxes[7].
2. It defines the competent institution as the one from which the beneficiary receives social provision. In case the beneficiary receives social provision outside the competent state the medical care offered is not in accordance with the medical care standards of the competent state but with the standards of the state the patient receives the care[8].

The four main principles are:

1. Equal treatment. workers and self-employed persons from other Member States must have the same rights as the competent State's own nationals. In other words, a Member State may not confine social security benefits to its own nationals. The right to equal treatment applies unconditionally to any worker or self-employed person from another Member State having resided for a certain period of time.

---

[6] Benefits covered by Regulation EEC 1408/71 encompass: sickness and maternity benefits; invalidity benefits, including those intended for the maintenance or improvement of earning capacity; old-age benefits; survivors benefits; benefits in respect of accidents at work and occupational diseases; unemployment benefits; family benefits.

[7] Regulation EEC 1408/71 Art. 13, Paragraph 2, Letter (a): A person employed in the territory of one Member State shall be subject to the legislation of that State even if he resides in the territory of another Member State or if the registered office or place of business of the undertaking or individual employing him is situated in the territory of another Member State.

[8] Regulation EEC 1408/71 Art. 19: Residence in a Member State other than the competent State - General Rules: 1. An employed or self employed person residing in the territory of a Member State other than the competent State, who satisfies the conditions of the legislation of the competent State for entitlement to benefits, (taking account where appropriate of the provisions of Article 18) shall receive in the State in which he is resident: benefits in kind provided on behalf of the competent institution by the institution of the place of residence in accordance with the provisions of the legislation administered by that institution as though he were insured by it.

2. Aggregation. The aggregation principle means that the competent Member State must take account of periods of insurance and employment completed under another Member State's legislation in deciding whether a worker satisfies the requirement regarding the duration of the period of insurance or employment. The right to membership of sickness funds, for example, can be transferred directly from a fund in one Member State to a fund in another Member State.
3. Prevention of overlapping benefits.
4. Exportability. Benefits can be paid throughout the EU and Member States are prohibited from reserving the payment of benefits to people resident in the country[9].

Regulation EEC 1408/71 is not specific about medical goods. Nevertheless, it does contain some provision allowing cross-border consumer choice in prescribed medical goods, which would otherwise not be granted. The most obvious case are frontier workers. They may obtain health care in both the country of the competent state and the competent institution[10].

Regulation EEC 1408/71 also provides a legal basis for different ways of intentional cross-border care and therefore for consumer choice. The first procedure, outlined in Article 22(1)(a), was originally intended for health care during a temporary stay abroad, during which insurance with the competent institution is certified through an E111 form. Only certain groups of persons may receive healthcare services regardless of whether their condition is urgent. These are:

- pensioners and their families;
- unemployed persons and their families who go to another Member State to seek employment;
- employed or self-employed persons exercising their professional activity in another Member State;
- frontier workers (although their families must obtain prior authorisation for non urgent treatment if there is no agreement between the countries concerned);
- students and those undertaking professional training and their families.

All other persons are only entitled to receive goods and services if their condition urgently requires it, i.e. it is not the intention of Regulation 1408/71 to facilitate the crossing of borders to receive goods or services.

The second procedure, regulated in Article 22(1)(c), is outlining an option for al these "other" persons. It requires, however, pre-authorisation by the competent institution, which is certified through an E112 form[11]. According to the Regulation, only under certain circumstances and on very specific grounds in regard to the health status of the patient can

---

[9] This principle does not apply to all social security benefits. There are special rules for the unemployed.

[10] Regulation EEC 1408/71 Art. 20: A frontier worker may also obtain benefits in the territory of the competent State. Such benefits shall be provided by the competent institution in accordance with the provisions of the legislation of that State, as though the person concerned were resident in that State.

[11] Regulation EEC 1408/71 Art. 22: An employed or self-employed person who satisfies the condition of the legislation of the competent State for entitlement to benefits, taking account where appropriate of the provisions of Article 18, and: [...] who is authorised by the competent institution to go to the territory of another Member State to receive there the treatment appropriate to his condition, shall be entitled: to benefits in kind provided on behalf of the competent institution by the institution of the place of stay or residence in accordance with the provision of the legislation which it administers, as though he were insured with it; the length of the period during which benefits are provided shall be governed, however, by the legislation of the competent State; to cash benefits provided by the institution in accordance with the provision of the legislation which it administers. However, by agreement between the competent institution and the institution of the place of stay or residence, such benefits may be provided by the latter institution on behalf of the former, in accordance with the provisions of the legislation of the competent State.

this pre-authorisation be denied[12]. A denial of the pre-authorisation is categorically ruled out if the patient has to wait an unacceptable time for treatment[13].

The pre-authorisation procedure – although not intentionally designed for the purchase of goods – does not seem to preclude cross-border consumer choice. As a matter of fact, if the wording of Regulation EEC 1408/71 is strictly applied, the competent institution has no right to deny pre-authorisation for the purchase of a pair of glasses in another Member State. Despite the bureaucratic procedure, Regulation EEC 1408/71 already facilitates consumer choice[14].

4.2 Elements of consumer choice in the "Decker ruling"[15]

In principle, the Decker ruling is on consumer choice. But three restrictions have to be made. First of all, it applies explicitly only to the ambulatory sector. Although the Attorney General referred to the hospitals sector in his opinion, the ECJ did not follow the argument because the Decker case did not apply to it.

The ECJ did not only scrutinise the case according to the Articles 28 (ex 30) and 30 (ex 36) of the Treaty of the European Communities, which deal with the free movement of goods, but also according to the Council Regulation (EEC) 1408/71 in its amended and updated version by Council Regulation (EC) 118/97. The main question was if a national rule which demands a prior authorisation by a social security institution of a Member State as pre-condition for a reimbursement of a good purchased by an optician established in another Member State is compatible with the Articles 28[16] and 30[17] of the TEC.

First of all, the ECJ questioned the applicability of Art. 30 in regard to social provision and came to the clear conclusion that social security cannot exclude the application of the principle of free movement of goods[18].

In regard to the limits of 1408/71, the ECJ concluded that although 1408/71 regulates reimbursement procedures in case of prior authorisation, it does not apply to cross-border provision of services and goods without prior authorisation (par. 27-29).

---

[12]Regulation EEC 1408/71 Art. 22: The authorisation required under Paragraph 1 (b) may be refused only if it is established that movement of the person concerned would be prejudicial to his state of health or the receipt of medical treatment.

[13]The authorisation required under Paragraph 1 (c) may not be refused where the treatment in question is among the benefits provided for by the legislation of the Member State on whose territory the person concerned resided and where he cannot be given such treatment within the time normally necessary for obtaining the treatment in question in the Member State of residence taking account of his current state of health and the probable course of the disease.

[14]The gap - or better gulf - between theory and practice of regulation EEC 1408/71 will be analysed below.

[15]The question of the Luxembourg legal backgrounds will not be discussed here, but instead the focus will be directed at the aspects which are relevant for the health systems throughout Europe.

[16]TEC Article 28 (ex-Article 30): Quantitative restrictions on imports and all measures having equivalent effect shall be prohibited between Member States.

[17]TEC Article 30 (ex-Article 36): The provisions of Articles 28 and 29 shall not preclude prohibitions or restrictions on imports, exports or goods in transit justified on grounds of public morality, public policy or public security; the protection of health and life of humans, animals or plants; the protection of national treasures possessing artistic, historic or archaeological value; or the protection of industrial and commercial property. Such prohibitions or restrictions shall not, however, constitute a means of arbitrary discrimination or a disguised restriction on trade between Member States.

[18]Par. 24: "[...] that measures adopted by Member States in social security matters which may affect the marketing of medical products and indirectly influence the possibilities of importing those products are subject to the Treaty rules on the free movement of goods; and that the fact that the national rules at issue in the main proceedings fall within the sphere of social security cannot exclude the application of Article 30 of the Treaty."

In regard to the assumed conflict between the pre-authorisation procedure and the free movement of goods, the ECJ endorsed the view of Nicolas Decker. The Court held the opinion (par. 34-36) that the rules at issue encourage persons insured under the Luxembourg social security scheme to purchase their medical goods in Luxembourg and not abroad[19]. This was regarded to be a barrier to the free movement of goods.

In Article 36 of the Treaty of the European Communities some exceptions to the free movement of goods are permitted, for example if the financial balance of the social security system is endangered. A reimbursement at a flat-rate would have – according to the ruling (par. 38-40) – no effect on the financing or the balance of the social security system.

According to the opinion of the court (par. 43), an equal quality of goods purchased in another Member State is guaranteed due to the system for the recognition of professional education and training. Furthermore, the Court pointed out (par. 44) that the protection of public health was guaranteed because the spectacles were purchased using a prescription from an ophthalmologist.

In conclusion, the European Court of Justice ruled:

> "Articles 30 and 36 of the Treaty of the European Communities preclude national rules under which a social security institution of a Member State refuses to reimburse to an insured person on a flat-rate basis the costs of a pair of spectacles with corrective lenses purchased from an optician established in another Member State, on the ground that prior authorisation is required for the purpose of any medical product abroad."

5. Impact on national legislation

Unlike European directives, regulations such as EEC 1408/71 and preliminary rulings (like the Decker ruling) do not require a formal process of transposition. Regulations are addressed towards EU citizens, and they are generally and immediately in force.

Two reactions are possible: 1. Actors in the health policy arena may feel obliged to comply with the regulation or ruling instantly, even if the government is inactive. 2. The regulations and their contents are not generally known by citizens or other actors involved because they do not have to be transposed into national legislation through a process which, depending on the subject, will bring many details to light (as it is the case with directives).

Nevertheless, governments can feel obliged to amend existing legislation in order to bring it into line with the regulation or preliminary ruling.

Not all Member States adopted a formal position in regard to the Decker ruling or documented one in the course of a preparatory meeting in November 1998 for the German Presidency (Gobrecht 1999).

5.1 Impact of the "Decker ruling" in Germany

In Germany, the Decker ruling caused a sharp political response (Wismar & Busse 1998). With the 2nd SHI Restructuring Act of 1997 (i.e. before "Decker"), the previous conservative-liberal parliamentary majority had expanded the choice between the customary benefit in kind principle and the cost-reimbursement procedure to all insurees

---

[19] Par. 35: "While the national rules at issue [...] do not deprive insured persons of the possibility of purchasing medical product in another Member State, they do nevertheless make reimbursement of the costs incurred in that Member State subject to prior authorisation. Costs incurred in the State of insurance are not subject to that authorisation."

while it had previously been restricted to voluntary members (i.e. those who have a choice between SHI and substitutional private health insurance). The earlier restriction was re-introduced with the Act to Strengthen Solidarity in SHI which was passed by Parliament late in 1998, i.e. after "Decker". The objective was to roll-back all those market mechanisms which were believed to cause social inequalities or to undermine solidarity. This restriction met the firm criticism especially of the liberal party which did repeat its opposition to the measure even a year later during the debate of the Reform Act of SHI 2000 (Deutscher Bundestag 1999).

In a draft version of that Reform Act of SHI 2000, clarification in regard to the Decker ruling was planned, but for unknown reasons it was finally abandoned. The original amendment stated that insurees, who are eligible for cost-reimbursement in the domestic territory, could submit claims from all EU Member States. Additionally, there were plans to allow those (mandatory) insurees who had chosen the option of cost-reimbursement previously to be granted this right again. This was in reaction to the protest especially by pensioners who live for longer periods in the south without giving up Germany as country of residence.

5.2 Impact on pharmaceuticals in Germany

These legal activities limiting consumer choice of medical goods across borders can be contrasted against legal provisions made in regard to pharmacies and parallel and re-imports of pharmaceuticals[20]. Parallel and re-import pharmaceuticals do play a role in regard to consumer choice in prescribed medical goods. Parallel imports are those which were produced abroad by companies linked to German producers but imported by an independent import company parallel to the distribution channel of the resident company. Re-imported pharmaceuticals are those which were produced by a domestic company and exported to markets abroad and then re-imported to the market of origin by an independent company. The incentive for both parallel imports and re-imports is the pricing differences of pharmaceutical goods across Member States.

The Health Care Reform Act of 29th December 1988, which came into force on 1st of January 1989, required through §129 SCB that all pharmacies have to hold stocks of cheap imported pharmaceuticals for consumers. This rule was abolished due to doubts that such a legal provision might not comply with the rules of a free market. Nevertheless, the federal associations of sickness funds and the German Pharmacists' Organization (*Deutscher Apothekerverband*) agreed to have import pharmaceuticals in stock as long as they are at least DM 1 cheaper than the comparable product on the German market.

6. Outcome

6.1 The outcome of the "Decker ruling"

Despite the harsh reaction of the former German government in regard to the "Decker ruling", sickness funds felt obliged to comply with the new legal situation. The telephone

---

[20]In the strict sense, re-imports and parallel imports do not fall in the scope of this chapter, because it is not the consumer that moves across the border but the good. Nevertheless, it is briefly dealt with to draw a more complete picture from the consumers' point of view.

interviews conducted in 1998[21] produced evidence on the cost-reimbursement of costs incurred abroad[22].

According to the sickness funds, prescriptions issued by a physician can generally be used in every Member State, provided that foreign pharmacies, opticians or medical suppliers accept the prescription. The application of an E-form or the pre-authorisation procedure is necessary neither for acquisition nor for reimbursement of medical goods. Therefore, the German liaison office for SHI ("Deutsche Verbindungsstelle Krankenversicherung Ausland") is not involved.

Cross-border purchases of medical goods require the cost-reimbursement procedure because the sickness funds do not have a direct link to pharmacies, opticians or in the medical suppliers abroad and are therefore unable to clear the bill directly in terms of the "benefit in kind" procedure.

Obviously there are variations in the handling of cost-reimbursement. The Kaufmännische Krankenkasse Hannover (KKH) asks the foreign health insurance before reimbursing the patient which costs would have been reimbursed there in the same case and uses this amount as a measure for its payment. The Barmer Ersatzkasse (BEK) reimburses the costs at the price of the most favourable contract provider after individual case examination only. If a therapeutic aid is purchased abroad, maintenance and guarantee from the side of the health insurance and at the expense of the health insurance are excluded.

In regard to pharmaceuticals the patient also receives the equivalent quality and the same active substance in the other Member States, in accordance with European licensing regulations, and in addition, if possible, the same volume. However, differences in package size and in the appearance of the package are possible[23]. The German SHI funds only reimburse the costs of pharmaceuticals according to German law, the pharmaceutical guidelines and in accordance with the German contracted rates, i.e. minus a rebate of 5% which German pharmacies have to give to sickness funds and minus the patient's co-payment. Additionally, the patient has to cover costs above the German reference price.

The case of therapeutic appliances appears more complicated than pharmaceuticals. In the case of eyeglasses purchased abroad, the insuree receives the fixed subsidy for the eyeglass lens according to German reimbursable prices. Frames of eye glasses are generally not reimbursed, however. Payment occurs at maximum up to that German price level, yet never more than the invoice amount. That means that the insured can never make a profit but may save money by purchasing pharmaceuticals or eyeglasses abroad.

Most German SHI funds have a pool of therapeutic aids and appliances which need not be made up for each insured person individually (wheel-chairs, walking aids etc.). The patient only borrows the appliance from this pool, i.e. they do not pass into the possession of the patient. Generally, the permission of the sickness fund must be given first, as in Germany, before medically prescribed therapeutic aids or appliances can be purchased. The legal requirements for cost-reimbursement of therapeutic aids or appliances are laid out in the SGB V. According to § 13 and § 126, the dispensary supplying the therapeutic aids has to be a contracting party of the health insurance. Therefore, reimbursement of costs for therapeutic appliances acquired abroad might be possible merely in individual cases after precise examination.

---

[21] Telephone interviews were conducted in August 1998 with major SHI funds (Allgemeine Ortskrankenkasse, AOK; Techniker Krankenkasse, TK; Deutsche Angestellten Krankenkasse, DAK; Barmer Ersatzkasse, BEK; Innungskrankenkasse, IKK; Kaufmännische Krankenkasse Hannover, KKH; Gmünder Ersatzkasse, GEK). Local offices were chosen in order to get as close to operational business as possible.

[22] Question in the structured interview fell in four categories: pharmaceuticals, small appliances (eyeglasses), expensive appliances (wheel-chair), denture.

[23] This applies theoretically to eyeglasses and wheel-chairs, too, according to statements of sickness funds.

All sickness funds interviewed would grant the fixed cost subsidy – which was used at that time but has since been abolished in favour of co-insurance – for dentures purchased abroad only under certain conditions which again vary from sickness fund to sickness fund. The Techniker Krankenkasse (TK) grants the fixed cost subsidy only if the denture was made in Member or in countries with which a Social Security agreement exists to regulate the terms of settling the account. The Allgemeine Ortskrankenkasse AOK demands a certification that the dentures correspond to German high-quality standards (expert opinion, equivalence certification). The BEK excludes guarantees in the case of foreign dentures purchased at its expense.

One of the reasons to expect (more) cross-border consumer choice are price differentials. Yet, knowledge on pricing of medical goods across Europe is limited. But both patients and the competent financing institution may have an incentive for cross-border consumer choice as Table 5 suggests for dentures

Table 5: Price indices (purchasing power parity / average hourly wage in manufacturing industry) for selected dental care procedures in 1999 (Germany = 100)

	CH	D	DK	F	GB	NL	H
crown	149/161	100/100	178/149	199/290	44/49	100/111	72/183
cast metal bridge	140/150	100/100	264/221	278/405	n.a.**	144/161	145/365
full porcelain bonded bridge	88/95*	100/100	158/132	177/258	35/39	81/90	60/150
metal cast denture (frame prosthesis)	91/98*	100/100	130/109	207/302	42/46	99/111	49/123
total prosthesis	132/141	100/100	139/117	251/365	28/31	77/86	63/159

* only dentist's honorarium; **is not part of the benefit package and only asked for seldomly by private patients

Source: Kaufhold & Schneider 2000

6.2 Pharmaceuticals: parallel and re-imports

It is estimated, that parallel trade within the European Union could reach annual growth rates of up to 5-12%. In 1995, the Federal Constitutional Court in Germany ruled that wholesalers have to take parallel imports and that pharmacies also have to stock the cheapest product. As a result, importers and wholesalers save money, but they also have to spend extra money on licences for the import and the re-labelling of the drugs as well as for instruction leaflets.

According to information of the Statutory Health Insurance and pharmaceutical importers, the total amount of turnover of parallel- and re-importing is about DM 700 million per year. This is equivalent to a rate of less than 2% of the total amount of prescribing turnover. A survey of the Federal Association of Pharmaceutical Manufacturers (*Bundesfachverband der Arzneimittelhersteller*) – representing the non-prescription manufacturers – found that the most important countries of origin for parallel- and re-importing of pharmaceuticals are Greece and Portugal and then by a wide margin Belgium, Italy and Spain (cf. chapter on pharmaceutical market in Sweden). There has to be a minimum difference of 10% of the consumer price, for the importing to be profitable[24].

---

[24] Arzneimittel für Europa, published by Arzneimittel Zeitung, 11th Edition, 1998: 24-8.

6.3 Unintended effects

At Community level, two basic intentions can be distinguished, one relating to secondary legislation and the other one to the TEC.

In regard to the former, Regulation EEC 1408/71's main intention was to ensure that EU citizens who are eligible for health care provision under a national health service or an insurance system can obtain access to the health care system of the state where they reside. EU citizens should not be deterred from exercising their free movement because of a possible loss of social security rights. In this respect the intention of Regulation EEC 1408/71 was to facilitate in the first place a European labour market. The objective was to link national social protection systems so that they interact or provide the migrant with a constant social protection (van der Mei 1998). Nevertheless, it was demonstrated, that the legal provision laid out in regulation EEC 1408/71 goes – at least in theory – beyond the mere European labour market perspective. From that point of view, the development towards an extended consumer choice in prescribed medical goods was not intended.

Approaching the issue from the TEC, the conclusion in regard to unintended effects is somewhat different. From the point of view of Community policy the attack on the "benefit in kind" principle is probably the most important unintended effect of the current developments. Although economists who favour market-like organisation of health services have always argued that the "benefits in kind" principle blurs the financial transparency of service provision – and is a source of inefficiency and waste and restricts the consumer sovereignty of patients – throughout the Member States the benefit in kind principle is still favoured. The argument go that the patient usually meets the provider of services under circumstances which are characterised by various asymmetries and, probably more importantly that, due to contractual arrangements, the "benefits in kind" principle allows better expenditure control.

Although the previous German government had strong views in regard to the Decker ruling and the influence of European legislation and jurisdiction, the current coalition government in Germany was far more moderate – if not tentative in its conclusion. Its first Minister of Health, Andrea Fischer pointed out that the accelerating economic integration inevitably has a growing influence on the structures and contents of health care systems (Fischer 1999). In this respect, restriction of free choice between the benefit-in-kind and the cost-reimbursement principle with the Act to Strengthen Solidarity in SHI was not so much a reaction to the assumed growing influence of Brussels on the German health service. It was far more an attempt to roll-back policies introduced by her predecessor, such as the increase in co-payments, the exclusion of services covered by SHI etc. (Busse & Wismar 1997). The idea was to eliminate elements of health care legislation with market character in so far as they were suspected of undermining solidarity.

7. Comparison – Spain, Sweden and the UK

The outcome of the Decker ruling on the German health service was quiet unique compared to other countries for various reasons.

7.1 Cost-reimbursement

Among the Member States analysed in this project, Germany was the only one which endowed its insurees – at least for a certain span of time – with the universal right to cost-reimbursement. Therefore, the Decker ruling was directly relevant to Germany but to the other countries with NHS-type systems delivering medical goods in kind (or not at all).

In Spain, a 1967 Royal Decree permitted the reimbursement of costs in case of emergency and of unjustified refusal to provide health care. Today, the Spanish Royal Decree 63/1995 limits reimbursement to "cases of urgent, immediate and crucial health care for patients that have received care outside the National Health System. In these cases costs are reimbursed, once it has been proven that the National Health Services could not be used appropriately and that it is not an abuse or deviation of this exception".

From Sweden rather anecdotal evidence is reported from the handling of cost-reimbursement issues in regard to both 1408/71 and the Decker ruling. First of all, medically necessary treatment beyond the scope of E 111 (short term stay) seems to be ruled out. That implies that regulation EEC 1408/71 and especially the pre-authorisation procedure is handled very restrictively. In turn, cross-border consumer choice in prescribed medical goods is allegedly not taking place. According to information from the National Social Insurance Board, the Decker ruling was not regarded as providing a precedence. It was suggested rather that, if a patient should refer to the Decker case, this should be treated on an individual basis. Planned medical treatment, except in special cases – e.g. for dialysis or oxygen treatment – was more or less ruled out. However, an excessive waiting period for treatment could qualify for medical treatment abroad with cost reimbursement. Nevertheless, no reports on such cases were found.

In the UK cost reimbursement is literally unknown. At least until recently, the NHS lacked institutional, organisational and technical facilities to organise cost-reimbursement.

7.2 Benefit packages

A pre-condition for consumer choice of prescribed medical goods under 1408/71 is that the competent state and the Member State of the competent institution both have the desired item in their benefit packages. Yet, very little is known about what is in the benefit packages across Member States.

In Spain, the Royal Decree 63/1995 establishes a common frame for medical goods and services covered by the National Health System. In regard to dental care as specified in this catalogue, primary dental health care comprises: a) information and education regarding dental hygiene and health, b) preventive and care measures: administration of topical fluoride, obturations, seal of fissures with topical fluoride and other measures for children, according to the funding and the special dental programmes each year, c) acute orthodontic care including teeth extraction, d) preventive mouth exploration for pregnant women. On the basis of this catalogue, most dentures and prosthetics seem to be excluded from the benefit package (with the exception of the Basque Country where a more generous dental benefits' basket exists).

Dentures are, in principle, covered in the Swedish health service. Although, due to the decentralised organisation of the service, there seem to be some variation in access and user charges.

Table 6 shows that in many European countries dentures are not part of the benefit package, i.e. result in 100% user charges.

Table 6: User charges* in selected dental care procedures/goods (in per cent in 1999)

	CH	D	DK	F	GB	NL	H
crown	100 %	100 %	42-55%**	93 %	80 %	100 %	100 %
cast metal bridge	100 %	47-59 %	100 %	92 %	n.a.	100 %	100 %
full porcelain bonded bridge	100 %	78-84%**	100 %	93 %**	80 %	100 %	100 %
metal cast denture (frame prosthesis)	100 %	35-50 %	100 %	86 %	80 %	100 %	100 %
total prosthesis	100 %	35-50 %	100 %	89 %**	80 %	25 %	100 %

* without private complementary insurance; ** calculated per-cent

Source: Kaufhold & Schneider 2000

7.3 Distribution of prescribed medical goods

A further reason for the limitation of free consumer choice in prescribed medical goods is the specificity of the goods themselves. They are either only available in special shops, they do not always pass into possession of the patient or they need a national certificate to prove its quality.

In Germany, patients cannot buy their own dentures. The order for the denture is sent directly from the dentist to the dental laboratory which is accredited to the SHI. The dentist invoices the patient (for the co-insurance part) and the Regional Association of SHI Dentists (*Kassenzahnärztliche Vereinigung*) which in turn has contracts with the sickness funds. The cross-border purchase for denture or prosthetic parts by a German patient for his treatment in Germany is therefore impossible.

Therapeutic appliances may only be delivered to insured persons by authorised service providers. Authorisation is granted to service providers who guarantee a sufficient, expedient, functional and economical production, delivery and adaptation of therapeutic appliances and who recognise the declarations valid for supply to the insured (§ 126 SGB V). The federal associations of sickness funds are jointly drawing up a list of therapeutic appliances. In this register all therapeutic aids which must be provided by the SHI are listed and the intended reference prices are to be indicated (§128 SGB V). Only the products recorded in this list of therapeutic appliances can be prescribed at the cost of the SHI.

Quite similar distribution channels exist in Sweden. According to the Health and Medical Services Act appliances are tested individually. Most of the appliances do not pass into the possession of the consumer, but are owned by the county council. More than 90 per cent of all the appliances in Sweden are tested by a special institute. This institute also gives recommendations to the county councils which appliances should be used. But it is always the physician or the expert who helps the consumer to choose the appliances. Therefore, it is almost impossible to choose appliances across borders.

Reference List

Busse R. Health care systems in transition – Germany. Edited by A. Dixon. Copenhagen: European Observatory on Health Care Systems; 2000.

Busse R, Wismar M. Health care reform in Germany: the end of cost containment? eurohealth 1997;3(2):32-3.

Calnan M, Palm W, Sohy F, Quaghebeur D. Implementing a policy for cross-border use of health care: a case study of frontier worker's knowledge, attitudes and use. In Leidl R. (ed.) Health care and its financing in the single European market. Amsterdam-Berlin-Oxford-Tokyo-Washington DC: IOS Press; 1998. p. 306-11.

Deutscher Bundestag. Stenographischer Bericht, 66. Sitzung, Berlin, Donnerstag, den 4. November 1999. Plenarprotokoll 14/66.

Fischer A. A new public health policy in the European Union. In Bellach B-M, Stein H, editors. The new public health policy of the European Union. Past experience, present needs, future perspectives. München: Urban und Vogel; 1999. p. 10-22.

Gobrecht J. National reactions to Kohll and Decker. eurohealth 1999;5(1):16-7.

Hermans HEGM. Patient's rights in the European Union. Eur J Public Health 1997;7(3 Suppl.):11-7.

Hermesse J, Lewalle H, Palm W. Patient mobility within the European Union. Eur J Public Health 1997;7(3 Suppl.):4-10.

Hilfsmittelkatalog einschließlich Hilfsmittelverzeichnis [katalogue of appliances and aids including the appliances and aids inventory], Stand 1.11.1996

Kassenzahnärztliche Vereinigung. KZBV Jahrbuch 96. Statistische Basisdaten zur vertragszahnärztlichen Versorgung [German Federal Association of Sick Fund Dentists Yearbook 1996. Statistical data on the the service provision of statutory health insuarance dentists]. Köln: Kassenzahnärztliche Vereinigung 1996.

Kaufhold R, Schneider M. Preisvergleich zahnärztlicher Leistungen im europäischen Kontext [Price comparison of dental benefits in the European context]. IDZ - Information Institut der deutschen Zahnärzte 2000/1: 1-33.

Leder H. Internationale Sicherung [International social security]. In: Bundesministerium für Arbeit und Sozialordnung, editor. Übersicht über das Sozialrecht. Bonn: Bundesministerium für Arbeit und Sozialordnung, Referat Öffentlichkeitsarbeit; 1995. p. 697-721.

Leidl R, Rhodes G. Cross-border health care in the European Union. Eur J Public Health 1997;7(3 Suppl):1-3.

McKee D. Health care across borders: The scope for North-South cooperation in hospital services. eurohealth 1999;5(4):19-20.

Neumann-Duesberg R. Die EuGH-Position ist angreifbar [The ECJ's position is open to attack]. Gesundheit und Gesellschaft 1998;1(10):22-7.

Perleth M, Busse R, Schwartz FW. Regulation of health-related technologies in Germany. Health Policy 1999;46(2):105-26.

Schwartz FW, Wismar M. Planung und Management [Planning and management]. In: Schwartz FW, Badura B, Leidl R, Raspe H, Siegrist J. Hg.) Das Public-health-Buch - Gesundheit und Gesundheitswesen. München-Wien-Baltimore: Urban und Schwarzenberg; 1998. p. 558-73.

Tögel T. Draft opinion of Commission 5 for Social Policy, Public Health, Consumer Protection, Research and Tourism on the role of the local and regional authorities in the reform of European public health systems 1999. COM 5/021.

van der Mei AP. Cross-border access to medical care within the European Union - Some reflections on the judgements in Decker and Kohll. The Maastricht Journal of European and Comparative Law 1998;5(4):277-97.

The European Union and Health Services
R. Busse et al. (Eds.)
IOS Press, 2002

Consumer choice of healthcare services across borders

Reinhard BUSSE, Markus DREWS and Matthias WISMAR

Abstract. The chapter first explores access to healthcare services across borders, especially the E111 and attached administrative procedures in the case of Germany, cross-border patient flows and resulting expenditure under E106, E111 and E112, and the ECJ "Kohll" case which established a new procedure for cross-border care. It then analyses the various procedures in regard to consumer choice in four dimensions: range of benefits, degree of restrictions, choice among providers and rate of reimbursement. It demonstrates that E112 is strong on benefits and reimbursement but weak on restrictions while "Kohll/ Decker" is strong on choice but weak on benefits and reimbursement. The chapter concludes by outlining activities to improve access to services across borders, especially in the Euregios.

1. Introduction

Consumer choice for healthcare services across borders is a relatively new research topic. Until 1998, attention focused on the free movement of persons and their potential healthcare needs when on the "other side of the border". This was particular relevant for frontier workers, i.e. persons who live in one country but work in another on a daily basis. But, with the growing movement of workers from southern European countries to those further north, the issue of how to ensure their right to healthcare services while on holidays in their country of origin became an issue. The advent of mass tourism has added a third group of persons to those in need of access to healthcare services in other countries. It was with these groups in mind that, building on previous regulations as well as bi-lateral agreements, Regulation 1408/71 was passed. Regulation 1408/71's original intention was therefore not to facilitate the free movement of services or goods but to facilitate the free movement of persons, more specifically that of workers (for details see previous chapter). The practical consequences of Regulation 1408/71 for people travelling to and from Germany using the E111 process is analysed in Section 2.

From its inception, Regulation 1408/71 also contained, however, an element of the free movement of services, namely the procedure of pre-authorised care with the E112 form. Under this procedure, persons cross borders specifically to receive healthcare services in the other country. In economic terms, services are imported to the country which authorises the patient to go abroad while the country providing the service is exporting it. As the Regulation does not mention that it is based on the free movement of services, this can therefore be considered an unintentional effect. Section 3 will briefly summarise the existing research on the amount of such imported/exported healthcare services.

The famous "Kohll" ruling is dealt with in Section 4. In brief, Raymond Kohll had argued that a restriction of consumer choice for healthcare services across borders – under Regulation 1408/71 and the respective procedures in Luxembourg – would violate Articles 49 and 50 of the TEC. As this conflict was new, the "Cour de cassation" in Luxembourg referred it to the ECJ which agreed with the plaintiff's interpretation of the Treaty, basing consumer choice of healthcare services across borders directly on the Treaty, and not on secondary legislation (Table 1).

Table 1: Major European sources and interventions analysed and discussed

Legal source	Articles, paragraphs or rulings
TEC	Art. 28-30 (ex-Art. 30, 34, 36), Prohibition of quantitative restrictions between Member States
	Art. 49-50 (ex-Art. 59-60), Free movement of services
Secondary legislation	EEC 1408/71 (Art. 13, 19, 22), modified/ extended by EEC 1390/81 [self-employed], 2791/81 [modification following the Pierik cases] and 1606/98 [civil servants]
	EEC 574/72
ECJ	C-117/77 & C-182/78 Pierik I & II
	C-158/96 Kohll
	C-368/98 Vanbraekel
	C-157/99 Geraets-Smits/ Peerbooms
	currently pending at the ECJ: C-385/99-1 Müller-Fauré/ van Riet

Section 5 analyses the resulting new "Kohll/ Decker" procedure to obtain healthcare services as well as the E111 and E112 procedures in respect of four dimensions relevant to consumer choice – range of benefits, degree of restrictions, choice among providers and reimbursement. Finally, explicit measures to facilitate a higher choice of healthcare services across borders in the "Euregios" will be briefly summarised in Section 6.

The following chapter looks at future scenarios concerning the development of consumer choice in respect of the four dimensions. This chapter also includes a section on the latest rulings, namely "Geraets-Smits/ Peerbooms" and "Vanbraekel".

2. Choice of healthcare services under Regulation 1408/71

2.1 E111 in practice: the case of foreigners coming to Germany

A person coming to Germany from an EEA country who seeks medical help and who produces an E111 is entitled only to healthcare services that are of "immediate necessity" and in accordance with the existing regulations within German statutory health insurance.[1] Apart from the E111 no further document is required, although an identity card or passport may be requested. The patient is accepted as being a member of the health insurance/national health system of the country of origin. The same applies to family members who are included on the E111 form. The foreign health authority decides in accordance with local laws and regulations which family members are insured and includes these persons on the E111. In regard to entitlements and actual treatment, no difference is made between the insured persons and their dependants included on the E111.

Equally, no difference is made with respect to employment status – with one exception. Members of the social insurance scheme of Belgium who are self-employed have only limited access to benefits. They receive the form E111 "B" in Belgium which only entitles them to hospital treatment in Germany (as well as in other countries), while they have to pay privately for ambulatory care services.

There is no specific time span within which holders of an E111 can claim benefits other than the period of validity of the E111 itself as issued by the health authority of the country

---

[1] Certain groups, such as the unemployed seeking a job, are exempted from the principle of "immediate necessity" and use a different form, i.e. the E119.

of origin (section 3.1 of the form). In some countries, for example the United Kingdom, E111 forms are frequently issued without any expiry date (as possible under section 3.2 of the form). If a long period of time has passed between the day the E111 was issued and the day when it is actually being used, it is likely that the sickness fund will check whether the holder of the document should be insured under the regulations of the German health insurance system. This is the case when anyone taking up work in Germany earns less than the current (2002) threshold of Euro 3375 per month. Students, artists, handicapped living in specialized institutions and others are also compulsory members of one of the legal sickness funds when they start work or enroll at university etc. If there is no reason to believe that the person should be insured in Germany, the form will be accepted as valid.

If a citizen of another Member State wishes to obtain health care services and benefits in Germany, the formal process would be to see an office of one of the approximately 420 statutory sickness funds. The visitor will show his E111 and the official will check formal criteria of the document such as validity, name of patient's insurance company in his country, signature, falsification (handwritten additions possibly made by holder, e.g. adding family members). A frequently occuring problem seems to be that handwritten forms are presented which, depending on the handwriting, seem to be more or less illegible. The foreign visitor with a valid E111 will then receive a document called a "Krankenschein" which substitutes for the German insurance card. This document is essential if a physician in the ambulatory care sector is to claim reimbursement from the sickness fund via the ambulatory physicians' association. The document will carry a note made by the sickness fund official about restrictions of EU regulations to "immediate illness", which by definition excludes health promotion and prevention services. The foreigner will then be able to present this "Krankenschein" to the physician of his/her choice. Should he/she need treatment in a hospital or from a specialist physician he/she will then have to go back to the sickness fund he originally chose with a document from the physician to obtain another such "Krankenschein".

In reality, the experience is that neither the patient nor the physician really knows how to deal with the E111 process, and frequently the patient will not even possess an E111 form. In practice, therefore, the ambulatory care physician will probably telephone one of the legal sickness funds requesting information about the procedure. He will then mail the patient's E111 to the sickness fund, provided the patient is in possession of one. The fund, in turn, will post the "Krankenschein" for this patient. If no E111 is available, the physician has to bear the financial risk of treating the patient. In emergency cases, he is obliged by law to treat the patient. After treatment, the sickness fund will assist both the patient and the doctor to acquire an E111 form from the responsible authority in the patient's country of origin.

If the E111 holder seeks treatment in a hospital directly, he/she will, generally speaking, be in need of very urgent attention, such as in cases of traffic accidents or suspected heart attack (as German hospitals do not regularly have outpatient departments). He/she might even have to be taken to hospital by an ambulance (which is covered by the German SHI benefits catalogue). In practice he/she will not have had time to consult a sickness fund office. If he/she presents an E111, the hospital official will know (or find out) what to do. If the patient is not in possession of an E111, the hospital will give the relevant data to a sickness fund which in turn requests the E111 from the patient's sickness fund or national health service in the country of origin.

German sickness fund officials will not issue any E111 to foreigners, as the form may only be issued by the relevant authority in the country of insurance affiliation (often at the request of the German sickness fund). There are no specific lists of physicians or hospitals for E111 holders – they can receive medical attention for immediate illness at any of the institutions or practices contracted by the sickness funds. Under the current system of collective contracts of sickness funds and providers, these include about 97 % of all hospitals and practices. As the non-contracted hospitals are specialised and small, it is extremely unlikely that a foreigner will seek treatment by a non-contracted provider.

After treatment has ended (involving possibly more than one consultation) and/or at the end of every quarter, the service provider will claim reimbursement from the German sickness fund, in the case of hospitals directly, in the case of ambulatory care physicians via the regional physicians' association. The fund or the physicians' association will pay the provider and in turn will request reimbursement from the German liaison office for SHI ("Deutsche Verbindungsstelle Krankenversicherung Ausland") by posting all relevant information (name, date of birth, services given, amount of fees) to this institution. The German liaison office will forward the claim and debit the charges to the insurance company or national health service of the patient's country of origin. The United Kingdom and Ireland have, in relation to Germany, bilaterally waived their right for refund concerning E111 cases (except dialysis). This agreement has recently been terminated by Germany as it feels that the waiver is to its disadvantage. A similar waiver agreement exists between Denmark and Germany in respect to unemployed persons using the E119, but not for E111-related cases.

There are two considerations involved in accepting or refusing foreigners' "consumption" of healthcare services. The competent authority – the statutory sickness fund – must first decide on the formal criteria (such as EU regulations and German laws as outlined above). In cases of doubt the German sickness fund will get in contact with the foreign authority. The extent of benefits a foreigner may receive in respect of "immediate illness" and "immediate necessity for treatment" is primarily decided by the provider treating the patient. The sickness fund may, in turn, check whether any "unnecessary" treatment has been given before reimbursing the treatment. In case of doubt, the fund will ask the Medical Review Board to re-evaluate the treatment before withholding reimbursement. Only suspicious cases would be considered for two reasons. First, the sickness fund official is not a physician and will probably not become aware of questionably urgent cases. Second, the additional costs arising from the re-evaluation cannot be claimed from the foreign competent authority. In practice, the sickness fund checks the E111 document, getting into contact with the issuing institution if considered necessary, and the physician in his practice or in the hospital decides about the necessary treatment. Apart from the restriction to immediately necessary treatment, foreign visitors are dealt with in the same way as Germans (appointments etc.). Obviously this depends very much on the individual physician and the special circumstances applying to the foreign visitor through his short stay, the type of illness, and the slightly different formal procedures.

An illness that has existed before the claimant arrives in Germany is an exclusion criterion for obtaining healthcare benefits if a patient presents with such an illness without a need for immediate treatment. A different situation arises if the cause for seeking help is a worsening of a preexisting illness (e.g. onset of pain). The patient will then be able to make use of E111 benefits. It is not possible for the German liaison office to estimate how often patients are not aware or purposely violate this restriction and how often, if at all, their intention to receive treatment for a preexisting illness with the E111 is rejected. In general there is no indication of obvious abuse of the E111 process or fraud on a regular basis. Individual cases cannot be excluded because there is no institutionalized report system of abuse.

Patients needing dialysis receive it with the E111. Dialysis is considered a treatment of immediate necessity, although in conjunction with a preexisting illness. These patients are well informed about their situation and dependence on treatment. Normally, they will arrange treatment in Germany prior to leaving their home country.

Benefits under the provisions of the E111 for pregnancy depend on the stage of pregnancy. If a woman falls pregnant while in Germany she is able to claim full benefits from the German statutory health insurance scheme. With the exception of Finland, a woman already pregnant at the time when leaving her country of insurance affiliation will normally not receive benefits, unless the pregnancy gives rise for immediate necessity of treatment (incuding birth) while the woman is staying in Germany. In practice, a pregnant woman visiting a foreign country will probably only visit a doctor if she gets worried that something is wrong. Should her situation not fall within the limits set by the regulations for the E111, the German fund contact the foreign authority.

As a general rule visitors presenting an E111 form do not have to pay any fees before being treated especially since there will normally be some element of urgency. The visitor can claim all benefits in kind, including medication, which a German patient would receive. There is the limitation to these benefits in kind for a visitor in that he can claim only what is needed until his intended return to his home country. For example, he will only receive a small pack of a necessary medication. Additionally, the E111 holders are required to pay all co-payments that are applicable in the German SHI system.

2.2 E111 in practice: the case of Germans going abroad[2]

In Germany, E111 forms are issued by the statutory sickness fund with which the person is insured. Some sickness funds have changed their practice and now issue blank E111 forms with instructions on how to complete it. The funds usually also issue information brochures about the the health services and possible pitfalls in country to be visited.

German sickness funds will cover all costs for treatment of immediate necessity which were provided and invoiced by the foreign provider or the statutory health insurance/national health service. If a person insured with one of the German funds has been treated by a private practitioner or a private hospital, only those costs will be reimbursed directly to the patient that the treatment would have costed if the patient had been treated in Germany. Therefore tourists are advised to insure themselves privately in addition to the E111. Costs arising through repatriation will not be reimbursed, a further reason to have additional insurance.

A somewhat unusual institution has been introduced In Mallorca with the opening of an information service by the AOK (Allgemeine Ortskrankenkasse), the General Regional Sickness Fund. About 2.5 million Germans visit Mallorca annually, of whom approximately 2 million are insured with the AOK. It therefore made sense to open a branch since many visitors need help with translation or when choosing a hospital or physician. Many difficulties, initially for the tourist and subsequently for the AOK, can be avoided before they arise, e.g. the problem that apparently many taxi drivers and tour guides bring tourists who become ill only to private physicians and private hospitals.

Problems of a similar kind have been reported about Austria. Physicians and hospitals seem to be unwilling to treat patients according to EU regulations upon presentation of an E111. They advise patients to pay directly and to claim refund from their sickness fund in Germany. As such a private bill is almost always higher, the patient then has to cover that part which the German fund does not reimburse.

As only 88 % of the population living in Germany is insured with a statutory sickness fund and is thus entitled to receiving an E111, the question arises of how the others are covered for healthcare services across borders. Nine per cent of the population are covered by private health insurance, 2 % by free governmental health care (i.e. police officers,

---

[2] This section complements the chapter on "The mobility of citizen - a case study and scenario on the health service of the Costa del Sol".

soldiers and those on welfare who have not been a sickness fund member previously) while only 0.1 % are not insured.

Persons with a private health insurance pay their fees directly to the provider and will be reimbursed by their private insurer. They do not use the E111. The latest Standard Insurance Regulations, which state the minimal set of regulations and which apply to all German private health insurance companies, provide coverage for all EU countries for an unlimited period in respect to length of stay in that country (as long as the place of residence of the insured person remains within Germany). As the insurers also do not limit reimbursement to a certain number of (contracted) providers but allow access to all providers, persons covered by full-cover private health insurance clearly have a larger degree of "consumer choice" than E111 holders. There are, however, some differences depending on the insurance company and the tariff/scheme chosen by the insured person.

About one third of those with private insurance are civil servants who also receive "Beihilfe" (governmental financial support) covering between 50 and 100 % of costs (i.e. they are privately insured only for the remainder). In case of treatment outside Germany, "Beihilfe" only reimburses the types of treatment and up to the value that would paid for in Germany. All costs that are not covered by the "Beihilfe" have to be paid privately or by an additional insurance.

Some people, who are fully dependent on social welfare, are not insured with one of the sickness funds. Their treatment is covered by the community of residence and they receive the same benefits in kind as do members of one of the legal sickness funds. They do not receive an E111, yet should they travel to another EU Member State, become sick and identify themselves as dependent on social welfare, according to the European Convention on Social and Medical Assistance they should receive the same help as citizens of that country.

3. Cross-border patient flows

Knowledge on the actual cross-border movement of persons receiving healthcare services remains rather limited. In quantitative terms, it is mainly based on one study on the amounts and flows of financial transfers for cross-border care within the EU (Hermesse et al. 1997), which has been updated to 1998 (Palm et al. 2000).

According to these figures, the total amount for claims for reimbursement of cross border healthcare rose from 461 million Euro in 1989 to 1103 million Euro in 1993, but then fell to 894 million in 1997 and 758 million in 1998. In relation to public spending on healthcare in the European Union, these values are in the 0.1 %-0.2 % range of overall expenditure. The study carried out research into the flow of the three most important forms for cross-border mobility: E106 (migrant workers), E111 (temporary stay, e.g. tourism and business travel) and E112 (pre-authorised care). Pre-authorised care accounted for nearly 60 % of the total cost of cross border care, while the transfer for temporary stay and migrant workers were financially less important with 25 % and 16 % respectively of the total expenditure. In terms of the number of forms submitted the ranking was in reverse order. With a share of 53 %, the E106 form (migrant workers) was most applied, while E111 (temporary stay) accounted for 33 % and E112 (pre-authorised care) only for 14 %. Only 9 % of the forms referred to hospital care.

Table 2 summarises the expenditure on imported services, i.e. on patients going abroad. Consistently, Luxembourg had the highest per-capita expenditure, but this fell in line with the EU average from 1993. Other countries with above-average expenditures are especially Belgium, Italy and Portugal. Low expenditure figures can be seen particularly in the Nordic countries.

According to the same study, France has been the main exporter of services (= importer of patients) with a share of at least 40 %. It receives its money from the other Member States exclusively through invoiced credits, i.e. does not use lump-sum payments. The latter method is, for example, favoured by Spain.

Table 2: Expenditure on patients receiving healthcare services in other EU Member States in Euro per capita (= volume of imported healthcare services per capita)

	1989	1993	1997	1998
Belgium	3.62	8.93	8.93	4.38
Denmark	-	0.16	0.83	0.63
France	0.79	1.87	1.21	1.05
Germany	1.77	1.83	2.08	2.21
Greece	0.95	2.51	2.68	3.15
Ireland	0.18	0.65	1.68	0.93
Italy	2.99	8.36	3.52	2.89
Luxembourg	58.01	149.55	135.29	116.00
Netherlands	1.95	0.26	1.98	2.85
Portugal	0.82	3.76	6.81	7.00
Spain	0.33	1.48	1.03	1.11
United Kingdom	0.33	1.61	1.92	0.36
Austria	-	-	0.48	1.87
Finland	-	-	0.49	0.52
Sweden	-	-	0.65	0.96
AVERAGE	1.31	2.95	2.37	1.99

Source: Palm et al. 2000

Certain limitations have to kept in mind when interpreting the data, however. First, there are (or have been) waiver agreements between several countries, for example between Germany and the United Kingdom, so that healthcare services provided on that basis do not appear in the expenditure data. Second, France was the claimant for more than half of all money in 1993 (57.6 %) while Italy was the debtor for 43.1% which can either be explained by an extensive cross-border movement of patients from Italy to France or simply by incomplete, and therefore misleading, statistics. Third, expenditure per capita seems to be decreasing, even though public awareness of the issue has increased, especially in 1998 (see below).

The case of Italy has been studied in some depth (France 1997, Mountford 2000). Italian doctors seem to refer patients to specific healthcare providers outside Italy quite often and feel justification for doing so because of the perceived low quality of their own healthcare system. In addition, authorisation by the regional health authorities for care outside Italy did not have any financial consequences for the regional health authorities until 1997 as expenditure was paid directly by the Ministry of Health. Only since 1998 have such expenditures been deducted from the money allocated to the regions.

In regard to the double access eligibility of frontier workers (i.e. access to services both in the country of residence and in the country of work), a survey, conducted at the French-Belgian border in 1994/95, produced evidence that level of awareness of the arrangements for double access to health care was limited. Approximately one-fifth of both groups of frontier workers were unaware that this option was available. In regard to consumer choice, the results of the survey indicated that 64% of the Belgian and 42 % of the French frontier workers used the option for cross border health care occasionally or usually for goods such as drugs' 38 % and 20 % respectively used it for specialist care, and 27 %, and 23 % respectively for hospital care. Both groups reported problems with reimbursement, of which the most common problem was "expenses not being covered" (Calnan et al. 1998).

4. Unfolding a new dimension of consumer choice: the "Kohll" case[3]

4.1 The issues

In its judgment of 25 April 1996, the Luxembourg Cour de Cassation (Court of Cassation) referred to the Court for a preliminary ruling two questions on the interpretation of Articles 59 and 60 of the TEC in the Maastricht version (now Articles 49 and 50). Those questions arose in proceedings between Mr Kohll, a Luxembourg national, and the Union des Caisses de Maladie (UCM), with which he is insured, concerning a request by a doctor established in Luxembourg for authorisation for Mr. Kohll's daughter, who is a minor, to receive treatment from an orthodontist established in Trier (Germany).

In a decision on 7 February 1994, following a negative opinion of the social security medical supervisors, the request was rejected on the grounds that the proposed treatment was not urgent and that it could be provided in Luxembourg. That decision was confirmed on 27 April 1994 in a decision of the UCM board. Mr Kohll appealed against that decision to the Conseil Arbitral des Assurances Sociales (Social Insurance Arbitration Council), arguing that the provisions relied on were contrary to Article 59 of the Treaty. The appeal was dismissed in a decision dated 6 October 1994.

Mr Kohll appealed against the latter decision to the Conseil Supérieur des Assurances Sociales (Higher Social Insurance Council) which, in its judgment of 17 July 1995, upheld the contested decision on the ground that Article 20 of the Luxembourg Codes des Assurances Sociales (Social Insurance Code) and Articles 25 and 27 of the UCM statutes were consistent with Council Regulation (EEC) No 1408/71.

It appears from Article 20(1) of the Code des Assurances Sociales, that with the exception of emergency treatment received in the event of illness or accident abroad, insured persons may be treated abroad or use a treatment centre or centre providing ancillary facilities abroad only after obtaining the prior authorisation of the competent social security institution. Under Article 27, authorisation will be granted only after a medical assessment and on production of a written request from a doctor established in Luxembourg indicating the doctor or hospital centre recommended and the facts and criteria which make it impossible for the treatment in question to be carried out in Luxembourg.

Mr Kohll appealed against the judgment of the Conseil Supérieur des Assurances Sociales, arguing in particular that it had considered only whether the national rules were consistent with Regulation No 1408/71, and not whether they were consistent with Articles 59 and 60 of the Treaty. Since it considered that this argument raised a question concerning the interpretation of Community law, the Cour de Cassation stayed the proceedings and referred the following two questions to the Court for a preliminary ruling:

1. Are Articles 59 and 60 of the Treaty establishing the EEC to be interpreted as precluding rules under which reimbursement of the cost of benefits is subject to

---

[3] As there have been numerous articles dealing with the judgement (see the chapter on "The European Union and health services - the context"), this section will concentrate on the facts and follows closely the text provided by the ECJ in its ruling.

authorisation by the insured person's social security institution if the benefits are provided in a Member State other than the State in which that person resides?

2. Is the answer to Question 1 any different if the aim of the rules is to maintain a balanced medical and hospital service accessible to everyone in a given region?

Through these questions, the national court was essentially asking whether Articles 59 and 60 of the Treaty preclude the application of social security rules such as those at issue in the main proceedings. Mr Kohll submitted that Articles 59 and 60 of the Treaty preclude such national rules which make reimbursement of the cost of dental treatment provided by an orthodontist established in another Member State, in accordance with the scale of the Member State of insurance, subject to authorisation by the insured person's social security institution. UCM and the Luxembourg, Greek and United Kingdom Governments contended that those provisions are not applicable or, alternatively, do not preclude the rules in question from being maintained. The German, French and Austrian Governments agreed with the alternative submission.

The questions to be considered concerned first the application of the principle of freedom of movement in the field of social security, then the effect of Regulation No 1408/71, and finally the application of the provisions on freedom to provide services.

In the proceedings before the ECJ, Mr Kohll submitted that he sought reimbursement by UCM of the amount he would have been entitled to if the treatment had been carried out by the only specialist established in Luxembourg. On that point, UCM considered that the principle that a person is subject to one social security tariff only would indeed be complied with if the Luxembourg tariff were applied, but claimed that Regulation No 1408/71 would compel it to reimburse expenditure according to the tariffs in force in the State in which the service was provided.

4.2 The ruling

The European Court of Justice ruled as follows (Kohll ruling, paragraphs 4-6):

"The fact that national rules fall within the sphere of social security cannot exclude the application of Articles 59 and 60 of the Treaty. While Community law does not detract from the powers of the Member States to organise their social security systems, they must nevertheless comply with Community law when exercising those powers, i.e. the fact that a national measure may be consistent with a provision of secondary legislation, in this case Article 22 of Regulation No 1408/71, does not have the effect of removing that measure from the scope of the provisions of the Treaty.

Article 22 of Regulation No 1408/71 is intended to allow an insured person, authorised by the competent institution to go to another Member State to receive there treatment appropriate to his condition, to receive sickness benefits in kind, on account of the competent institution but in accordance with the provisions of the legislation of the State in which the services are provided, in particular where the need for the transfer arises because of the state of health of the person concerned, without that person incurring additional expenditure. It is not intended to regulate and hence does not in any way prevent the reimbursement by Member States, at the tariffs in force in the competent State, of costs incurred in connection with treatment provided in another Member State, even without prior authorisation.

Articles 59 and 60 of the Treaty preclude national rules under which reimbursement, in accordance with the scale of the State of insurance, of the cost of dental treatment provided by an orthodontist established in another Member State is subject to authorisation by the insured person's social security institution. Such rules deter insured persons from approaching providers of medical services established in another Member State and constitute, for them and their patients, a barrier to freedom to provide services. They are not justified by the risk of seriously undermining the financial balance of the social security system, since reimbursement of the costs of dental treatment provided in other Member States in accordance with the tariff of the State of insurance has no significant effect on the financing of the social security system, nor are they justified on grounds of public health within the meaning of Articles 55 and 66 of the Treaty in order to protect the quality of medical services provided to insured persons in other Member States and to maintain a balanced medical and hospital service open to all. Since the conditions for taking up and pursuing the profession of doctor and dentist have been the subject of several coordinating or harmonising directives, doctors and dentists established in other Member States must be afforded all guarantees equivalent to those accorded to doctors and dentists established on national territory, for the purposes of freedom to provide services. …"

4.3 Impact on national legislation

Following the judgements of the ECJ, only Luxembourg, Belgium and Denmark amended their legislation and established administrative procedures for the unconditional reimbursement of certain out-patient services and health care products purchased in another Member State. In Austria, even before the *Kohll* and *Decker* rulings, socially insured persons were entitled to reimbursement of health care from a non-contracted provider in Austria or abroad at a rate of 80 % of the amount paid for the same treatment from a contracted provider. As explained in the previous chapter, eight months after "Kohll and Decker" Germany abolished the option for all sickness fund members to choose patient reimbursement (instead of the customary benefits-in-kind) which had been introduced shortly before and which facilitated the possibility to receive healthcare services in other EU countries. In summary, impact upon legislation in EU Member States as a whole was negligible.

5. Analysis: degree of consumer choice of cross-border healthcare

The Kohll and Decker rulings of the ECJ (Decker C-120/95; Kohll C-158/96) established, probably unintentionally, a new type of cross-border access to healthcare. European citizens covered by a statutory social protection scheme in one country (CoI = country of insurance affiliation) now have, in principle, three ways to receive healthcare services in another EEA country (CoS = country of service provision), namely

- the procedure outlined in Article 22(1)(a) of Regulation 1408/71, i.e. access to immediately necessary care during short-term stays using the E111 form
- the procedure outlined in Article 22(1)(c) of Regulation 1408/71, i.e. pre-authorisation to receive care in another Member State using the E112 form
- the "Kohll/ Decker" procedure, i.e. "free access" to ambulatory services (and goods) with retrospective reimbursement.

For the purposes of comparison, "consumer choice" is intended to demonstate maximum benefit for the consumer, i.e.

- to have access to the fullest range of medical goods and services ("benefits"),
- to have these benefits with the minimum restrictions (such as necessary referral patterns or prescriptions),
- to have maximum choice between different providers, and
- to have full reimbursement for any amount charged by the provider.

This description does not imply that a maximum of consumer choice is a preferable situation. Table 3 examines the degree of choice for each of the four dimensions mentioned earlier for each of the three cross-border options in comparison to the statutory social protection/ insurance system inside the CoI.

Table 3: Applicability and degrees of consumer choice in accessing health services

	Inside country of insurance (CoI)	Short-term stay (E111)	Preauthorisation (E112)	"Kohll/ Decker" procedure
Countries in which applicable	CoI	Non-CoI EEA countries plus others with E111-agreement	Non-CoI EEA countries plus others with E112-agreement	Non-CoI EU coun-tries if CoI uses patient reimburse-ment system (incl. Austria)
Benefits available	Benefits catalogue of CoI	Benefits catalogue of CoS, provided the condition necessi-tates immediate care	Legally benefits catalogue of CoS, de facto often that of CoI	Ambulatory benefits of CoI
Condition to get service	Referral/ prescription/ rationing measures if necessary/ existing in CoI	Referral/ prescription if necessary in CoS (possibly plus further hurdles)	Pre-authorisation for particular service by responsible CoI-payer (but through certain rationing measures in CoI, e.g. waiting lists, patient has right to E112)	Referral/ prescription if necessary in CoI
Service providers available	Those contracted by CoI-payers (all providers in Austria and Belgium)	Those contracted by CoS-payers	Those contracted by CoS-payers	Wide availability as no contracts with CoI- or CoS-payers necessary
Rate of reimbursement	As agreed with CoI-payers, with possible reductions (e.g. 20% for non-contracted providers in Austria)	Usually as agreed with CoS-payers (CoI-rate if no CoS-rate exists or with consent of patient)	As agreed with CoS-payers	Price charged by provider, limited to patient/ provider re-imbursement in CoI

CoI = country of insurance (or other social security) affiliation; CoS = country of service provision

Benefits in country of insurance

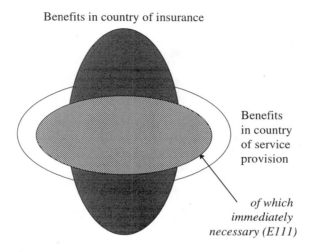

Benefits
in country
of service
provision

*of which
immediately
necessary (E111)*

Fig. 1: Extension of available benefits (vs. country of insurance) through E111

None of the options provides the highest degree of choice in all dimensions. Figures 1 to 3 explore the range of benefits available. All figures show two overlapping circles, the vertical one symbolises the benefits available in the country of insurande (CoI) and the horizontal one those in any other EEA country. If the range of benefits is larger than in the CoI, the appropriate area is marked.

Benefits in country of insurance
(= de facto available with E112)

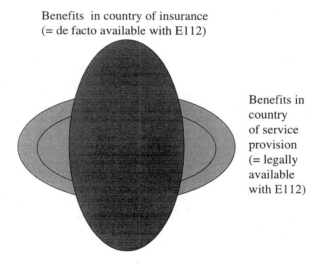

Benefits in
country
of service
provision
(= legally
available
with E112)

Fig. 2: Extension of available benefits (vs. country of insurance) through E112

If the benefits' catalogue in an EEA country during a short-term stay is larger than in the CoI, than the insured person has, under E111, access to additional benefits as Article 22(1)(a) of Regulation 1408/71 provides that a patient is treated according to the regulations of the CoS. However, as the availability of services under E111 is generally limited to those that are immediately necessary, the availability of the additional benefits will be restricted. Additionally, benefits included in the catalogue of the CoI will not be available in the CoS (Figure 1).

A good example of increased access to benefits under E111 are Norwegians travelling in Germany. In Norway, in contrast to Germany, dental care is not part of the statutory benefits package, but a Norwegian visitor in Germany will receive dental treatment on presentation with toothache. It is possible that there is some abuse although this is likely to be limited, since travelling from Norway to Germany for the sole purpose of abusing the system seems rather unlikely.

The benefits available with E112 under Article 22(1)(c) of Regulation 1408/71 are less clear. These have been subject, more than 20 years ago, to two important ECJ cases: Pierik I (C-117/77) and Pierik II (C-182/78). Pierik was a Dutch citizen insured in the Netherlands applying for authorisation to receive a treatment in Germany which was not included in the Dutch benefits catalogue. The ECJ confirmed her right to get the authorisation and in a second ruling, this positive discrimination was confirmed by the ECJ (and Regulation 1408/71 was subsequently amended through Regulation 2791/81).

Since then, the benefits catalogue available under Article 22(1)(c) of Regulation 1408/71 is actually larger than that in the CoI only (Figure 2) – even though de facto this is not usually the case (either because patients do not seek treatment abroad for services that are not available in the CoI, or because they do not sue the competent authorities when refused such treatment).

In contrast to these extensions of available benefits under E111 and E112, the widely publicised Kohll and Decker cases did not lead to an extension of available benefits. Under the resulting "Kohll/ Decker" procedure, the range of benefits is not only limited to those covered in the CoI, but is even limited to a subset of benefits, namely ambulatory services (Figure 3).

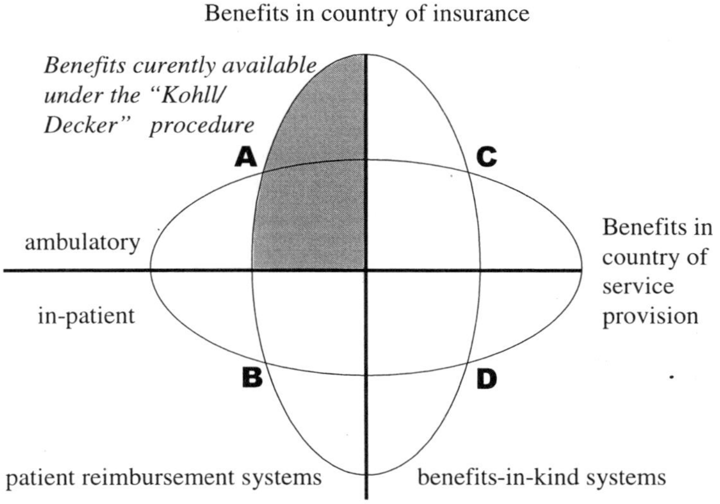

Fig. 3: Benefits available under the "Kohll/ Decker" procedure (early 2001)

In addition, based on the interpretation of the Member States, the benefits are largely limited to countries which routinely use patient reimbursement (Belgium, France,

Luxembourg) or as an alternative to the provision of benefits in kind (Austria). In some other countries, it is restricted to certain special groups (group 2 persons in Denmark; voluntarily insured with patient reimbursement agreement in Germany) or certain services (Denmark for group 1 and 2).

Figure 3 tries to capture these double restrictions by dividing the two overlapping circles into four parts, symbolising ambulatory care in patient reimbursement systems ("A") and in benefits-in-kind systems ("C") as well as in-patient services in these two types of systems ("B" and "D" respectively).

In respect to the other dimensions of choice, differences between the various procedures are especially striking in regard to the range of service providers available (Table 3):

– Regarding the conditions to obtain a service, an E111 patient has to conform with the conditions in the CoS which might be better or worse than at home. E112 has mixed effects; on the one hand, it provides another hurdle (i.e. to get the E112 authorisation), on the other hand, it improves the situation in comparison to within the CoI as it provides a way to circumvent waiting lists.
– E111 and E112 procedures limit the choice of providers to those contracted by the responsible third-party payers in the CoS, i.e. systematically it neither decreases nor increases choice. It will, rather, depend on a comparison between the circumstances in the CoI vs. the CoS. Patients coming to Belgium, for example, will find their choice increased while it will be the other way around for Belgian patients who go to, for example, Spain.
– Under the "Kohll/ Decker" procedure, the choice of provider is virtually unlimited. This definite advantage is, however, counterbalanced by a potentially higher patient cost-sharing due to a difference between the price paid in the CoS and the price reimbursed by the responsible third-party payer in the CoI (while there are currently no savings to be made if the price differential is the other way around).

6. Activities to improve access to healthcare services across borders

As shown in the previous sections, consumer choice across borders is quite restricted under the two main options provided by Regulation 1408/71, mainly through administrative hurdles. However, the new "Kohll/ Decker" procedure also has its limitations. A potentially serious limitation is that direct payment is required and that a lower rate of reimbursement in the country of insurance affiliation may lead to a co-payment which would otherwise not arise (and which does not arise under the E111 and E112 procedures due to the benefit in kind principle).

Two promising options to improve access to healthcare services across borders are therefore to ease the administrative procedures and to extent contracts for providing benefits-in-kind across borders. Both options have been and are used in certain border regions within the EU, most notably in the context of the Euregios.

Euregios which have included health services arrangement in their activities include Meuse-Rhine (involving Belgium, Germany and the Netherlands), Rhine-Waal (Germany and the Netherlands), Scheldemond (Belgium and the Netherlands), Hainaut/Nord-Pas-de-Calais (Belgium and France), Schleswig/Südjütland (Denmark and Germany), Eems-Dollart and Rhine-Eems-Ijssel (both Germany and the Netherlands) (Palm et al. 2000).

Long before the term "Euregio" was created or the Euregio Scheldemond established, the Dutch Zeeland-Flanders and West Brabant Sickness Fund (OZ) established contracts with two Belgish hospitals in Ghent and Bruges in 1978. Currently, about 4 % of CZ insurees make use of these contracts. Another example of a contractual arrangement is the one on cross-border ambulance transport from the Belgish municipality of Riemst to the AZ hospital in Maastricht, the Netherlands, as part of the Euregio Meuse-Rhine (see below).

Classical examples of easing the administrative burden for patients can be found in the Euregios Scheldemond and Hainaut/Nord-Pas-de-Calais. In the former, a simplified E112 procedure using a form called E112+ is used. This idea was then adapted in the latter region where an E112TF form can be printed using the French insured person's *Vitale* card or the Belgish insured person's S/S card. Form E112TF is then filled out by the hospital where the insured person seeks treatment and is send directly with the request for payment to a sickness fund in the country of the hospital (which then reimburses the hospital and handles reimbursement by the patient's country of insurance). The project demonstrated that social security cards can be used from one country to another.

Activities in the Euregio Meuse-Rhine started with an analysis of cross-border patient flows in 1991/92 to four large hospitals in the three-country zone. Flows were quite small, ranging from 0.01 % German patients in Liege (Belgium) to 1.7 % Belgish patients in Maastricht (The Netherlands) (Starmans et al. 1997). Since spring 1997, the project has sought to improve cooperation between hospitals and health insurance funds in the three countries. "Zorg op Maat" enabled Dutch patients to access Belgish and German ambulatory care specialists with the E112+ form. This activity was extended to a trilateral project named "Integration Zorg op Maat" from 2000 (Table 4).

Table 4: Cross-border care activities in the Euregio Meuse-Rhine

Name	Features	Period
AOK office in Vaals (The Netherlands)	An office of the German sickness fund AOK provides support to insured living in the Netherlands	Since 1995
Zorg op Maat	Access to Belgish and German ambulatory specialists for Dutch patients using the E112+ form	Ended 1999
Integration Zorg op Maat	Specialist treatment and therapy	Since spring 2000
	Prescription of pharmaceuticals	
	Hospital treatment	
	Therapeutic appliances (requires E112/E114)	
	Centres of excellence (requires E112/E114)	
Rescue and Emergency	Under the Interreg II Programme planning for Interreg III	
Transparency in therapeutic appliances (hearing aids)	Under the Interreg II Programme cost-utility analysis for cross-border service provision	
Co-operation with health insurance funds	Co-operations and co-ordination	

A similarly wide array of activities can be found in the Euregio Rhine-Waal (Table 5), ranging from sickness fund offices in the other country to arrangements enabling patients to access both outpatient and inpatient specialist care across borders (in this case, Germans to access the hospital in Nijmegen).

Table 5: Cross-border care activities in the Euregio Rhine-Waal

Name	Features	Time
Office Service at the Dutch coast for holiday makers	Germans insured with AOK Rheinland receive support in Middleburg and Vlissingen/Zelland from CZ Groep	Since 1996
Patient treatment without borders	Heart surgery	Since 1997
	Radio therapy	
	Renal transplantation	
	Neurosurgery/Traumatology	
Zorg op Maat	See the Zorg op Maat in the Euregio Rhine-Maas	Since 1999
Needs and quality analysis	Needs for cross-border care	
	Quality of service provision	
	Humanitarian aspects	
	Patient/Insuree satisfaction	
	Impact on planning	
	Economic aspects	
Traumatology	Emergency care	Until 1999
HealthCard international	Like Integration Zorg op Maat, but with a Smart card	Since summer 2000

All these activities, with the exception of Scheldemond, involve rather small numbers of patients, usually not exceeding a few hundred. Their evaluation, however, implies some important lessons: First, waiting lists are cited as the major factor contributing to cross-border care (Coheur 2001) which might become an even more relevant factor in the future. Second, proximity of the provider to the place of residence of the patient is another major factor stimulating cross-border care. In the case of Rhine-Waal, for example, the university hospital in Nijmegen is less than 15 km from the German border, whereas comparable hospitals in Germany are up to 100 km away. Using a rather narrow definition of border areas, i.e. all those counties within a 20 km strip along the borders, it becomes clear that the potential for patients seeking access to healthcare services is quite large – but will vary between ambulatory and hospital as well emergency and elective care (Table 6).

The topic of easier access to healthcare services across borders is gaining increasing attention also outside the Euregios: In Germany, the Working Group of Federal Associations of Sickness Funds, which comprises all groups of sickness funds, is urging the government to amend social legislation in order to allow German sickness funds to selectively contract providers in the EEA (Arbeitsgemeinschaft der Spitzenverbände der gesetzlichen Krankenkassen 2000). The reasons for this are threefold. First of all, sickness funds do not appreciate a "Decker/Kohll solution" since this would entail the abolition of the benefit in kind principle. The benefit in kind principle establishes a close link between payers and providers not only on prices and volumes but also on quality. The price issue is not of primary concern since reimbursement would be limited to the domestic level (even though keeping budgets for healthcare sectors will become more difficult). And the volume issue does not matter much, since cross border care still occurs in rather small numbers. The quality issue seems to be more tricky because it assumes that quality abroad is lower than in Germany, an assumption which is difficult to base on evidence. The political reason for the contracting solution is to evade the collective contracts sickness funds hold with providers inside Germany. Provider associations, especially associations of statutory health insurance-affiliated physicians, would loose power if German sickness funds could contract providers abroad.

Table 6: Potential cross-border patients in German *Länder* (population in countries within 20 km of border with EU countries)

Land	Absolute number in million and percentage of population	
	Currently	After accession of Czech Republic and Poland
Baden-Württemberg	1.69 (16 %)	1.69 (16 %)
Bavaria	1.68 (14 %)	2.42 (20 %)
Berlin	0	0
Brandenburg	0	0.93 (36 %)
Bremen	0	0
Hamburg	0	0
Hesse	0	0
Mecklenburg-Western Pomerania	0	0.20 (11 %)
Lower Saxony	0.64 (8 %)	0.64 (8 %)
North Rhine-Westphalia	2.20 (12 %)	2.20 (12 %)
Rhineland-Palatinate	0.67 (17 %)	0.67 (17 %)
Saarland	0.83 (77 %)	0.83 (77 %)
Saxony	0	1.46 (32 %)
Saxony-Anhalt	0	0
Schleswig-Holstein	0.44 (16 %)	0.44 (16 %)
Thuringia	0	0
GERMANY	7.52 (9 %)	11.74 (13 %)

Source: own calculations based on data from Federal Statistical Office

Moreover it is suggested that the opportunities inherent in Article 22(1)(c) of Regulation 1408/71 (E112 procedure) should be used more often and more intensely for healthcare provision in border regions, holiday regions and for specific indications (Arbeits-gemeinschaft der Spitzenverbände der gesetzlichen Krankenkassen 2000). The sickness funds suggest to engage in a debate on the European level to agree on common standards in regard to quality, planning, cross-border contracting and financing, which should facilitate an easier cross-border service provision. The strategy of the sickness funds is to expand European collaboration under the control of the payers. The Working Group of Federal Associations of Sickness Funds suggests to amend Art. 34 par. 4 of Regulation 574/72. The article entitles sickness funds to reimburse costs in exceptional cases to the medical fee schedule of the country of insurance. Currently, the ceiling for this is Euro 500. It is suggested to raise this ceiling. It would make reimbursement procedures easier and quicker since the sickness funds would not need to inquire into the medical fee schedules of other Member States.

The Federal Chamber of Physicians (representing all physicians and not only the SHI-affiliated ones) is also supporting a more liberal approach to cross-border care according to a resolution ratified at the annual congregation in 2000. German physicians (or at least their representatives) do not seem to be afraid of cross-border patient mobility. On the contrary, they rather seem to expect a net-win since Germany has a very comprehensive healthcare basket and no severe capacity problem.

References

Arbeitsgemeinschaft der Spitzenverbände der gesetzlichen Krankenkassen. Strategischer Umgang der GKV mit den aktuellen europarechtlichen Entwicklungen – Herausforderung Europa annehmen und gestalten [Strategy of the statutory health insurance in regard to current European legal developments - tackling the European challenge and shaping the future]. 2000.

Calnan M, Palm W, Sohy F, Quaghebeur D. Implementing a policy for cross-border use of health care: a case study of frontier worker's knowledge, attitudes and use. In: Leidl R, editor. Health care and its financing in the single European market. Amsterdam-Berlin-Oxford-Tokyo-Washington DC: IOS Press; 1998. p. 306-11.

Coheur A. Integrating care in border regions. An analysis of the Euregio projects. eurohealth 2001;7(4):10-2.

France G. Cross-border flows of Italian patients within the European Union. An international trade approach. Eur J Public Health 1997;7(3 Suppl.):18-25.

Hermans HEGM. Patient's rights in the European Union. Eur J Public Health 1997;7(3 Suppl.):11-7.

Hermesse J, Lewalle H, Palm W. Patient mobility within the European Union. Eur J Public Health 1997;7(3 Suppl.):4-10.

Palm W, Nickless J, Lewalle H, Coheur A. Implications of recent jurisprudence on the co-ordination of health care protection systems. General report produced for the Directorate-General for Employment and Social Affairs of the European Commission. Brussels: Association Internationale de la Mutualité (AIM); 2000.

Starmans B, Leidl R, Rhodes G. A comparative study on cross-border hospital care in the Euregio Meuse-Rhine. Eur J Public Health 1997;7(3 Suppl.):33-41.

The European Union and Health Services
R. Busse et al. (Eds.)
IOS Press, 2002

249

Scenarios on the development of consumer choice for healthcare services

Reinhard BUSSE and Matthias WISMAR

Abstract. This chapter explores future options for the development of consumer choice for healthcare across borders. It analyses the effects of various verdict options of current ECJ cases (i.e. Geraets-Smits/Peerbooms, Müller-Fauré/van Riet and Vanbraekel) in regard to four dimensions relevant for choice, namely range of benefits, degree of restrictions, choice among providers and reimbursement. It demonstrates that important policy questions arise, no matter whether the decisions will freeze the status-quo, open up new opportunities for consumer choice or lie somewhere in between. Finally, it presents the actual rulings in the Geraets-Smits/Peerbooms and Vanbraekel cases and analyses them in the light of the scenario outcomes.

For the purposes of the scenarios developed in this chapter, "consumer choice" is intended to demonstate maximum benefit for the consumer, i.e.

- to have access to the fullest range of medical goods and services ("benefits"),
- to have these benefits with the minimum restrictions (such as necessary referral patterns or prescriptions),
- to have maximum choice between different providers, and
- to have full reimbursement for any amount charged by the provider.

This description does not imply that the maximum consumer choice is the preferred situation. It is not the intention of the scenario to direct the discussion in one particular direction nor to find the "one possible solution". Rather, it is intended to steer a discussion, based on current status as developed under EU law and as interpreted by the ECJ, taking into account the possible outcomes of currently pending ECJ cases. The base line, i.e. how much consumer choice the three procedures E111, E112 and "Kohll/ Decker" allow for each of the four dimensions (range of benefits, degree of restrictions, choice among providers and reimbursement), has been developed in the previous chapter.

As the scenario was originally developed early in 2001 (i.e. before the verdicts on Geraets-Smits/Peerbooms (C-157/99) and Vanbraekel (C-368/98) in July 2001), sections 1 to 3 do not take account of the actual verdicts on these cases. However, these are addressed in section 4.

1. Issues and outcomes forecasted in the scenarios

These scenarios are based on different possible verdicts to current ECJ cases (Geraets-Smits/Peerbooms [C-157/99]; Müller-Fauré/van Riet [C-385/99-1]; Vanbraekel [C-368/98]). These deal primarily – simplified for the sake of the scenario – with the following four issues:
1. Extension of the "Kohll/ Decker" procedure to in-patient services;

2. Application of the "Kohll/ Decker" procedure from patient reimbursement systems to systems of benefits-in-kind;
3. Extension of the "Kohll/ Decker" procedure to goods and services which are not included in the benefits catalogue in the country of insurance affiliation ("CoI"), i.e. the country where the citizen has his/her health insurance;
4. Right to be reimbursed at most favourable rate.

The first three issues relate directly to the available benefits and are therefore dealt with jointly (while issue 4 will be introduced in Section 2).

Issue 1 (extension of "Kohll/ Decker" procedure to in-patient services) relates to the question which was left unresolved in the Kohll and Decker judgements, namely "For which healthcare services (and goods) has the principle of free movement as established in the TEC priority over healthcare values such as the financial sustainability of social protection systems or the health of the population?" Possible outcomes are:

A. The right to choose in-patient services across borders is denied as it would interfere with national capacity planning (which in this outcome is given high importance).
B. The right to choose in-patient services across borders is accepted but, at the same time, the necessity for national capacity planning is acknowledged, especially for certain high-technology services, so that Member States may limit the free choice to non-high technology services, i.e. general in-patient services.
C. The free choice of in-patient services is considered a higher value than national capacity planning.

Issue 2 (application of the "Kohll/ Decker" procedure from patient reimbursement systems to systems of benefits-in-kind) relates to a fundamental question regarding the application of the TEC, namely "Are any methods of organising access to healthcare excluded from the application of the principles governing the free movement of goods and services and, if so, which methods?" Possible outcomes are:

A. Healthcare services in benefit in kind systems are not considered "services" under the TEC. Therefore, the ECJ denies any freedom of choice to cross-border care for persons covered under social security systems operating on the benefits-in-kind principle.
B. Healthcare services in benefit in kind systems are considered "services" under the TEC, but the right of Member States to organize their social protection systems is also acknowledged, meaning in effect that they have the right to limit the freedom of choice if it endangers the financial sustainability of the system or the health of the population.
C. Healthcare services in benefit in kind systems are considered as "services" under the TEC. The freedom of services (and goods) is therefore fully applicable.

Issue 3 (extension of "Kohll/ Decker"-procedure to services which are not included in the benefits catalogue of the CoI) is one which was already dealt with in relation to E112, but which is now more generally at stake as it relates to at least two underlying questions: "What powers do Member States have to make access to services subject to certain conditions (e.g. age as in the Peerbooms case) or processes (gate-keeping or waiting periods as in the Van Riet case)? And, more generally, what powers do they have to limit the benefits covered by their statutory health protection system?" Possible outcomes are:

A. An extension to the Kohll/ Decker rulings is not made, i.e. the choice of services across borders is limited to those included in the benefits catalogue of the CoI and the necessity of which is certified through a prescription.

B. Access to services which are not included in the national benefits catalogue is principally accepted, but is made dependent on certification by physicians in the CoI that the benefits available in that country are insufficient and that a different treatment (which is available in another EU country) is indicated – in effect this would mean an extension of E112 principles to the "Kohll/ Decker" procedure.

C. Choice is extended to services which are not included in the benefits catalogue of the CoI, i.e. implicitly to all services included in one of the Member States' benefits catalogues.

The arrows in Figure 1 indicate the possible extensions for consumer choice for these three issues.

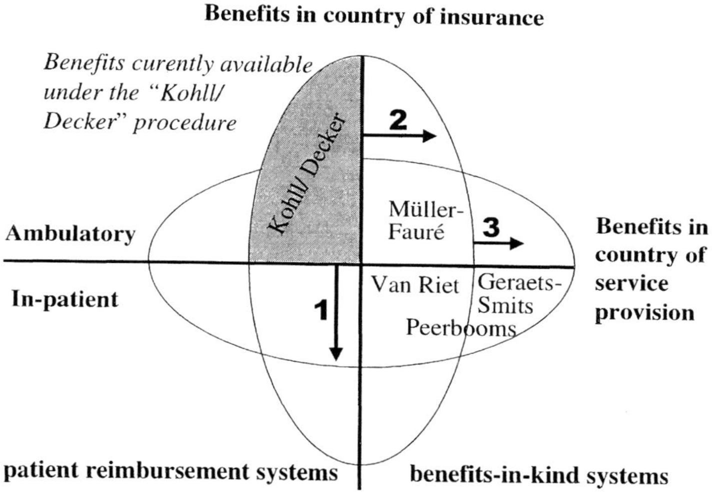

Fig. 1: Benefits available under the "Kohll/ Decker" procedure (early 2001), current ECJ cases and pending extension issues, indicated by arrows for 1. extension to in-patient services, 2. benefits in kind systems and 3. benefits outside the catalogue of the country of insurance

2. Possible general outcomes

Taken together, four general outcomes are possible. Three of them are based on the assumption that the ECJ has a clear line when deciding upon the various cases. These possible general lines – building on the three options A to C above – are "no increase in European patient choice" (Table 1), "more patient choice but also stability for the social protection systems" (Table 2) and "freedom of services and goods is highest value" (Table 3). The result of only "pro-freedom" decisions on the range of services which would then be available under the all-encompassing "Kohll/ Decker" procedure is also demonstrated in Figure 2.

Table 1: General outcome "no increase in European patient choice"

Consumer choice issue	Decision		
	Anti consumer choice	Middle way	Pro consumer choice
In-patient services	A	B	C
Benefits-in-kind systems	A	B	C
Services not included in benefits catalogue	A	B	C

Table 2: General outcome "more patient choice but also stability for the social protection systems"

Consumer choice issue	Decision		
	Anti consumer choice	Middle way	Pro consumer choice
In-patient services	A	B	C
Benefits-in-kind systems	A	B	C
Services not included in benefits catalogue	A	B	C

Table 3: General outcome "freedom of services and goods is highest value"

Consumer choice issue	Decision		
	Anti consumer choice	Middle way	Pro consumer choice
In-patient services	A	B	C
Benefits-in-kind systems	A	B	C
Services not included in benefits catalogue	A	B	C

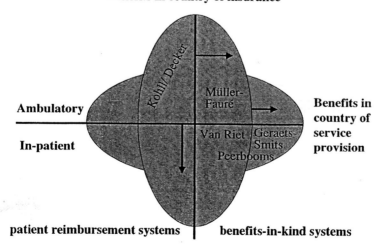

Benefits in country of insurance

Ambulatory

In-patient

Benefits in country of service provision

Kohll/ Decker

Müller-Faure

Van Riet Geraets-Smits

Peerbooms

patient reimbursement systems   **benefits-in-kind systems**

Fig. 2: Benefits available under the "Kohll/ Decker" procedure under the general outcome "freedom of services and goods is highest value"

Taking into consideration that the ECJ has not yet (visibly) found a consistent approach to dealing with these issues, it is possible that such an apparently inconsistent approach will continue. In this case, the various issues could be decided quite differently in regard to their effect on choice, as Table 4 exemplifies. In this example, the "Kohll/ Decker" procedure would be restricted to ambulatory services but be made available to entitled persons in all EEA countries. The availability of benefits not included in the catalogue of the CoI would be made dependant upon certain conditions.

Table 4: General outcome without clear orientation (example)

Consumer choice issue	Decision		
	Contra consumer choice	Middle way	Pro consumer choice
In-patient services	A	B	C
Benefits-in-kind systems	A	B	C
Services not included in benefits catalogue	A	B	C

Issue 4. Clearly, the real effect on patient choice and mobility will also depend to a large degree on the outcome of the ECJ rulings regarding issue 4, i.e. the right to be reimbursed at the most favourable rate. In this respect, possible outcomes are:

A. The ECJ upholds its view that any reimbursement is limited to the actual bill in the country of service provision ("CoS") as well the reimbursement used in the CoI (i.e. whatever is lower).
B. The ECJ considers a limitation of reimbursement to the CoI rate as an impediment to free movement and mandates that the responsible third-party payer has to cover the costs incurred in the CoS if they are higher than in the CoI (limited to the reimbursement which applies to persons insured and treated in that country).
C. The ECJ comes to the conclusion that for full freedom of services and goods the patient should be reimbursed independently of the place of service (i.e. de facto at the rate used in the CoI).

3. Discussion of scenarios

The most likely outcome of the scenarios is some intermediate form rather than the two extremes of "no increase in European patient choice" or "freedom of services and goods is highest value". Whether an intermediate outcome will, however, result from a consistent "middle way" approach or from an apparently inconsistent "muddling through" approach is less clear.

These various outcomes will not, however, lead to a stable situation for European health care systems as new problems will have to be tackled – either because of new European health policy initiatives or (possibly more likely) additional cases submitted to the ECJ.

The "freedom of services and goods is highest value" outcome would lead to an almost unrestricted access to services and providers outside the borders of the CoI. This in turn would pose serious questions for national policy making:

– How can Member States deny certain dimensions of choice inside their country (e.g. to restrict access to a limited number of contracted providers) if these limitations do not exist for cross-border care?

– How can equivalence be applied between services belonging to different health care systems where they are integrated and financed according to different rules?
– (and possibly most importantly:) To what extent would the new situation weaken or even cancel out national health policy measures, especially regarding cost containment?

It is important to recognise that one apparently obvious solution – i.e. to restrict access to a defined minimum standard benefits package – is not a real solution if this done individually by each Member State, as access to excluded services which are included in any other Member State would remain (for those patients who are willing/ able to go there). This, in turn, leads to the ultimate question:

– Will Member States need to design a uniform benefits catalogue, to fix uniform reimbursement rates and to develop a uniform system of accrediting/ contracting/paying providers to regain the political power to steer the – then European – health care system?

The most restricted general outcome "No increase in European patient choice" equally generates a set of questions:

– How can it be justified that the alternative methods of accessing healthcare services across borders (E111, E112, "Kohll/ Decker") enable the European citizen to receive such different options of benefits, service provider and reimbursement, in particular as the third method is available only to those insured under certain healthcare systems?
– If it is regarded as not justified, will this lead to a cut-back of certain freedoms granted in Regulation 1408/71 to reach a status of equality, but at the lowest possible level?

While at first sight the "middle way" outcome ("more patient choice, but restricted") appears promising, it would also fail to provide a stable situation. Quite to the contrary, many details resulting from the ECJ decisions would be unresolved:

– Will the recognition that certain high-technology services require national planning necessitate an EU-wide list of such technologies? If so, who should decide on such a list?
– Will the recognition that restrictions on access for the sake of financial sustainability necessitate a common understanding of what restrictions are tolerable?
– Is the extension of national contracting systems across borders, which may result in overlapping provider networks, really an effective solution?

4. Developments through the Smits-Geraets/ Peerbooms and Vanbraekel rulings

Before discussing the directions for future development that the rulings point towards, a summary of the cases will be presented. On the Geraets-Smits/Peerbooms case (C-157/99), the ECJ reported the ruling under the heading of "The conditions for obtaining prior authorisation to receive hospital treatment in another Member State must not give rise to an arbitrary refusal" as follows (ECJ Press Release No 32/2001):

> "Mrs Geraets-Smits, who is of Netherlands nationality, suffers from Parkinson's disease. She was treated in a specialist clinic in Germany without obtaining prior authorisation from her Netherlands sickness insurance fund. When she sought reimbursement of the costs incurred, her sickness insurance fund refused

to reimburse her on the ground that satisfactory and adequate treatment for that disease was available in the Netherlands and that the treatment provided in Germany conferred no additional advantage.

Mr Peerbooms, who is of Netherlands nationality, fell into a coma following a road accident. He received special intensive therapy in an Austrian clinic, which proved beneficial. Mr Peerbooms did not satisfy the requirements for admission to two Netherlands establishments offering the same medical technique on an experimental basis (as this technique was available in the Netherlands only to persons under the age of 25 years). Mr Peerbooms was also refused reimbursement by his Netherlands sickness insurance fund of the costs incurred, since, according to the authority dealing with his claim, the treatment given to the comatose patient in Austria had no advantage over the treatment available in the Netherlands.

Under the Netherlands social security legislation, a patient can receive medical treatment, either in the Netherlands or abroad, at an establishment which has not entered into agreement with his sickness insurance fund only after obtaining prior authorisation. The Netherlands court hearing the disputes between the persons concerned and their sickness insurance funds has asked the Court of Justice whether legislation of that type is compatible with the principle of freedom to provide services.

The Court observes that Member States are free to organise their social security systems. In the absence of harmonisation at Community level, it is for the legislation of each Member State to determine the conditions concerning the right or duty to be insured with a social security scheme and the conditions for entitlement to benefits. Nevertheless, the Member States must comply with Community law and in particular with the principle of freedom to provide services. Medical activities, even taking into consideration the particular nature of the services concerned (benefits-in-kind, for which the hospital establishment is paid by the fund with which the person concerned is insured), do indeed fall within the scope of freedom to provide services.

The Court then considers whether the effect of the rules in question is to restrict freedom to provide services. By subjecting reimbursement of costs to authorisation, which is granted only where two conditions are satisfied (the treatment must be regarded as normal in the professional circles concerned; and the treatment abroad must be necessary), the rules in question constitute an obstacle to freedom to provide services. Is there any justification for that obstacle? The Court recalls that a risk of seriously undermining a social system's financial balance and the maintenance of a balanced medical and hospital service open to all constitute financial and public-health requirements capable of justifying an obstacle to freedom to provide services.

In the Court's view, the need to have resort to a system of prior authorisation, in the context of a system of agreements to provide health care, makes it possible to ensure that there is sufficient and permanent access to a balanced range of high-quality hospital treatment on the national territory, to ensure that costs are controlled and to prevent any wastage of financial, technical and human resources. None the less, any conditions, such as those applied in the Netherlands, which must be satisfied in order to obtain prior authorisation must be justified and must satisfy the principle of proportionality.

Thus, the condition that the proposed hospital treatment in another Member State must be regarded as normal is acceptable only in so far as it refers to what is sufficiently tried and tested by international medical science.

The second condition, namely the necessity of the proposed treatment, that is to say the requirement that the insured person receive treatment in a foreign establishment owing to his medical state, must mean that authorisation can be refused only if the patient can receive the same or equally effective treatment without undue delay from an establishment with which his sickness insurance fund has contractual arrangements."

On the Vanbraekel case (C-368/98), the ECJ reported the ruling as follows (ECJ Press Release No 33/2001):

"Mrs Descamps, a Belgian national residing in Belgium, requested authorisation from her sickness insurance fund to undergo orthopaedic surgery in France. That authorisation was initially refused: her request was deemed insufficiently supported in the absence of the opinion of a doctor from a Belgian university. Mrs Descamps none the less went ahead with the operation in April 1990. She brought an action against her sickness insurance fund before the Belgian courts for reimbursement of the costs incurred on the basis of the tariffs applied in Belgium (FRF 49,935.44) and not those applied in France (FRF 38,608.89). In December 1994, a report by a medical expert designated by the Cour du travail de Mons confirmed that the surgery was not currently performed in Belgium and that the restoration of Mrs Descamps's health did indeed necessitate hospital treatment abroad. As Mrs Descamps had died in the course of the proceedings, her heirs, Mr Vanbraekel and her children, pursued the action.

The Cour du travail de Mons has asked the Court of Justice of the European Communities whether, once it has been established that hospital treatment in another Member State should have been authorised, reimbursement of the costs of hospital treatment must be made in accordance with the scheme of the State of the competent institution (here the Belgian institution) or in accordance with that organised by the State on whose territory the hospital treatment has taken place (in the present case the French scheme). Last, the Court has been asked about the rules on assumption of costs to be followed when the authorisation provided for in the Community rules to obtain hospital treatment in another Member State has been obtained, by declaration of a court where appropriate.

The Court recalls that the Community rules established a system which ensures that a person covered by social insurance who is authorised to receive medical benefits-in-kind in a Member State other than the State in which he is insured enjoys in the Member State in which the treatment is provided conditions as favourable as those enjoyed by insured persons covered by the legislation of that State. The Court therefore considers that the applicable rules on assumption of costs are those applied in the State in which treatment is provided.

The costs of benefits-in-kind are borne, in principle, by the institutions of the State in which the treatment is provided and are subsequently refunded by the institution with which the person concerned is insured. The Court rules that where the costs were not assumed owing to an unjustified refusal to grant authorisation by the institution with which the person concerned is insured, the latter institution must guarantee directly to the person concerned reimbursement of an amount equivalent to that which it would ordinarily have assumed if authorisation had been properly granted.

Taking the view that medical activities do indeed fall within the scope of the rules on freedom to provide services, the Court also considers that national legislation must guarantee that an insured person who has been authorised to receive hospital treatment abroad receives a level of payment comparable to that which he would have received if he had received hospital treatment in his own Member State.

In those circumstances, the Court considers that the principle of freedom to provide services defined in the Treaty precludes rules which prevent additional reimbursement corresponding to the difference between the lower tariff of reimbursement of the State of stay in which the hospital treatment was carried out and the more favourable tariff laid down in the social insurance scheme of the State of registration.

Although the risk of seriously undermining the financial balance of the social security system may constitute an overriding reason in the general interest capable of justifying a barrier to the principle of freedom to provide services, in the Court's view there is no reason to consider that payment of the additional reimbursement in question would entail an additional financial burden for the sickness insurance scheme of the State in which the person concerned was originally insured capable of preventing the maintenance of treatment capacity or medical competence on national territory."

When these two rulings are analysed in relation to the four issues explored in section 1 (in-patient services; benefits-in-kind systems; goods and services not included in the benefits catalogue; reimbursement), some clear answers become apparent. Regarding the first two issues, the ECJ decided that both hospital services as well as healthcare services delivered as benefits-in-kind are clearly services under the TEC. This is all the more surprising as the Advocate General in his opinion of 18th May 2000 had originally stated the opposite:

"Overriding reasons for maintaining the financial balance of the compulsory sickness insurance scheme of the Netherlands, which provides only benefits-in-kind, justify restrictions on the freedom to provide hospital care within the Union. In any event, the Advocate General, Mr Ruiz-Jarabo, considers that medical care, provided as a benefit in kind, does not constitute a service and therefore is not subject to the Treaty."

Regarding the third issue, the Court confirmed, in line with its earlier Pierik rulings, the fact that benefits are not covered within a country does not preclude them from being covered if provided in another Member State – though the Court attached certain conditions (see below). The same is true for the generally consumer-friendly Vanbraekel verdict on reimbursement which should not be misinterpreted as an invitation to profit financially from accessing healthcare services across borders.

In regard to the four dimensions of consumer choice, the "post-Peerbooms" situation can therefore now be assessed as follows:

– *Access to a range of medical goods and services ("benefits"):* The range of benefits has definitely increased. While the Court confirms that Member States are free to organise their social security systems (and therefore also to limit the benefits available under those systems), they cannot restrict cross-border access to healthcare services if they are "sufficiently tried and tested by international medical science". Clearly, this will have serious implications for national benefits catalogues and may very well be a powerful driver towards a European benefits catalogue (cf. next chapter). Assuming, for example, that the emerging activities in the area of evidence-based dental care will produce favourable results, it will be difficult for countries which have excluded such services from their benefits catalogues to maintain this non-coverage unless all countries agree to exclude these services.

–   *Restrictions to access healthcare services:* Restrictions to access healthcare services will be lessened for two principal reasons. First, in the Geraets-Smits/Peerboms case, the Court stated that authorisation may be refused only if the patient can receive the same or equally effective treatment without "undue delay" from a contracted provider. While the ECJ has not yet defined how an "undue" delay is to be determined (which it will probably do in the pending Müller-Fauré/van Riet case), maximum waiting times as currently accepted for certain specialities in certain countries should definitely qualify. Second, a refusal to authorise a patient to receive cross-border care may prove costly for the competent authority, as the Vanbraekel case has demonstrated. Increasing consumer-friendliness can therefore be expected.

–   *Choice among providers:* Two aspects have to be distinguished. On the one hand, choice will certainly increase considerably with the availability of providers in other countries. On the other hand, the Court does not suggest the simple extension of the "Kohll/ Decker" procedure to hospital services (which would have the potentially serious "side-effect" that it would be difficult to withhold payment for non-contracted providers within the country while allowing it for services delivered outside the country) but rather the modification of the pre-authorisation rules. These, however, generally allow access to contracted providers only.

–   *Reimbursement:* A further result of the attempt by the ECJ to integrate consumer choice-driven access to cross-border hospital services into the scope of Regulation 1408/71 is that patients will not have to face – potentially high – costs which are not reimbursed. This could have been the case if the "Kohll/ Decker" procedure had simply been copied. Compared to that advantage, the possibility for patients of making a "profit" is of minor importance as it is only possible if two conditions are met – 1. the pre-authorisation has been refused on unjustified grounds and 2. the tariff in the country of insurance is higher than in the country of service provision – and, more importantly, it could also turn out that the refusal was well-founded and the patient has to cover the full costs.

Meanwhile, Peerbooms-induced change is already visible for European citizens, at least in the United Kingdom where the recent rulings had an almost immediate impact on the NHS. On 26th August 2001, The Sunday Times had an article titled "Patients win fight for surgery abroad" on its cover page, stating that "Alain Milburn, the health secretary, [...] would change the law to let health authorities sign contracts with providers of medical care in other European Union countries", something that "could spark one of the biggest shake-ups of the National Health Service since its inception in 1948." Milburn also announced that he would review the E112 system to make it "simpler, more transparent and available to everyone."

Part V

The future

The European Union and Health Services
R. Busse et al. (Eds.)
IOS Press, 2002

261

Scenarios on the future of healthcare in Europe

Matthias WISMAR and Reinhard BUSSE

Abstract. In this chapter three scenarios on the future of European integration in healthcare are developed and analysed. Scenario A is based on the assumption that healthcare should remain entirely in the competencies of the Member States and their regions. Scenario B is based on two assumptions. First, the free movement of individuals, goods, services and capital has to be applied to all structures and processes of healthcare. Second, it is acknowledged that healthcare is part of the European Social Model and therefore the SEM has to be contained in a social framework to ensure that a basic set of rules on equity and solidarity is not undermined. Scenario C is characterised by the absence of an overarching or consensual policy vision.

1. Introduction

In this chapter, three scenarios on the future of European integration in healthcare are developed and analysed. The scenarios are not designed to predict the future. They aim at discussing "ideal types" and their consequences. According to Max Weber, ideal types do not necessarily have to be identical with current or future settings but resemble typical features which are based on the logical development of basic assumptions.

The purpose of these scenarios is to distance the debate from the short term political, economic and social interest in regard to European integration and healthcare. By developing scenarios it is intended

– to facilitate a debate on the vision on European integration and healthcare,
– to discuss consequences of theses visions and
– to identify the technical, economic, juridical, social and political requirements of these visions.

The scenario approach as presented here does not start from the political will or the interest of stakeholders as currently expressed, nor from current institutional settings and their developmental tendencies. Not even intensely debated European visions such as a federal Europe will guide these scenarios. The common starting point is an assumed tension between the Single European Market (SEM) which is universal across Europe on the one hand and the European welfare states – which are unique to each Member State – on the other. The scenarios are not designed either to abolish welfare states nor to abolish the SEM.

Each scenario is developed by starting with a policy vision, based on a number of assumptions and characterised by some key features. From that policy vision, the consequences of the scenario are explored in terms of the distribution of competencies and accountability as well as the financing and delivery of services.

In a second step the scenarios will be assessed in terms of their inherent conflicts, the winners and losers they produce, and the likelihood that they will occur.

Finally, the lines of argument will be drawn together to specify key issues of the role of European integration in healthcare and the role of healthcare in European integration.

2. Scenario A: bi-lateral and multi-lateral agreements

Scenario A is based on the assumption that healthcare should remain entirely within the competencies of Member States and their regions. A functional extension of cross-border care and service provision is in principle feasible but is not a task of the European Union. The development of a further "internationalisation" of healthcare is based, rather, on bi-lateral or multi-lateral agreements between Member States and their regions. Regulation 1408/71 on the coordination of social systems should only be applied very closely to the purpose of the free movement of people. This regulation should not be applied beyond this purpose and therefore it should not serve any health or healthcare related activities.

Functional requirements of cross-border care in densely populated border areas or in typical tourist regions should be met by bi-lateral or multi-national agreements and contracts. The key features underpinning these agreements and contracts are networks, interfaces and co-ordinating systems.

A universal right for European citizens to the use of healthcare facilities or health-related goods across the Member States of the EU is not intended. Any legal provision, whether in the Treaty Establishing the European Community (TEC) or in secondary legislation which is ambivalent in this respect has to be clarified in order to give the domestic courts and the European Court of Justice (ECJ) a clear account of the political will concerning the extent of European integration in regard to healthcare, and to prevent rulings like those on Decker and Kohll or Geraets-Smits/Peerbooms.

According to the health policy vision, European integration in this scenario is neither a matter of principle nor a vehicle for thorough reform or reorientation of health policy in the Member States.

2.1 Distributing competencies and accountabilities

The intended political order of Scenario A entails a return to an ideal type "classic" domestic responsibility and accountability for health policy making – a return to pre-TEC times.

But for some Member States, especially the smaller ones, this "classic" order in regulating and developing health services has never existed and, for the larger Member States in some border regions, close social, economic and cultural ties have always existed – making cross-border healthcare a valuable endeavour. Nevertheless, the argument is made that health policy in terms of health services should not be a Community or EU responsibility. That is not to say that the Community has no role to play in health. On the contrary, it is conceivable that, as the perfect complement to the exclusive right of the Member States to regulate all affairs in regard to health services, a more effective integration of public health considerations into all community policies would be desired. The Community's role would therefore be restricted to a very specific public health domain. Problems such as BSE would be dealt with on the European level. But to interfere with health services in Member States is entirely out of question.

The Community's role in health policy making will be very restricted. It will focus exclusively on those policy areas where the Community has a legislative right – including public health, the free movement of goods and services (as long as healthcare is not concerned) and agricultural policies.

To prevent ambiguities, the Community is held responsible for disentangling those policies where the four freedoms may overlap with health service provision – particularly in the complex areas of the health professions, pharmaceuticals and medical devices (see appropriate chapters). Due to the policy vision and the derived political order, the right of free movement and establishment may be restricted. The same applies to cases when certain mechanisms are interpreted in a more "pro-EU" way by the ECJ.

The Member States regain their undisputed sovereignty on health service policy, they are free to use their competencies to intensify cross-border collaboration – whether in the area of patient care or, for example, on a joint strategy on pharmaceutical reimbursement.

Some of the regions, especially those with long and relatively densely populated borders with other Member States, have an intrinsic interest in developing co-ordinated services and in facilitating the establishment of networks or integrated care arrangements as part of a regional social and economic development strategy. As long as domestic legislation is not violated, they are certainly free to develop those cross-border relations. But in their attempts to do so they may not refer to the Treaty, to Regulation 1408/71 or to any other source of European law.

Nevertheless, the different political status of regions across Member States may form an impediment to setting up cross-border ties. Some will find it extremely difficult to articulate their interest, let alone to become actively involved in planning and negotiating bi- and multilateral agreements.

Due to the bi- or multi-lateral development in cross-border care, the provider and purchaser organisations stay in contact Europe-wide but do not implement solutions according to any universal principle. Each solution to cross-border care will be unique.

2.2 Providing and financing health services

In terms of service provision, the territorial boundaries of health services are not superseded by European legislation insofar as no payer or provider may invest in health service institutions across the border or engage in a joint-venture on the basis of the TEC. Still, if domestic legislation allows cross-border ownership, they are free to do so. The cross-border use of facilities by patients relies entirely on contractual relations between competent institutions or governments in the Member States or regions.

Harmonisation of the scope of services provided by Member States or regions is not intended. Healthcare baskets – as far as they are explicitly defined – remain entirely in the accountability of the competent institutions and political bodies. However, the contractual partners are free to adjust services as long as domestic legislation is not interfered with.

Each contractual partner is held responsible to keep in line with domestic legislation or funds. An unbalanced transfer of money or even an extra income for service providers is not intended, since this may result in a loss of resources for domestic providers. Nevertheless, the uneven distribution of holiday travel may cause – in small quantities – net transfers.

2.3 Ensuring co-ordination

Member States realise that existing regulations like 1408/71 leave gaps in terms of access to health services. Rather than implementing new rules at the EU level, they are addressing the problems bilaterally if appropriate. Sweden and Spain will probably sign an agreement to define access and benefits for each other's citizens, but Estonia and Portugal probably not.

Equally, the improvement of cross-border care for workers who reside in one country but work across the border in another country is addressed where it is relevant. Some

Member States also allow cross-border choice of care for residents in defined areas without working in the other country and therefore extend the legal provision, but these agreements are strictly based on bi-lateral contracts.

Some border regions try to improve cross-border resource management. Co-ordination in border regions might be of value in terms of allowing rescue services in both border regions, of using jointly hospital capacities or to overcome short-term bottlenecks with specialist services. In terms of centres of excellence cross-border coordination could be useful both for patients if they are not required to travel far and for more efficient use of spare capacities.

2.4 Designing interfaces

Individual interfaces will be designed to allow cross-border service provision for patients in areas such as Euregios. In each particular case, they will be designed to regulate eligibility to cross-border services, cross-border transfer of money and transfer of patient records or other patient data.

Robust interfaces require a solid juridical foundation which is designed to serve them. Questions of data-exchange in regard to the patient records, their usage and the resulting expenditure have to be clarified, especially if the patient flow using the interface is substantial or asymmetric.

Interfaces often use smart card technology. This technology can be introduced to facilitate cross-border care – e.g. through an EU-wide patient card. This is, however, against the spirit of Scenario A and will not be pursued. Rather, it could be used to allow a seamless integration of the chain of service provision across borders in particular areas or between certain countries which agree to do so. Moreover, the technology may be used to improve efficient use of capacities either in border areas or for highly specialised centres of excellence. Smaller countries might be able to avoid unnecessary investment in facilities which could be available in neighbouring countries, if usage abroad is possible without bureaucratic complexity – especially if post-operative treatment could be carried out in the domestic environment.

3. Scenario B: regulated European competition

This scenario is based on two assumptions. First, it is acknowledged that the free movement of individuals, goods, services and capital has to be applied to all structures and processes of healthcare. Second, it is the common understanding in the EU that healthcare is part of the European Social Model and therefore the SEM has to be contained in a social framework to ensure that a basic set of rules on equity and solidarity is not undermined. The desired competition aims at efficiency and not at profits.

Consequently, free access to basic healthcare and to different competing competent financing institutions across all Member States is an established right of EU-citizenship but at the same time, a tight European regulatory framework is put in place to contain their competition.

European integration in this scenario is a matter of principle. Furthermore, it is used as a vehicle both to develop healthcare provision attuned to the preferences of patients and to introduce more competition between both payers and provider of healthcare not on a merely regional or national level but on a European scale. Competition takes place in three dimensions: 1) European competition for citizens by payers; 2) European competition for payers by providers; and 3) direct competition between providers for patients. The key elements are pooling mechanisms to allow a socially acceptable competition, a European

Basic Benefit Package which will clearly define the services and goods in the competition and a contribution/tax collecting system, which allows both tax based and social insurance systems to operate in the SEM.

3.1 Designing a "European Basic Benefit Package"

One of the basic principles of the competition-based European Social Model is the equality of available benefits throughout the Union for two reasons. First, if access to healthcare is an universal right for citizens which goes beyond rhetoric, it is essential that patients are aware of their rights and informed on what these rights entail. Second, competition can only be carried out if the product or the service is specified. Following the direction set by the ECJ in its "Peerbooms" ruling, all healthcare services and medical goods (e.g. pharmaceuticals) which are internationally sufficiently tried and tested are included in the European Basic Benefit Package (EuBasicBP). Any financing institution has to offer the whole scope of benefits services defined within the EuBasicBP.

3.2 Setting up a system of European accreditation and certification

In order to guarantee the quality of services and goods provided, a European system to accredit healthcare facilities and to certify health professionals will enhance transparency. This system builds on existing domestic institutional settings by harmonising goals and criteria but not necessarily means.

Accreditation and certification gain overwhelming importance in the light of the future enlargement of the EU. An effective system would both improve quality and raise trust in healthcare institutions in other countries. In regard to the patient, it is a question of consumer protection, and in regard to regulated competition, it is question of transparency.

3.3 Earmarking taxes for health

Tax-based systems are, in Scenario B, in a somewhat awkward situation, whether the tax is levied nationally, regionally or locally. To allow them to compete with SHI-based countries, the health-portion of taxes has at least to be earmarked. During preparatory negotiations, Member States will have to decide among various options how to handle the situation. One option is that the earmarked part is directly passed into the European Healthcare Finance Pool (see below). A second option is that those citizens who wish to change from the competent financing institution, currently called the NHS, to another receive an equivalent allowance or are freed from the "health tax" altogether.

A possible compromise between Beveridge and Bismarck countries could be that taxes will be reduced (in the tax-based systems) but introduced in all Member States as a financial basis for funding healthcare which does not only rely on the contributions of individuals. The tax-part could be spend on population-based health activities (e.g. prevention) or included in the pooled financial resources to be allocated to the competent financing institutions.

3.4 Pooling financial resources

The systems of collecting the financial resources remain largely intact, but to prevent competition based on cream-skimming for low risk and high income citizens which would put less wealthier (or less healthier) European regions at a disadvantage, a pooling mechanism – the European Healthcare Finance Pool (EuHFiP) – is introduced. Each competent financing institution pays the collected contributions into the pool and in turn receives a European Standardised Per-Capita Allocation (EuSCAl) for each enrolled citizen. The standardisation of the EuSCAl aims at levelling out differences in morbidity as well as income and regional purchasing power parity on an EU-wide level. The EuSCAl guarantees each purchaser the average costs of patient care. But a purchaser which manages its affairs efficiently would gain a surplus. Since all purchasers remain non-profit organisations, the surplus can only be used for refunds or to offer additional services.

To guarantee that extremely costly patients are equally well treated, the EuHFiP also manages an European High Risk Pool (EuHiRiP), out of which parts of the costs for patients suffering from diseases like AIDS, cancer etc. is covered directly.

3.5 Ensuring Europe-wide choice, preferences and service provision

Citizens have in principle a free choice of doctors, specialists and – within given restrictions – a free choice of hospitals. Yet, competent financing institutions are free to tie the provision of services included in the EuBasicBP to specified settings and to organise the chain of service provision according to patient preferences and efficiency criteria. A financing institution could, for example, offer various forms of integrated care including primary healthcare and gate keeping. If that would result in a more efficient service provision, the financing institution could offer additional services beyond the EuBasicBP or pay back part of the contributions. If services cannot be financed out of the EuSCAl (plus possibly the EuHiRiP), the competent financing institution has to raise additional contributions from its insured.

3.6 Distributing competencies and accountabilities

Inevitably, Europe-wide regulated competition entails a redistribution of competencies and accountabilities. The political aspect of the health policy vision is not based on a hierarchical understanding of regulating health services but on a European multi-layer system, where the various layers (EU, national, regional, self-government and local levels) are linked and dove-tailed in various ways.

The Community's role in health and healthcare is changed completely and made more explicit. The EuBasicBP, the EuHFiP and the EuHiRiP will not have to be embedded in a revised Treaty directly, though. Alternatively, they could be the result of a coordination process among Member States. It is also possible that, as with the Euro, not all Member States will initially participate. But EU citizens will win a new benefit since access to healthcare will be established as a universal right.

More practically, Community institutions – existing (e.g. Eurostat) or newly established – will handle the data needed to facilitate the regulated European competition in healthcare. Nevertheless, in most areas the Community does not become involved in managing health services.

The Member States will largely lose their right to define the healthcare basket independently, although they can still influence the basket. In order to limit the EuBasicBP, each Member State has the right to commission Health Technology Assessment (HTA) reports in order to find out whether a given service in the benefit package is inadequate. If that is the case, the service will be taken out of the EuBasicBP. The competent financing institution is free to keep those services on offer for an additional premium. It will be an important marketing instrument for the financing institution to serve preferences which go beyond conventional medicine and expand to those based on social values or tradition. Clearly, some of the services which are at stake have been in Member States' benefit baskets for a long time because of social values attached to them and not because of their effectiveness – an issue which will have to be dealt with at European level as well.

For some of the regions, regulated European competition provides the opportunity to develop a strategic health profile and to make health, healthcare and related products and services the centre piece of their regional economic strategy. This is a reaction to the high relevance of healthcare in terms of the GDP and employment.

3.7 Providing and financing health services

Almost everything seems to be possible. Investment across-border, joint ventures, contractual co-operation and co-ordination. In terms of the healthcare basket, beyond the evidence-based EuBasicBP, financing institutions are free to offer extra services which go beyond the narrow definition of academic medicine and may offer complementary medicine, wellness, comfort healthcare and esoteric health following demands of patients who are willing to pay more for their preferences.

4. Scenario C: muddling through

This scenario is characterised by the absence of an overarching or consensual policy vision. It extends today's status quo on the role of European integration in healthcare to the future. Clearly, the different players in the emerging European health policy arena do hold different incompatible policy visions, often in stark contrast with their national governments.

But this will become more difficult since the health systems do not fall into two categories like the Bismarck and the Beveridge model but there are also mixed systems. Moreover, some of these systems are subject to rapid changes. And these changes may not be in line with the rulings of the courts since it becomes increasingly difficult to understand Europe's position on health services.

In the absence of a coherent political will in a policy field which is not yet politically defined, domestic courts and the ECJ are frequently called upon in order to interpret secondary European law in the light of the TEC. Without a explicit policy vision established in the TEC, the courts have to "read between the lines" and provide a policy surrogate. Yet, due to political pressure and the complexity of the subject as well as the fact that Advocates General and Judges are neither specialised on social law or healthcare law and certainly have only a basic understanding of the health services in the Community, rulings will appear insufficient, inadequate and incongruent.

This poses a difficulty to the actors in national health services, because the interpretation of a given case is unpredictable. Health management, which is always carried out under the circumstances of insufficient information, will find it more difficult to act in a proactive way. This is a highly relevant issue since the European legislation beyond Decker and Kohll has severe consequence for health services. This is, for example, the case for competition law.

Healthcare managers will be urged to use these inconsistencies in order to gain benefits for their organisations. They may try to use inconsistencies in ECJ rulings to have some legal backing for action which would otherwise not be allowed by the Member State. For example it remains questionable whether Regulation 1408/71 is a proper legal foundation to organise cross-border care beyond matters of urgency. Managers will use Regulation 1408/71 as a legal lever against domestic law, which would not allow cross-border activities.

Like managers, patients will try to use the uncertainties and inconsistencies to receive the services abroad. Without an established "safety valve" they will use cross border care and will put their competent financing institution under pressure. They will try to use the E111 procedure under Article 22(1)(a) of Regulation 1408/71 to obtain medical goods and services for free which are not in the healthcare basket of their country. Another strategy will be to pretend that they need urgent treatment in order to meet the criteria for the application of Article 22(1)(c) of Regulation 1408/71. Others will go abroad to by-pass waiting lists and will demand reimbursement, threatening the competent financing institution with public exposure to personal hardship and unfairness for withholding treatment which is readily available elsewhere. This has already proven to be a strategy that works in healthcare systems which have introduced competition between purchasers.

5. Assessing the scenarios

In this section the conflicts inherent to the scenarios and technical and political aspects will be discussed.

5.1 Inherent conflicts

Obviously, none of the three scenarios offer a conflict free or instantly convincing solution in terms of combining SEM dynamics with health services of Member States. But the scenarios serve to make explicit these conflicts. Some of them are already at work today.

To restrict the TEC and secondary European legislation to areas not related healthcare, as suggested in Scenario A on bi- and multi-lateral agreements, is – if possible – a difficult task. But even if it was possible, the question of the consequences remains. For the health services, the consequences are relatively small. Those institutions which enjoy the legal right to establish cross-border care will have an advantage in their domestic systems. Yet, they will establish links across borders for their own purposes and will not necessarily pursue their patients' interests. The result would be a patchwork of different pilots and projects. Existing differences in service provision, usage and probably outcomes would increase both on a European and domestic level. Instead of an economic convergence, the (regionalised) healthcare sectors would diverge also in economic terms in regard to expenditure and employment. The heterogeneity of interests in healthcare would increase. Eventually, this development would contribute to a disintegration and fragmentation of the medical, political and economic aspects of healthcare both on a European and domestic level.

Scenario B on regulated European competition establishes more problems than solutions. First, it is clear that insurance systems are at an advantage compared to tax-based systems. The changes necessary for tax-based systems in terms of financing and organising the systems would be enormous. In many Member States, health services are financed out of a variety of sources combining contributions, user charges, general taxation and earmarked taxes. Fair European competition would need to disentangle these sources or to find mechanisms of compensation – a task which would be highly complicated if not impossible on a mere technical level.

Moreover, it is likely that sickness funds might find it easier to develop a business approach to healthcare provision than health authorities. Strategic thinking, investments, joint-ventures, mergers and the development of new business-ideas will be easier for them, at least if they are based in countries which have already opened up such opportunities. That will disadvantage health authorities and sickness funds which currently have monopolies based on geography or occupational factors. While certain sickness funds may aggressively enter European competition and may even invade the territory of national health services, others will face severe competitive disadvantages.

Open competition across Europe would be difficult for other reasons too. While the EuSCAl aims at levelling out discrepancies in the level of contribution due to differences in wealth and possibly healthcare needs, it is difficult to assess the role of medical fee schedules. Should there be a unified European medical fee schedule or none at all? Should the reimbursement level in the fee schedule vary from region to region or should it just establish a ceiling?

Clearly, the diversity between regions and systems is – despite convergence in some areas of health systems – still too large to find an easy solution. But the differences in systems are not only a matter of historical or technical settings. To have – and to keep – a national health service instead of a statutory health insurance is also a matter of values. Regulated European competition would be indifferent in regard to such national values. Systems which find it easier to operate in a competitive context will be at an advantage and will expand over borders. Even if it were conceivable to implement such competition, a European health service would emerge not on the basis of what European citizen desire politically but on the basis of aggregate consumer preferences. That would put an end to health policy-making in the "European sense" by political interest mediation and would entirely surrender system-development of health services to market or quasi-market forces.

Moreover, it will be extremely difficult to define a EuBasicBP. As experience in various countries has shown, politically restricting benefit packages is very difficult. It is therefore likely that the EuBasicBP would include all in-patient services. Areas which in some health services are already excluded – such as dental care – could be reintroduced. Another difficulty will be to bridge cultural gaps. Some health services, for example, refer to the concept of solidarity to define both the distribution of financial burden and the right to healthcare, while others are based on equity. As a result it is likely that - instead of a restriction - an upward dynamic could be triggered which would put a high financial burden particularly on some tax-based systems.

At first glance, Scenario C on muddling through seems to be the most convenient way to handle the inherent conflict between the SEM and the territoriality of Member State based health services. The political costs appear to be the lowest, compared to the other scenarios since no decision has to be made whether to go down the road of further integration or reverse the process and to erect firewalls between the health services by excluding them entirely from the TEC. Political rhetoric may pay lip-services to both the protagonists of integration and those of segregation. If something undesired happens it is always possible to put on the blame on the ECJ or the Brussels bureaucrats, neglecting that they act on behalf of the political will once articulated by the Member State governments as manifested in the TEC.

For organisations in the Member States it will, however, be very difficult to adjust themselves to the uncertainty of European integration. Moreover it could happen that Member States with statutory health insurance systems are hit harder by European competition law than others, because they are detached from the state and come almost instantly under the suspect of acting as undertakings.

5.2 From today's health services to scenarios

In terms of technical and organisational aspects already at work – whether fully developed or just at an embryonic stage – almost nothing is inconceivable. In fact the race to define the future of healthcare in European integration has already started on a technical and organisational basis too.

There are a variety of cross-border agreements or pilot agreements involving the Netherlands, Belgium, Grand-Duchy of Luxembourg, the UK, Ireland and various European Regions (see the chapters on context and consumer choice of healthcare services). Additionally, some regions and organisations have been very active the recent years to establish cross-border care. These pilots may be considered a testing lab for European integration in healthcare.

The quest for efficiency in healthcare provision by inserting market mechanisms into the institutional settings of health services has been the hallmark of healthcare reform during the 1990s across Member States in rhetoric and to a certain degree in reality. To create competition inside socially financed health services has become an acceptable instrument to develop health services. Competition between payers has been introduced in some Member States. And in others, competition between providers for payers has also been introduced.

The idea to extend this competition beyond national borders is no longer an intellectual consideration. A German company based sickness fund, the Siemens BKK, tried in 1999 to alter its statute to allow cost-reimbursement across all Member States. This was denied by the competent authority but the sickness fund took the case to the Social Court in Munich where it is currently pending (file S 18 KR 367/00). Moreover, this sickness fund is developing a far reaching European strategy which entails selective contracting abroad for integrated care, the right to establish new funds abroad (according to domestic rules) and, eventually, the free choice of insurer for European citizens. It appears, therefore, that actors are beginning to appear in the emerging European health policy arena that have an intrinsic interest into Europe-wide competition for insurees and a Europe-wide competition between providers for payers.

A (possible) paradox becomes evident: While the "drivers" for pan-European healthcare are trying to escape from some of the perceived restrictions of regulated competition on the national level, the development this triggers might end up with similar mechanisms on a European-wide scale, as the Scenario B suggests.

6. Concluding remarks

If we knew the final outcome of European integration, it would be far easier to develop a vision on the future of healthcare in Europe. But since European integration is an open process of conflicting concepts and interest, we can only assess what the role of Europe in healthcare – and vice versa – could be in relation to the three scenarios.

Only scenario B on regulated European competition gives Europe a definite role in healthcare. All actors in healthcare shall enjoy the freedoms established in the TEC. But although the scenario is based on the assumption that these freedoms should take place in a framework of a solidarity and equity, the political dimension of healthcare seems to vanish. As far as system development is concerned, market forces would probably be dominant. In Scenario A on bi- and multi-lateral agreements, there is no role for Europe in healthcare. The competent financing institutions may use the opportunity of cross-border service provision according to their own interest. Scenario C on muddling through remains neutral in relation to the role that Europe has to play in healthcare.

In regard to European citizens all three scenarios produce severe conflicts. The regulated competition scenario B endows the European citizen with a (slightly restricted) universal right to healthcare across Europe. But this implies a citizenship in terms of the "Bourgeois" based on economic freedom and liberalism, transferring the patient into a consumer, needs into preferences, planning into competition and policy into strategic marketing. But at the same time – due to the overwhelming role of competition – citizens may be stripped of their political powers. Competition will drive system development at the expense of health policy reform. New developments will not be a matter of different values, political concepts or democratic interest mediation. The "Bourgeois" is not accompanied by the "Citoyen", who is not only the sovereign of market decisions but also of political decisions. The process of moving European integration from a mere market based approach into a political and social Union would be reversed in the area of healthcare.

A positive statement on the role of healthcare in Europe can only be derived from the regulated competition scenario, under which convergence will occur over time. Convergence is enforced by those organisations which will operate most successfully. The scenario on bi- and multi-lateral agreements offers no role for healthcare in Europe, at least not in terms of the Community. And again the muddling through scenario is neutral.

But this again poses a paradox. There is a growing awareness that healthcare is not only an economic burden in terms of welfare state expenditure but also an economic asset as a major source of employment and a necessity for sunrise industries such as telematics, e-business, new pharmaceuticals. It is almost inconceivable that healthcare should not, sooner or later, play a role in European integration.

From the previous chapters and these three scenarios, it is clear that new challenges to research, the establishment of a European health policy arena and domestic legislation arise.

Some of the pilots in cross-border regions have already produced evaluation reports of their activities. While some of the data on the extent and direction of patient flows is interesting, it is far more important to assess the political, technical, juridical and managerial issues involved in setting up those interfaces. The evaluation will help to assess what needs to be changed in order to make cross-border care managerially effective and efficient.

Comparative research in benefit packages has to be commissioned very soon for a variety of reasons. In all three scenarios – to different degrees – a growing need to know what is provided on "the other side of the border" becomes evident. The scenario on regulated European competition requires the knowledge of healthcare basket for the merger into the EuBasicBP. For the scenario on bi- and multilateral agreements, some substantial knowledge on what is provided abroad is also important, in order to find partners and reach sensible agreements. Even the muddling through scenario will require some understanding of the benefit packages from abroad since patients may want to know whether it is possible to go abroad intentionally for treatment.

At the same time, the chain of service provision and the institutional setting in which healthcare is provided appears on the research agenda. While it is on one the hand "only" a descriptive task to portrait service provision in other Member States and regions, it could also be an analytical task for HTA to expand from "stand alone technologies" to "complex technologies". The assessment of the effectiveness and efficiency of the complete chain of service provision from preventive, ambulatory, hospital and rehabilitative services in regard to a given indication in different healthcare settings would be both a good argument for (or against) integrated care across borders and could, at the same time, trigger a convergence by learning from best solutions.

The issue of social values embedded in healthcare institutions and health services seems to be a much neglected issue in comparative terms. Nevertheless, the Commission claims, for example, that there is a common "European Social Welfare Model" which is based on values and which makes Europe distinct from other places around the world. If convergence or integration will take place at least to some degree, it will become important to understand the commonalities and differences between the values and belief-systems embedded in health services of Member States and regions.

Last but not least, we know little about what the European citizen or patient thinks and desires in relation to the European dimension in healthcare. There is some research, for example on the knowledge of frontier workers on their healthcare rights. Other studies have tried to quantify the potential willingness of (healthy) patients going abroad when sick. But little is known about experiences in other health services or, for example, pensioners living abroad.

According to the three scenarios, Europe is at the same time a threat, a challenge and a opportunity for patients, providers and financiers. To prevent the worst and promote the best, it will be necessary for all actors to become more involved into European politics both at informal and at official levels. It will be crucial that health managers on the operational level will also be involved both in terms of understanding European issues and transferring institutional and operational knowledge into the political process.

On the one hand, existing legal provisions, such as Regulation EEC 1408/71, clearly do not sufficiently serve the careful development of pilot projects and interfaces. At the European level it should be acknowledged that cross border care may not only be a matter of facilitating the free movement of workers but, at the same time, a desirable end in itself.

On the other hand, a complete and thoughtless application of SEM legislation to healthcare would be devastating and has not been explored here as a scenario. The scenario on regulated European competition takes into account that acknowledging the SEM in health services necessitates the setting of new, European rules if the European Social Model should be preserved.

Logically, all scenarios demand as a first step a European health policy – not the least to address openly the question of the EU's healthcare future.

Author Index

Berman, Philip C.	1,17,31
Busquin, Philippe	v
Busse, Reinhard	1,17,31,41,49,213,231,249,261
Byrne, David	vii
Drews, Markus	231
Gobrecht, Jens	213
Jinks, Clare	63
Ong, Bie Nio	1,31,63,91
Paton, Calum	1,31,49,63,91
Prieto Rodríguez, Maria Angeles	49,97,179
Rehnberg, Clas	1,131
Renck, Barbro	1,49,109
Romo Avilés, Nuria	1,49,97,179
Silió Villamil, Fernando	1,49,97,179
Sundh, Mona	1,49,109,159
Wismar, Matthias	1,17,31,41,49,213,231,249,261